I0425630

Classic Yoga Collection

A Collection on Developing your Spiritual Consciousness

Includes the following works:

A SERIES OF LESSONS IN RAJA YOGA

A SERIES OF LESSONS IN GNANI YOGA

THE HATHA YOGA PRADIPIKA

For inquiries, please contact us at ilifeebooks@gmail.com

Table of Contents: **Page**

INDEX

A SERIES OF LESSONS IN RAJA YOGA

By YOGI RAMACHARAKA

"*When the soul sees itself as a Center surrounded by its circumference—when the Sun knows that it is a Sun, surrounded by its whirling planets-then is it ready for the Wisdom and Power of the Masters*."

PUBLISHERS' NOTICE

The lessons which compose this volume, originally appeared in the shape of monthly lessons, the first of which was issued in October, 1905, and the twelfth in September, 1906. These lessons met with a hearty and generous response from the public, and the present volume is issued in response to the demand for the lessons in a permanent and durable form. There have been no changes made in the text.

The publishers take the liberty to call the attention of the reader to the great amount of information condensed within the space given to each lesson. Students have told us that they have found it necessary to read and study each lesson carefully, in order to absorb the varied information contained within its pages. They have also stated that they have found it advisable to re-read the lessons several times, allowing an interval between each reading and that at each re-reading they would discover information that had escaped them during the course of the previous study. This has been repeated to us so often that we feel justified in mentioning it, that other readers might avail themselves of the same course and plan of study.

Following his usual custom, the writer of the lessons has declined to write a preface for this book, claiming that the lessons speak for themselves, and that those for whom they are intended will receive the message contained within them, without any prefatory talk.

THE YOGI PUBLICATION SOCIETY.

INDEX

THE FIRST LESSON.

THE "I."

In India, the Candidates for Initiation into the science of "Raja Yoga," when they apply to the Yogi Masters for instruction, are given a series of lessons designed to enlighten them regarding the nature of the Real Self, and to instruct them in the secret knowledge whereby they may develop the consciousness and realization of the real "I" within them. They are shown how they may cast aside the erroneous or imperfect knowledge regarding their real identity.

Until the Candidate masters this instruction, or at least until the truth becomes fixed in his consciousness, further instruction is denied him, for it is held that until he has awakened to a conscious realization of his Actual Identity, he is not able to understand the source of his power, and, moreover, is not able to *feel* within him the power of the Will, which power underlies the entire teachings of "Raja Yoga."

The Yogi Masters are hot satisfied if the Candidate forms merely a clear intellectual conception of this Actual Identity, but they insist that he must *feel* the truth of the same—must become *aware* of the Real Self—must enter into a consciousness in which the realization becomes a part of his everyday self—in which the realizing consciousness becomes the prevailing idea in his mind, around which his entire thoughts and actions revolve.

To some Candidates, this realization comes like a lightning flash the moment the attention is directed toward it, while in other cases the Candidates find it necessary to follow a rigorous course of training before they acquire the realization in consciousness.

The Yogi Masters teach that there are two degrees of this awakening consciousness of the Real Self. The first, which they call "the Consciousness of the 'I'," is the full consciousness of *real* existence that comes to the Candidate, and which causes him to *know* that he is a real entity having a life not depending upon the body—life that will go on in spite of the destruction of the body—*real* life, in fact. The second degree, which they call "the Consciousness of the 'I AM'," is the consciousness of one's identity with the Universal Life, and his relationship to, and "in-touchness" with all life, expressed and unexpressed. These two degrees of consciousness come in time to all who seek "The Path." To some it comes suddenly; to others it dawns gradually; to many it comes assisted by the exercises and practical work of "Raja Yoga."

The first lesson of the Yogi Masters to the Candidates, leading up to the first degree, above mentioned, is as follows: That the Supreme Intelligence of the Universe—the Absolute—has manifested the being that we call Man—the highest manifestation on this planet. The Absolute has manifested an infinitude of forms of life in the Universe, including distant worlds, suns, planets, etc., many of these forms being unknown to us on this planet, and being impossible of conception by the mind of the ordinary man. But these lessons have nothing to do with that part of the philosophy which deals with these myriad forms of life, for our time will be taken up with the unfoldment in the mind of man of his true nature and power. Before man attempts to solve the secrets of the Universe without, he should master the Universe within—the Kingdom of the Self. When he has accomplished this, then he may, and should, go forth to gain the outer knowledge as a Master demanding its secrets, rather than as a slave begging for the crumbs from the table of knowledge. The first knowledge for the Candidate is the knowledge of the Self.

Man, the highest manifestation of the Absolute, as far as this planet is concerned, is a wonderfully organized being—although the average man understands but little of his real nature. He comprises within his physical, mental and spiritual make-up both the highest and the lowest, as we have shown in our previous lessons (the "Fourteen Lessons" and the "Advanced Course"). In his bones he manifests almost in the form of mineral life, in fact, in his bones, body and blood mineral substances actually exist. The physical life of the body resembles the life of the plant. Many of the physical desires and emotions are akin to those of the lower animals, and in the undeveloped man these desires and emotions predominate and overpower the higher nature, which latter is scarcely in evidence. Then Man has a set of mental characteristics that are his own, and which are not possessed by the lower animals (See "Fourteen Lessons"). And in addition to the mental faculties common to all men, or rather, that are in evidence in a greater or lesser degree among all men, there are still higher faculties latent within Man, which when manifested and expressed render Man more than ordinary Man. The unfoldment of these latent faculties is possible to all who have reached the proper stage of development, and the desire and hunger of the student for this instruction is caused by the pressure of these unfolding latent faculties, crying to be born into consciousness. Then there is that wonderful thing, the Will, which is but faintly understood by those ignorant of the Yogi Philosophy—the Power of the Ego—its birthright from the Absolute.

But while these mental and physical things *belong* to Man, they are *not* the Man himself. Before the Man is able to master, control, and direct the things belonging to him—his tools and instruments—he must awaken to a realization of Himself. He must be able to distinguish between the "I" and the "Not I." And this is the first task before the Candidate.

That which is the Real Self of Man is the Divine Spark sent forth from the Sacred Flame. It is the Child of the Divine Parent. It is Immortal—Eternal—Indestructible—Invincible. It possesses within itself Power, Wisdom, and Reality. But like the infant that contains within itself the sometime Man, the mind of Man is unaware of its latent and potential qualities, and does not know itself. As it awakens and unfolds into the knowledge of its real nature, it manifests its qualities, and realizes what the Absolute has given it. When the Real Self begins to awaken, it sets aside from itself those things which are but appendages to it, but which it, in its half-waking state, had regarded as its Self. Setting aside first this, and then that, it finally discards all of the "Not I," leaving the Real Self free and delivered from its bondage to its appendages. Then it returns to the discarded appendages, and makes use of them.

In considering the question: "What is the Real Self?" let us first stop to examine what man usually means when he says "I."

The lower animals do not possess this "I" sense. They are conscious of the outer world; of their own desires and animal cravings and feelings. But their consciousness has not reached the Self-conscious stage. They are not able to think of themselves as separate entities, and to reflect upon their thoughts. They are not possessed of a consciousness of the Divine Spark—the Ego—the Real Self. The Divine Spark is hidden in the lower forms of life—even in the lower forms of human life—by many sheaths that shut out its light. But, nevertheless, it is there, always. It sleeps within the mind of the savage—then, as he unfolds, it begins to throw out its light. In you, the Candidate, it is fighting hard to have its beams pierce through the material coverings When the Real Self begins to arouse itself from its sleep, its dreams vanish from it, and it begins to see the world as it is, and to recognize itself in Reality and not as the distorted thing of its dreams.

The savage and barbarian are scarcely conscious of the "I." They are but a little above the animal in point of consciousness, and their "I" is almost entirely a matter of the consciousness of the wants of the body; the satisfaction of the appetites; the gratification of the passions; the securing of personal comfort; the expression of lust, savage power, etc. In the savage the lower part of the Instinctive Mind is the seat of the "I." (See "Fourteen Lessons" for explanation of the several mental planes of man.) If the savage could analyze his thoughts he would say that the "I" was the physical body, the said body having certain "feelings," "wants" and "desires." The "I" of such a man is a physical "I," the body representing its form and substance. Not only is this true of the savage, but even among so-called "civilized" men of to-day we find many in this stage. They have developed powers of thinking and reasoning, but they do not "live in their minds" as do some of their brothers. They use their thinking powers for the gratification of their bodily desires and cravings, and really live on the plane of the Instinctive Mind. Such a person may speak of "my mind," or "my soul," not from a high position where he looks upon these things from the standpoint of a Master who realizes his Real Self, but from below, from the point-of-view of the man who lives on the plane of the Instinctive Mind and who sees above *himself* the higher attributes. To such people the body is the "I." Their "I" is bound up with the senses, and that which comes to them through the senses. Of course, as Man advances in "culture" and "civilization," his senses become educated, and are satisfied only with more refined things, while the less cultivated man is perfectly satisfied with the more material and gross sense gratifications. Much that we call "cultivation" and "culture" is naught but a cultivation of a more refined form of sense gratification, instead of a real advance in consciousness and unfoldment. It is true that the advanced student and Master is possessed of highly developed senses, often far surpassing those of the ordinary man, but in such cases the senses have been cultivated under the mastery of the Will, and are made servants of the Ego instead of things hindering the progress of the soul—they are made servants instead of masters.

As Man advances in the scale, he begins to have a somewhat higher conception of the "I." He begins to use his mind and reason, and he passes on to the Mental Plane—his mind begins to manifest upon the plane of Intellect. He finds that there is something within him that is higher than the body. He finds that his mind seems more *real* to him than does the physical part of him, and in times of deep thought and study he is able almost to forget the existence of the body.

In this second stage, Man soon becomes perplexed. He finds problems that demand an answer, but as soon as he thinks he has answered them the problems present themselves in a new phase, and he is called upon to "explain his explanation." The mind, even although not controlled and directed by the Will, has a wonderful range, but, nevertheless, Man finds himself traveling around and around in a circle, and realizes that he is confronted continually by the Unknown. This disturbs him, and the higher the stage of "book learning" he attains, the more disturbed does he become. The man of but little knowledge does not see the existence of many problems that force themselves before the attention of the man of more knowledge, and demand an explanation from him. The tortures of the man who has attained the mental growth that enables him to see the new problems and the impossibility of their answer, cannot be imagined by one who has not advanced to that stage.

The man in this stage of consciousness thinks of his "I" as a mental thing, having a lower companion, the body. He feels that he has advanced, but yet his "I" does not give him the answer to the riddles and questions that perplex him. And he becomes most unhappy. Such men often develop into Pessimists, and consider the whole of life as utterly evil and disappointing—a curse rather than a blessing. Pessimism belongs to this plane, for neither the Physical Plane man or the Spiritual Plane man have this curse of Pessimism. The former man has no such disquieting thoughts, for he is almost entirely absorbed in gratifying his animal nature, while the latter man recognizes his mind as an instrument of himself, rather than as *himself*, and knows it to be imperfect in its present stage of growth. He knows that he has in himself the key to all knowledge—locked up in the Ego—and which the trained mind, cultivated, developed and guided by the awakened Will, may grasp as it unfolds. Knowing this the advanced man no longer despairs, and, recognizing his real nature, and his possibilities, as he awakens into a consciousness of his powers and capabilities, he laughs at the old despondent, pessimistic ideas, and discards them like a worn-out garment. Man on the Mental Plane of consciousness is like a huge elephant who knows not his own strength. He could break down barriers and assert himself over nearly any condition or environment, but in his ignorance of his real condition and power he may be mastered by a puny driver, or frightened by the rustling of a piece of paper.

When the Candidate becomes an Initiate—when he passes from the purely Mental Plane on to the Spiritual Plane—he realizes that the "I," the Real Self—is something higher than either body or mind, and that both of the latter may be used as tools and instruments by the Ego or "I." This knowledge is not reached by purely intellectual reasoning, although such efforts of the mind are often necessary to help in the unfoldment, and the Masters so use it. The real knowledge, however, comes as a special form of consciousness. The Candidate becomes "aware" of the real "I," and this consciousness being attained, he passes to the rank of the Initiates. When the Initiate passes the second degree of consciousness, and begins to grow into a realization of his relationship to the Whole—when he begins to manifest the Expansion of Self—then is he on the road to Mastership.

In the present lesson we shall endeavor to point out to the Candidate the methods of developing or increasing the realization of this "I" consciousness—this first degree work. We give the following exercises or development drills for the Candidate to practice. He will find that a careful and conscientious following of these directions will tend to unfold in him a sufficient degree of the "I" consciousness, to enable him to enter into higher stages of development and power. All that is necessary is for the Candidate to feel within himself the dawn of the awakening consciousness, or awareness of the Real Self. The higher stages of the "I" consciousness come gradually, for once on the Path there is no retrogression or going backward. There may be pauses on the journey, but there is no such thing as actually losing that which is once gained on The Path.

This "I" consciousness, even in its highest stages, is but a preliminary step toward what is called "Illumination," and which signifies the awakening of the Initiate to a realization of his actual connection with and relation to the Whole. The full sight of the glory of the "I," is but a faint reflected glow of "Illumination." The Candidate, once that he enters fully into the "I" consciousness, becomes an "Initiate." And the Initiate who enters into the dawn of Illumination takes his first step upon the road to Mastery. The Initiation is the awakening of the soul to a knowledge of its real existence—the Illumination is the revelation of the real nature of the soul, and of its relationship with the Whole. After the first dawn of the "I" consciousness has been attained, the Candidate is more able to grasp the means of developing the consciousness to a still higher degree—is more able to use the powers latent within him; to control his own mental states; to manifest a Centre of Consciousness and Influence that will radiate into the outer world which is always striving and hunting for such centres around which it may revolve.

Man must master himself before he can hope to exert an influence beyond himself. There is no royal road to unfoldment and power—each step must be taken in turn, and each Candidate must take the step himself, and by his own effort. But he may, and will, be aided by the helping hand of the teachers who have traveled The Path before him, and who know just when that helping hand is needed to lift the Candidate over the rough places.

We bid the Candidate to pay strict attention to the following instruction, as it is all important. Do not slight any part of it, for we are giving you only what is necessary, and are stating it as briefly as possible. Pay attention, and follow the instruction closely. This lesson must be mastered before you progress. And it must be practiced not only now, but at many stages of the journey, until full Initiation and Illumination is yours.

RULES AND EXERCISES DESIGNED TO AID THE CANDIDATE IN HIS INITIATION.

The first instruction along the line of Initiation is designed to awaken the mind to a full realization and consciousness of the individuality of the "I." The Candidate is taught to relax his body, and to calm his mind and to meditate upon the "I" until it is presented clearly and sharply before the consciousness. We herewith give directions for producing the desired physical and mental condition, in which meditation and concentration are more readily practiced. This state of Meditation will be referred to in subsequent exercises, so the Candidate is advised to acquaint himself thoroughly with it.

STATE OF MEDITATION. If possible, retire to a quiet place or room, where you do not fear interruption, so that your mind may feel secure and at rest. Of course, the ideal condition cannot always be obtained, in which case you must do the best you can. The idea is that you should be able to abstract yourself, so far as is possible, from distracting impressions, and you should be alone with yourself—in communion with your Real Self.

It is well to place yourself in an easy chair, or on a couch, so that you may relax the muscles and free the tension of your nerves. You should be able to "let go" all over, allowing every muscle to become limp, until a feeling of perfect peace and restful calm permeates every particle of your being. Rest the body and calm the mind. This condition is best in the earlier stages of the practice, although after the Candidate has acquired a degree of mastery he will be able to obtain the physical relaxation and mental calm whenever and wherever he desires.

But he must guard against acquiring a "dreamy" way of going around, wrapped in meditation when he should be attending to the affairs of life. *Remember this*, the State of Meditation should be entirely under the control of the Will, and should be entered into only deliberately and at the proper times. The Will must be master of this, as well as of every other mental state. The Initiates are not "day dreamers," but men and women having full control of themselves and their moods. The "I" consciousness while developed by meditation and consciousness, soon becomes a fixed item of consciousness, and does not have to be produced by meditation. In time of trial, doubt, or trouble, the consciousness may be brightened by an effort of the Will (as we shall explain in subsequent lessons) without going into the State of Meditation.

THE REALIZATION OF THE "I." The Candidate must first acquaint himself with the reality of the "I," before he will be able to learn its real nature. This is the first step. Let the Candidate place himself in the State of Meditation, as heretofore described. Then let him concentrate his entire attention upon his Individual Self, shutting out all thought of the outside world, and other persons. Let him form in his mind the idea of himself as a *real* thing—an actual being—an individual entity—a Sun around which revolves the world. He must see himself as the Centre around which the whole world revolves. Let not a false modesty, or sense of depreciation interfere with this idea, for you are not denying the right of others to also consider themselves centres. You are, in fact, a centre of consciousness—made so by the Absolute—and you are awakening to the fact. Until the Ego recognizes itself as a Centre of Thought, Influence and Power, it will not be able to *manifest* these qualities. And in proportion as it recognizes its position as a centre, so will it be able to manifest its qualities. It is not necessary that you should compare yourself with others, or imagine yourself greater or higher than them. In fact, such comparisons are to be regretted, and are unworthy of the advanced Ego, being a mark and indication of a lack of development, rather than the reverse. In the Meditation simply ignore all consideration of the respective qualities of others, and endeavor to realize the fact that YOU are a great Centre of Consciousness—a Centre of Power—a Centre of Influence—a Centre of Thought. And that like the planets circling around the sun, so does your world revolve around YOU who are its centre. It will not be necessary for you to argue out this matter, or to convince yourself of its truth by intellectual reasoning. The knowledge does not come in that way. It comes in the shape of a realization of the truth gradually dawning upon your consciousness through meditation and concentration. Carry this thought of yourself as a "Centre of Consciousness—Influence—Power" with you, *for it is an occult truth,* and in the proportion that you are able, to realize it so will be your ability to manifest the qualities named.

No matter how humble may be your position—no matter how hard may be your lot—no matter how deficient in educational advantages you may be—still you would not change your "I" with the most fortunate, wisest and highest man or woman in the world. You may doubt this, but think for a moment and you will see that we are right. When you say that you "would like to be" this person or that, you really mean that *you* would like to have their degree of intelligence, power, wealth, position, or what not. What you want is something that is theirs, or something akin to it. But you would not for a moment wish to merge your *identity* with theirs, or to exchange *selves*. Think of this for a moment To *be* the other person you would have to let *yourself* die, and instead of *yourself* you would be the other person. The real *you* would be wiped out of existence, and you would not be *you* at all, but would be *he.*

If you can but grasp this idea you will see that not for a moment would you be willing for such an exchange. Of course such an exchange is impossible. The "I" of you cannot be wiped out. It is eternal, and will go on, and on, and on, to higher and higher states—but it always will be the same "I." Just as you, although a far different sort of person from your childhood self, still you recognize that the same "I" is there, and always has been there. And although you will attain knowledge, experience, power and wisdom in the coming years, the same "I" will be there. The "I" is the Divine Spark and cannot be extinguished.

The majority of people in the present stage of the race development have but a faint conception of the reality of the "I." They accept the statement of its existence, and are conscious of themselves as an eating, sleeping, living creature—something like a higher form of animal. But they have not awakened to an "awareness" or realization of the "I," which must come to all who become real centres of Influence and Power. Some men have stumbled into this consciousness, or a degree of it, without understanding the matter. They have "felt" the truth of it, and they have stepped out from the ranks of the commonplace people of the world, and have become powers for good or bad. This is unfortunate to some extent, as this "awareness" without the knowledge that should accompany it may bring pain to the individual and others.

The Candidate must meditate upon the "I," and recognize it—*feel* it—to be a Centre. This is his first task. Impress upon your mind the word "I," in this sense and understanding, and let it sink deep down into your consciousness, so that it will become a part of you. And when you say "I," you must accompany the word with the picture of your Ego as a Centre of Consciousness, and Thought, and Power, and Influence. See yourself thus, surrounded by your world. Wherever you go, there goes the Centre of your world. YOU are the Centre, and all outside of you revolves around that Centre. This is the first great lesson on the road to Initiation. Learn it!

The Yogi Masters teach the Candidates that their realization of the "I" as a Centre may be hastened by going into the Silence, or State of Meditation, and repeating their first name over slowly, deliberately and solemnly a number of times. This exercise tends to cause the mind to centre upon the "I," and many cases of dawning Initiation have resulted from this practice. Many original thinkers have stumbled upon this method, without having been taught it. A noted example is that of Lord Tennyson, who has written that he attained a degree of Initiation in this way. He would repeat his own name, over and over, and the same time meditating upon his identity, and he reports that he would become conscious and "aware" of his reality and immortality—in short would recognize himself as a *real* center of consciousness.

We think we have given you the key to the first stage of meditation and concentration. Before passing on, let us quote from one of the old Hindu Masters. He says, regarding this matter: "When the soul sees itself as a Centre surrounded by its circumference—when the Sun knows that it is a Sun, and is surrounded by its whirling planets—then is it ready for the Wisdom and Power of the Masters."

THE KNOWLEDGE OF THE INDEPENDENCE OF THE "I" FROM THE BODY. Many of the Candidates find themselves prevented from a full realization of the "I" (even after they have begun to grasp it) by the confusing of the reality of the "I" with the sense of the physical body. This is a stumbling block that is easily overcome by meditation and concentration, the independence of the "I" often becoming manifest to the Candidate in a flash, upon the proper thought being used as the subject of meditation.

The exercise is given as follows: Place yourself in the State of Meditation, and think of YOURSELF—the Real "I"—as being independent of the body, but using the body as a covering and an instrument. Think of the body as you might of a suit of clothes. Realize that you are able to leave the body, and still be the same "I." Picture yourself as doing this, and looking down upon your body. Think of the body as a shell from which you may emerge without affecting your identity. Think of yourself as mastering and controlling the body that you occupy, and using it to the best advantage, making it healthy, strong and vigorous, but still being merely a shell or covering for the real "You." Think of the body as composed of atoms and cells which are constantly changing, but which are held together by the force of your Ego, and which you can improve at Will. Realize that you are merely inhabiting the body, and using it for your convenience, just as you might use a house.

In meditating further, ignore the body entirely, and place your thought upon the Real "I" that you are beginning to feel to be "you," and you will find that your identity—your "I"—is something entirely apart from the body. You may now say "my body" with a new meaning. Divorce the idea of your being a physical being, and realize that you are above body. But do not let this conception and realization cause you to ignore the body. You must regard the body as the Temple of the Spirit, and care for it, and make it a fit habitation for the "I." Do not be frightened if, during this meditation, you happen to experience the sensation of being out of the body for a few moments, and of returning to it when you are through with the exercise. The Ego is able (in the case of the advanced Initiate) of soaring above the confines of the body, but it never severs its connection at such times. It is merely as if one were to look out of the window of a room, seeing what was going on outside, and drawing in his head when he wishes. He does not leave the room, although he may place his head outside in order to observe what is doing in the street. We do not advise the Candidate to try to cultivate this sensation—but if it comes naturally during meditation, do not fear.

REALIZING THE IMMORTALITY AND INVINCIBILITY OF THE EGO. While the majority accept on faith the belief in the Immortality of the Soul, yet but few are aware that it may be demonstrated by the soul itself. The Yogi Masters teach the Candidates this lesson, as follows: The Candidate places himself in the State of Meditation, or at least in a thoughtful frame of mind, and then endeavors to "imagine" himself as "dead"—that is, he tries to form a mental conception of himself as dead. This, at first thought, appears a very easy thing to imagine, but as a matter of fact it is *impossible* to do so, for the Ego refuses to entertain the proposition, and finds it impossible to imagine it. Try it for yourself. You will find that you may be able to imagine your *body* as lying still and lifeless, but the same thought finds that in so doing *You* are standing and looking at the body. So you see that *You* are not dead at all, even in imagination, although the body may be. Or, if you refuse to disentangle yourself from your body, in imagination, you may think of your body as dead but *You* who refuse to leave it are still *alive* and recognize the dead body as a thing apart from your Real Self. No matter how you may twist it you *cannot* imagine yourself as dead. The Ego insists upon being *alive* in any of these thoughts, and thus finds that it has within itself the sense and assurance of Immortality. In case of sleep or stupor resulting from a blow, or from narcotics or anaesthetics, the mind is apparently blank, but the "I" is conscious of a continuity of existence. And so one may imagine himself as being in an unconscious state, or asleep, quite easily, and sees the possibility of such a state, but when it comes to imagining the "I" as dead, the mind utterly refuses to do the work. This wonderful fact that the soul carries within itself the evidence of its own immortality is a glorious thing, but one must have reached a degree of unfoldment before he is able to grasp its full significance.

The Candidate is advised to investigate the above statement for himself, by meditation and concentration, for in order that the "I" may know its true nature and possibilities, it must realize that it cannot be destroyed or killed. It must know what it is before it is able to manifest its nature. So do not leave this part of the teaching until you have mastered it. And it is well occasionally to return to it, in order that you may impress upon the mind the fact of your immortal and eternal nature. The mere glimmering of this conception of truth will give you an increased sense of strength and power, and you will find that your Self has expanded and grown, and that you are more of a power and Centre than you have heretofore realized.

The following exercises are useful in bringing about a realization of the invincibility of the Ego—its superiority to the elements.

Place yourself in the State of Meditation, and imagine the "I" as withdrawn from the body. See it passing through the tests of air, fire and water unharmed. The body being out of the way, the soul is seen to be able of passing through the air at will—of floating like a bird—of soaring—of traveling in the ether. It may be seen as able to pass through fire without harm and without sensation, for the elements affect only the physical body, not the Real "I." Likewise it may be seen as passing through water without discomfort or danger or hurt.

This meditation will give you a sense of superiority and strength, and will show you something of the nature of the real "I." It is true that you are confined in the body, and the body may be affected by the elements, but the knowledge that the Real "I" is superior to the body—superior to the elements that affect the body—and cannot be injured any more than it can be killed, is wonderful, and tends to develop the full "I" consciousness within you. For You—the Real "I"—are not body. You are Spirit. The Ego is Immortal and Invincible, and cannot be killed and harmed. When you enter into this realization and consciousness, you will feel an influx of strength and power impossible to describe. Fear will fall from you like a worn-out cloak, and you will feel that you are "born again." An understanding of this thought, will show you that the things that we have been fearing cannot affect the Real "I," but must rest content with hurting the physical body. And they may be warded off from the physical body by a proper understanding and application of the Will.

In our next lesson, you will be taught how to separate the "I" from the mechanism of the mind—how you may realize your mastery of the mind, just as you now realize your independence of the body. This knowledge must be imparted to you by degrees, and you must place your feet firmly upon one round of the ladder before you take the next step.

The watchword of this First Lesson is "I." And the Candidate must enter fully into its meaning before he is able to progress. He must realize his real existence—independent of the body. He must see himself as invincible and impervious to harm, hurt, or death. He must see himself as a great Centre of Consciousness—a Sun around which his world revolves. Then will come to him a new strength. He will feel a calm dignity and power, which will be apparent to those with whom he comes in contact. He will be able to look the world in the face without flinching, and without fear, for he will realize the nature and power of the "I." He will realize that he is a Centre of Power—of Influence. He will realize that nothing can harm the "I," and that no matter how the storms of life may dash upon the personality, the real "I"—the Individuality—is unharmed. Like a rock that stands steadfast throughout the storm, so does the "I" stand through the tempests of the life of personality. And he will know that as he grows in realization, he will be able to control these storms and bid them be still.

In the words of one of the Yogi Masters: "The 'I' is eternal. It passes unharmed through the fire, the air, the water. Sword and spear cannot kill or wound it. It cannot die. The trials of the physical life are but as dreams to it. Resting secure in the knowledge of the 'I,' Man may smile at the worst the world has to offer, and raising his hand he may bid them disappear into the mist from which they emerged. Blessed is he who can say (understandingly) 'I'."

So dear Candidate, we leave you to master the First Lesson. Be not discouraged if your progress be slow. Be not cast down if you slip back a step after having gained it. You will gain two at the next step. Success and realization will be yours. Mastery is before. You will Attain. You will Accomplish. Peace be with you.

MANTRAMS (AFFIRMATIONS) FOR THE FIRST LESSON.

"I" am a Centre. Around me revolves my world.

"I" am a Centre of Influence and Power.

"I" am a Centre of Thought and Consciousness.

"I" am Independent of the Body.

"I" am Immortal and cannot be Destroyed.

"I" am Invincible and cannot be Injured.

[Illustration: "I"]

THE SECOND LESSON.

THE EGO'S MENTAL TOOLS.

In the First Lesson we gave instruction and exercises designed to awaken the consciousness of the Candidate to a realization of the real "I." We confined our instructions to the preliminary teachings of the reality of the "I," and the means whereby the Candidate might be brought to a realization of his real Self, and its independence from the body and the things of the flesh. We tried to show you how you might awaken to a consciousness of the reality of the "I"; its real nature; its independence of the body; its immortality; its invincibility and invulnerability. How well we have succeeded may be determined only by the experience of each Candidate, for we can but point out the way, and the Candidate must do the real work himself.

But there is more to be said and done in this matter of awakening to a realization of the "I." So far, we have but told you how to distinguish between the material coverings of the Ego and the "I" itself. We have tried to show you that you had a real "I," and then to show you what it was, and how it was independent of the material coverings, etc. But there is still another step in this self analysis—a more difficult step. Even when the Candidate has awakened to a realization of his independence of the body, and material coverings, he often confounds the "I" with the lower principles of the mind. This is a mistake. The Mind, in its various phases and planes, is but a tool and instrument of the "I," and is far from being the "I" itself. We shall try to bring out this fact in this lesson and its accompanying exercises. We shall avoid, and pass by, the metaphysical features of the case, and shall confine ourselves to the Yogi Psychology. We shall not touch upon theories, nor attempt to explain the cause, nature and purpose of the Mind—the working tool of the Ego—but instead shall attempt to point out a way whereby you may analyze the Mind and then determine which is the "not I" and which is the real "I." It is useless to burden you with theories or metaphysical talk, when the way to prove the thing is right within your own grasp. By using the mind, you will be able to separate it into its parts, and force it to give you its own answer to the questions touching itself.

In the second and third lessons of our "*Fourteen Lessons*," we pointed out to you the fact that man had three Mental Principles, or subdivisions of mind, all of which were below the plane of Spirit. The "I" is Spirit, but its mental principles are of a lower order.

Without wishing to unduly repeat ourselves, we think it better to run hastily over these three Principles in the mind of Man.

First, there is what is known as the Instinctive Mind, which man shares in common with the lower animals. It is the first principle of mind that appears in the scale of evolution. In its lowest phases, consciousness is but barely perceptible, and mere sensation is apparent. In its higher stages it almost reaches the plane of Reason or Intellect, in fact, they overlap each other, or, rather, blend into each other. The Instinctive Mind does valuable work in the direction of maintaining animal life in our bodies, it having charge of this part of our being. It attends to the constant work of repair; replacement; change; digestion; assimilation; elimination, etc., all of which work is performed below the plane of consciousness.

But this is but a small part of the work of the Instinctive Mind. For this part of the mind has stored up all the experiences of ourselves and ancestors in our evolution from the lower forms of animal life into the present stage of evolution. All of the old animal instincts (which were all right in their place, and quite necessary for the well-being of the lower forms of life) have left traces in this part of the mind, which traces are apt to come to the front under pressure of unusual circumstances, even long after we think we have outgrown them. In this part of the mind are to be found traces of the old fighting instinct of the animal; all the animal passions; all the hate, envy, jealousy, and the rest of it, which are our inheritances from the past. The Instinctive Mind is also the "habit mind" in which is stored up all the little, and great, habits of many lives, or rather such as have not been entirely effaced by subsequent habits of a stronger nature. The Instinctive Mind is a queer storehouse, containing quite a variety of objects, many of them very good in their way, but others of which are the worst kind of old junk and rubbish.

This part of the mind also is the seat of the appetites; passions; desires; instincts; sensations; feelings and emotions of the lower order, manifested in the lower animals; primitive man; the barbarian; and the man of today, the difference being only in the degree of control over them that has been gained by the higher parts of the mind. There are higher desires, aspirations, etc., belonging to a higher part of the mind, which we will describe in a few minutes, but the "animal nature" belongs to the Instinctive Mind. To it also belong the "feelings" belonging to our emotional and passional nature. All animal desires, such as hunger and thirst; sexual desires (on the physical plane); all passions, such as physical love; hatred; envy; malice; jealousy; revenge, etc., are part of this part of the mind. The desire for the physical (unless a means of reaching higher things) and the longing for the material, belong to this region of the mind. The "lust of the flesh; the lust of the eyes; the pride of life," belong to the Instinctive Mind.

Take note, however, that we are not condemning the things belonging to this plane of the mind. All of them have their place—many were necessary in the past, and many are still necessary for the continuance of physical life. All are right in their place, and to those in the particular plane of development to which they belong, and are wrong only when one is mastered by them, or when he returns to pick up an unworthy thing that has been cast off in the unfoldment of the individual. This lesson has nothing to do with the right and wrong of these things (we have treated of that elsewhere) and we mention this part of the mind that you may understand that you have such a thing in your mental make-up, and that you may understand the thought, etc., coming from it, when we start in to analyze the mind in the latter part of this lesson. All we will ask you to do at this stage of the lesson is to realize that this part of the mind, while *belonging* to you, is *not* You, yourself. It is *not* the "I" part of you.

Next in order, above the Instinctive Mind, is what we have called the Intellect, that part of the mind that does our reasoning, analyzing; "thinking," etc. You are using it in the consideration of this lesson. But note this: You are *using* it, but it is *not* You, any more than was the Instinctive Mind that you considered a moment ago. You will begin to make the separation, if you will think but a moment. We will not take up your time with a consideration of Intellect or Reason. You will find a good description of this part of the mind in any good elementary work on Psychology. Our only idea in mentioning it is that you may make the classification, and that we may afterward show you that the Intellect is but a tool of the Ego, instead of being the real "I" itself, as so many seem to imagine.

The third, and highest, Mental Principle is what is called the Spiritual Mind, that part of the mind which is almost unknown to many of the race, but which has developed into consciousness with nearly all who read this lesson, for the fact that the subject of this lesson attracts you is a proof that this part of your mental nature is unfolding into consciousness. This region of the mind is the source of that which we call "genius," "inspiration," "spirituality," and all that we consider the "highest" in our mental make-up. All the great thoughts and ideas float into the field of consciousness from this part of the mind. All the great unfoldment of the race comes from there. All the higher mental ideas that have come to Man in his upward evolutionary journey, that tend in the direction of nobility; true religious feeling; kindness; humanity; justice; unselfish love; mercy; sympathy, etc., have come to him through his slowly unfolding Spiritual Mind. His love of God and of his fellow man have come in this way. His knowledge of the great occult truths reach him through this channel. The mental realization of the "I," which we are endeavoring to teach in these lessons, must come to him by way of the Spiritual Mind unfolding its ideas into his field of consciousness.

But even this great and wonderful part of the mind is but a tool—a highly finished one, it is true, but still a tool—to the Ego, or "I."

We propose to give you a little mental drill work, toward the end that you may be able more readily to distinguish the "I" from the mind, or mental states. In this connection we would say that every part, plane, and function of the mind is good, and necessary, and the student must not fall into the error of supposing that because we tell him to set aside first this part of the mind and then that part, that we are undervaluing the mind, or that we regard it as an encumbrance or hindrance. Far from this, we realize that it is *by the use of* the mind that Man is enabled to arrive at a knowledge of his true nature and Self, and that his progress through many stages yet will depend upon the unfolding of his mental faculties.

Man is now using but the lower and inferior parts of his mind, and he has within his mental world great unexplored regions that far surpass anything of which the human mind has dreamed. In fact, it is part of the business of "Raja Yoga" to aid in unfolding these higher faculties and mental regions. And so far from decrying the Mind, the "Raja Yoga" teachers are chiefly concerned in recognizing the Mind's power and possibilities, and directing the student to avail himself of the latent powers that are inherent in his soul.

It is only by the mind that the teachings we are now giving you may be grasped and understood, and used to your advantage and benefit. We are talking direct to your mind now, and are making appeals to it, that it may be interested and may open itself to what is ready to come into it from its own higher regions. We are appealing to the Intellect to direct its attention to this great matter, that it may interpose less resistance to the truths that are waiting to be projected from the Spiritual Mind, which knows the Truth.

MENTAL DRILL.

Place yourself in a calm, restful condition, that you may be able to meditate upon the matters that we shall place before you for consideration. Allow the matters presented to meet with a hospitable reception from you, and hold a mental attitude of willingness to receive what may be waiting for you in the higher regions of your mind.

We wish to call your attention to several mental impressions or conditions, one after another, in order that you may realize that they are merely something *incident* to you, and *not* YOU yourself—that you may set them aside and consider them, just as you might anything that you have been using. You cannot set the "I" aside and so consider it, but the various forms of the "not I" may be so set aside and considered.

In the First Lesson you gained the perception of the "I" as independent from the body, the latter merely being an instrument for use. You have now arrived at the stage when the "I" appears to you to be a mental creature—a bundle of thoughts, feelings, moods, etc. But you must go farther. You must be able to distinguish the "I" from these mental conditions, which are as much tools as is the body and its parts.

Let us begin by considering the thoughts more closely connected with the body, and then work up to the higher mental states.

The sensations of the body, such as hunger; thirst; pain; pleasurable sensations; physical desires, etc., etc., are not apt to be mistaken for essential qualities of the "I" by many of the Candidates, for they have passed beyond this stage, and have learned to set aside these sensations, to a greater or lesser extent, by an effort of the Will, and are no longer slaves to them. Not that they do not experience these sensations, but they have grown to regard them as incidents of the physical life—good in their place—but useful to the advanced man only when he has mastered them to the extent that he no longer regards them as close to the "I." And yet, to some people, these sensations are so closely identified with their conception of the "I" that when they think of themselves they think merely of a bundle of these sensations. They are not able to set them aside and consider them as things apart, to be used when necessary and proper, but as things not fastened to the "I." The more advanced a man becomes the farther off seem these sensations. Not that he does not feel hungry, for instance. Not at all, for he recognizes hunger, and satisfies it within reason, knowing that his physical body is making demands for attention, and that these demands should be heeded. But—mark the difference—instead of feeling that the "*I*" is hungry the man feels that "*my body*" is hungry, just as he might become conscious that his horse or dog was crying for food insistently. Do you see what we mean? It is that the man no longer identifies himself—the "I"—with the body, consequently the thoughts which are most closely allied to the physical life seem comparatively "separate" from his "I" conception. Such a man thinks "my stomach, this," or "my leg, that," or "my body, thus," instead of "'I,' this," or "'I' that." He is able, almost automatically, to think of the body and its sensations as things *of* him, and *belonging to* him, which require attention and care, rather than as real parts of the "I." He is able to form a conception of the "I" as existing without any of these things—without the body and its sensations—and so he has taken the first step in the realization of the "I."

Before going on, we ask the students to stop a few moments, and mentally run over these sensations of the body. Form a mental image of them, and realize that they are merely incidents to the present stage of growth and experience of the "I," and that they form no real part of it. They may, and will be, left behind in the Ego's higher planes of advancement. You may have attained this mental conception perfectly, long since, but we ask that to give yourself the mental drill at this time, in order to fasten upon your mind this first step.

In realizing that you are able to set aside, mentally, these sensations—that you are able to hold them out at arm's length and "consider" them as an "outside" thing, you mentally determine that they are "not I" things, and you set them down in the "not I" collection—the first to be placed there. Let us try to make this still plainer, even at the risk of wearying you by repetitions (for you must get this idea firmly fixed in your mind). To be able to say that a thing is "not I," you must realize that there are two things in question (1) the "not I" thing, and (2) the "I" who is regarding the "not I" thing just as the "I" regards a lump of sugar, or a mountain. Do you see what we mean? Keep at it until you do.

Next, consider some of the emotions, such as anger; hate; love, in its ordinary forms; jealousy; ambition; and the hundred and one other emotions that sweep through our brains. You will find that you are able to set each one of these emotions or feelings aside and study it; dissect it; analyze it; consider it. You will be able to understand the rise, progress and end of each of these feelings, as they have come to you, and as you recall them in your memory or imagination, just as readily as you would were you observing their occurrence in the mind of a friend. You will find them all stored away in some parts of your mental make-up, and you may (to use a modern American slang phrase) "make them trot before you, and show their paces." Don't you see that they are not "You"—that they are merely something that you carry around with you in a mental bag. You can imagine yourself as living without them, and still being "I," can you not?

And the very fact that you are able to set them aside and examine and consider them is a proof that they are "not I" things—for there are two things in the matter (1) *You* who are examining and considering them, and (2) the thing itself which is the *object* of the examination and consideration at mental arm's length. So into the "not I" collection go these emotions, desirable and undesirable. The collection is steadily growing, and will attain quite formidable proportions after a while.

Now, do not imagine that this is a lesson designed to teach you how to discard these emotions, although if it enables you to get rid of the undesirable ones, so much the better. This is not our object, for we bid you place the desirable (at this time) ones in with the opposite kind, the idea being to bring you to a realization that the "I" is higher, above and independent of these mental somethings, and then when you have realized the nature of the "I," you may return and use (as a Master) the things that have been using you as a slave. So do not be afraid to throw these emotions (good and bad) into the "not I" collection. You may go back to them, and use the good ones, after the Mental Drill is over. No matter how much you may think that you are bound by any of these emotions, you will realize, by careful analysis, that it is of the "not I" kind, for the "I" existed before the emotion came into active play, and it will live long after the emotion has faded away. The principal proof is that you are able to hold it out at arm's length and examine it—a proof that it is "not I."

Run through the entire list of your feelings; emotions; moods; and what not, just as you would those of a well-known friend or relative, and you will see that each one—every one—is a "not I" thing, and you will lay it aside for the time, for the purpose of the scientific experiment, at least.

Then passing on to the Intellect, you will be able to hold out for examination each mental process and principle. You don't believe it, you may say. Then read and study some good work on Psychology, and you will learn to dissect and analyze every intellectual process—and to classify it and place it in the proper pigeon-hole. Study Psychology by means of some good text-book, and you will find that one by one every intellectual process is classified, and talked about and labeled, just as you would a collection of flowers. If that does not satisfy you, turn the leaves of some work on Logic, and you will admit that you may hold these intellectual processes at arm's length and examine them, and talk about them to others. So that these wonderful tools of Man—the Intellectual powers may be placed in the "not I" collection, for the "I" is capable of standing aside and viewing them—it is able to detach them from itself. The most remarkable thing about this is that in admitting this fact, you realize that the "I" is using these very intellectual faculties to pass upon themselves. Who is the Master that compels these faculties to do this to themselves? The Master of the Mind—The "I."

And reaching the higher regions of the mind—even the Spiritual Mind, you will be compelled to admit that the things that have come into consciousness from that region may be considered and studied, just as may be any other mental thing, and so even these high things must be placed in the "not I" collection. You may object that this does not prove that all the things in the Spiritual Mind may be so treated—that there may be "I" things there that can not be so treated. We will not discuss this question, for you know nothing about the Spiritual Mind except as it has revealed itself to you, and the higher regions of that mind are like the mind of a God, when compared to what *you* call mind. But the evidence of the Illumined—those in whom the Spiritual Mind has wonderfully unfolded tell us that even in the highest forms of development, the Initiates, yea, even the Masters, realize that above even their highest mental states there is always that eternal "I" brooding over them, as the Sun over the lake; and that the highest conception of the "I" known even to advanced souls, is but a faint reflection of the "I" filtering through the Spiritual Mind, although that Spiritual Mind is as clear as the clearest crystal when compared with our comparatively opaque mental states. And the highest mental state is but a tool or instrument of the "I," and is not the "I" itself.

And yet the "I" is to be found in the faintest forms of consciousness, and animates even the unconscious life. The "I" is always the same, but its apparent growth is the result of the mental unfoldment of the individual. As we described it in one of the lessons of the "*Advanced Course*" it is like an electric lamp that is encased in many wrappings of cloth.

As cloth after cloth is removed, the light seems to grow brighter and stronger, and yet it has changed not, the change being in the removal of the confining and bedimming coverings. We do not expect to make you realize the "I" in all its fullness—that is far beyond the highest known to man of to-day—but we do hope to bring you to a realization of the highest conception of the "I," possible to each of you in your present stage of unfoldment, and in the process we expect to cause to drop from you some of the confining sheaths that you have about outgrown. The sheaths are ready for dropping, and all that is required is the touch of a friendly hand to cause them to fall fluttering from you. We wish to bring you to the fullest possible (to you) realization of the "I," in order to make an Individual of you—in order that you may understand, and have courage to take up the tools and instruments lying at your hand, and do the work before you.

And now, back to the Mental Drill. After you have satisfied yourself that about everything that you are capable of thinking about is a "not I" thing—a tool and instrument for your use—you will ask, "And now, what is there left that should not be thrown in the "not I" collection." To this question we answer "THE 'I' ITSELF." And when you demand a proof we say, "Try to set aside the 'I' for consideration!" You may try from now until the passing away of infinities of infinities, and you will never be able to set aside the real "I" for consideration. You may think you can, but a little reflection will show you that you are merely setting aside some of your mental qualities or faculties. And in this process what is the "I" doing? Simply setting aside and considering things. Can you not see that the "I" cannot be both the *considerer* and the thing considered—the *examiner* and the thing examined? Can the sun shine upon itself by its own light? You may consider the "I" of some other person, but it is *your* "I" that is considering. But you cannot, as an "I," stand aside and see yourself as an "I." Then what evidence have we that there is an "I" to us? This: that you are always conscious of being the considerer and examiner, instead of the considered and examined thing—and then, you have the evidence of your consciousness. And what report does this consciousness give us? Simply this, and nothing more: "I AM." That is all that the "I" is conscious of, regarding its true self: "I AM," but that consciousness is worth all the rest, for the rest is but "not I" tools that the "I" may reach out and use.

And so at the final analysis, you will find that there is something that refuses to be set aside and examined by the "I." And that something is the "I" itself—that "I" eternal, unchangeable—that drop of the Great Spirit Ocean—that spark from the Sacred Flame.

Just as you find it impossible to imagine the "I" as dead, so will you find it impossible to set aside the "I" for consideration—all that comes to you is the testimony: "I AM."

If you were able to set aside the "I" for consideration, who would be the one to consider it? Who could consider except the "I" itself, and if it be *here*, how could it be *there?* The

"I" cannot be the "not I" even in the wildest flights of the imagination—the imagination with all its boasted freedom and power, confesses itself vanquished when asked to do this thing.

Oh, students, may you be brought to a realization of what you are. May you soon awaken to the fact that you are sleeping gods—that you have within you the power of the Universe, awaiting your word to manifest in action. Long ages have you toiled to get this far, and long must you travel before you reach even the first Great Temple, but you are now entering into the conscious stage of Spiritual Evolution. No longer will your eyes be closed as you walk the Path. From now on you will begin to see clearer and clearer each step, in the dawning light of consciousness.

You are in touch with all of life, and the separation of your "I" from the great Universal "I" is but apparent and temporary. We will tell you of these things in our Third Lesson, but before you can grasp that you must develop the "I" consciousness within you. Do not lay aside this matter as one of no importance. Do not dismiss our weak explanation as being "merely words, words, words," as so many are inclined to do. We are pointing out a great truth to you. Why not follow the leadings of the Spirit which even now—this moment while you read—is urging you to walk The Path of Attainment? Consider the teachings of this lesson, and practice the Mental Drill until your mind has grasped its significance, then let it sink deep down into your inner consciousness. Then will you be ready for the next lessons, and those to follow.

Practice this Mental Drill until you are fully assured of the *reality* of the "I" and the *relativity* of the "not "I" in the mind. When you once grasp this truth, you will find that you will be able to use the mind with far greater power and effect, for you will recognize that it is your tool and instrument, fitted and intended to do your bidding. You will be able to master your moods, and emotions when necessary, and will rise from the position of a slave to a Master.

Our words seem cheap and poor, when we consider the greatness of the truth that we are endeavoring to convey by means of them. For who can find words to express the inexpressible? All that we may hope to do is to awaken a keen interest and attention on your part, so that you will practice the Mental Drill, and thus obtain the evidence of your own mentality to the truth. Truth is not truth to you until you have proven it in your own experience, and once so proven you cannot be robbed of it, nor can it be argued away from you.

You must realize that in every mental effort You—the "I"—are behind it. You bid the Mind work, and it obeys your Will. You are the Master, and not the slave of your mind. You are the Driver, not the driven. Shake yourself loose from the tyranny of the mind that has oppressed you for so long. Assert yourself, and be free. We will help you in this direction during the course of these lessons, but you must first assert yourself as a Master of your Mind. Sign the mental Declaration of Independence from your moods, emotions, and uncontrolled thoughts, and assert your Dominion over them. Enter into your Kingdom, thou manifestation of the Spirit!

While this lesson is intended primarily to bring clearly into your consciousness the fact that the "I" is a reality, separate and distinct from its Mental Tools, and while the control of the mental faculties by the Will forms a part of some of the future lessons, still, we think that this is a good place to point out to you the advantages arising from a realization of the true nature of the "I" and the relative aspect of the Mind.

Many of us have supposed that our minds were the masters of ourselves, and we have allowed ourselves to be tormented and worried by thoughts "running away" with us, and presenting themselves at inopportune moments. The Initiate is relieved from this annoyance, for he learns to assert his mastery over the different parts of the mind, and controls and regulates his mental processes, just as one would a fine piece of machinery. He is able to control his conscious thinking faculties, and direct their work to the best advantage, and he also learns how to pass on orders to the subconscious mental region and bid it work for him while he sleeps, or even when he is using his conscious mind in other matters. These subjects will be considered by us in due time, during the course of lessons.

In this connection it may be interesting to read what Edward Carpenter says of the power of the individual to control his thought processes. In his book "*From Adam's Peak to Eleplumta*," in describing his experience while visiting a Hindu Gnani Yogi, he says:

"And if we are unwilling to believe in this internal mastery over the body, we are perhaps almost equally unaccustomed to the idea of mastery over our own inner thoughts and feelings. That a man should be a prey to any thought that chances to take possession of his mind, is commonly among us assumed as unavoidable. It may be a matter of regret that he should be kept awake all night from anxiety as to the issue of a lawsuit on the morrow, but that he should have the power of determining whether he be kept awake or not seems an extravagant demand. The image of an impending calamity is no doubt odious, but its very odiousness (we say) makes it haunt the mind all the more pertinaciously and it is useless to try to expel it.

"Yet this is an absurd position—for man, the heir of all the ages: hag-ridden by the flimsy creatures of his own brain. If a pebble in our boot torments us, we expel it. We take off the boot and shake it out. And once the matter is fairly understood it is just as easy to expel an intruding and obnoxious thought from the mind. About this there ought to be no mistake, no two opinions. The thing is obvious, clear and unmistakable. It should be as easy to expel an obnoxious thought from your mind as it is to shake a stone out of your shoe; and till a man can do that it is just nonsense to talk about his ascendancy over Nature, and all the rest of it. He is a mere slave, and prey to the bat-winged phantoms that flit through the corridors of his own brain.

"Yet the weary and careworn faces that we meet by thousands, even among the affluent classes of civilization, testify only too clearly how seldom this mastery is obtained. How rare indeed to meet a *man*! How common rather to discover a creature hounded on by tyrant thoughts (or cares or desires), cowering, wincing under the lash—or perchance priding himself to run merrily in obedience to a driver that rattles the reins and persuades him that he is free—whom we cannot converse with in careless *tete-a-tete* because that alien presence is always there, on the watch.

"It is one of the most prominent doctrines of Raja Yoga that the power of expelling thoughts, or if need be, killing them dead on the spot, *must* be attained. Naturally the art requires practice, but like other arts, when once acquired there is no mystery or difficulty about it. And it is worth practice. It may indeed fairly be said that life only begins when this art has been acquired. For obviously when instead of being ruled by individual thoughts, the whole flock of them in their immense multitude and variety and capacity is ours to direct and dispatch and employ where we list ('for He maketh the winds his messengers and the flaming fire His minister'), life becomes a thing so vast and grand compared with what it was before, that its former condition may well appear almost antenatal.

"If you can kill a thought dead, for the time being, you can do anything else with it that you please. And therefore it is that this power is so valuable. And it not only frees a man from mental torment (which is nine-tenths at least of the torment of life), but it gives him a concentrated power of handling mental work absolutely unknown to him before. The two things are co-relative to each other. As already said this is one of the principles of Raja Yoga.

"While at work your thought is to be absolutely concentrated in it, undistracted by anything whatever irrelevant to the matter in hand—pounding away like a great engine, with giant power and perfect economy—no wear and tear of friction, or dislocation of parts owing to the working of different forces at the same time. Then when the work is finished, if there is no more occasion for the use of the machine, it must stop equally, absolutely—stop entirely—no *worrying* (as if a parcel of boys were allowed to play their devilments with a locomotive as soon as it was in the shed)—and the man must retire into that region of his consciousness where his true self dwells.

"I say the power of the thought-machine itself is enormously increased by this faculty of letting it alone on the one hand, and of using it singly and with concentration on the other. It becomes a true tool, which a master-workman lays down when done with, but which only a bungler carries about with him all the time to show that he is the possessor of it."

We ask the students to read carefully the above quotations from Mr. Carpenter's book, for they are full of suggestions that may be taken up to advantage by those who are emancipating themselves from their slavery to the unmastered mind, and who are now bringing the mind under control of the Ego, by means of the Will.

Our next lesson will take up the subject of the relationship of the "I" to the Universal "I," and will be called the "Expansion of the Self." It will deal with the subject, not from a theoretical standpoint, but from the position of the teacher who is endeavoring to make his students actually *aware* in their consciousness of the truth of the proposition. In this course we are not trying to make our students past-masters of *theory*, but are endeavoring to place them in a position whereby they may *know* for themselves, and actually experience the things of which we teach.

Therefore we urge upon you not to merely rest content with reading this lesson, but, instead, to study and meditate upon the teachings mentioned under the head of "Mental Drill," until the distinctions stand out clearly in your mind, and until you not only *believe* them to be true, but actually are *conscious* of the "I" and its Mental Tools. Have patience and perseverance. The task may be difficult, but the reward is great. To become conscious of the greatness, majesty, strength and power of your real being is worth years of hard study. Do you not think so? Then study and practice hopefully, diligently and earnestly.

Peace be with you.

MANTRAMS (AFFIRMATIONS) FOR THE SECOND LESSON.

"I" am an entity—my mind is my instrument of expression.

"I" exist independent of my mind, and am not dependent upon it for existence or being.

"I" am Master of my mind, not its slave.

"I" can set aside my sensations, emotions, passions, desires, intellectual faculties, and all the rest of my mental collection of tools, as "not I" things—and still there remains something—and that something is "I," which cannot be set aside by me, for it is my very self; my only self; my real self—"I." That which remains after all that may be set aside *is* set aside is the "I"—Myself—eternal, constant, unchangeable.

[Illustration: "I am"]

THE THIRD LESSON.

THE EXPANSION OF THE SELF.

In the first two lessons of this course we have endeavored to bring to the candidate a realization in consciousness of the reality of the "I," and to enable him to distinguish between the Self and its sheaths, physical and mental. In the present lesson we will call his attention to the relationship of the "I" to the Universal "I," and will endeavor to give him an idea of a greater, grander Self, transcending personality and the little self that we are so apt to regard as the "I."

The keynote of this lesson will be "The Oneness of All," and all of its teachings will be directed to awakening a realization in consciousness of that great truth. But we wish to impress upon the mind of the Candidate that we are *not* teaching him that he is the Absolute. We are not teaching the "I Am God" belief, which we consider to be erroneous and misleading, and a perversion of the original Yogi teachings. This false teaching has taken possession of many of the Hindu teachers and people, and with its accompanying teaching of "Maya" or the complete illusion or non-existence of the Universe, has reduced millions of people to a passive, negative mental condition which undoubtedly is retarding their progress. Not only in India is this true, but the same facts may be observed among the pupils of the Western teachers who have embraced this negative side of the Oriental Philosophy. Such people confound the "Absolute" and "Relative" aspects of the One, and, being unable to reconcile the facts of Life and the Universe with their theories of "I Am God," they are driven to the desperate expedient of boldly denying the Universe, and declaring it to be all "an illusion" or "Maya."

You will have no trouble in distinguishing the pupils of the teachers holding this view. They will be found to exhibit the most negative mental condition—a natural result of absorbing the constant suggestion of "nothingness"—the gospel of negation. In marked contrast to the mental condition of the students, however, will be observed the mental attitude of the teachers, who are almost uniformly examples of vital, positive, mental force, capable of hurling their teaching into the minds of the pupils—of driving in their statements by the force of an awakened Will. The teacher, as a rule, has awakened to a sense of the "I" consciousness, and really develops the same by his "I Am God" attitude, because by holding this mental attitude he is enabled to throw off the influence of the sheaths of the lower mental principles, and the light of the Self shows forth fiercely and strongly, sometimes to such an extent that it fairly scorches the mentality of the less advanced pupil. But, notwithstanding this awakened "I" consciousness, the teacher is handicapped by his intellectual misconception and befogging metaphysics, and is unable to impart the "I" consciousness to his pupils, and, instead of raising them up to shine with equal splendor with himself, he really forces them into a shadow by reason of his teachings.

Our students, of course, will understand that the above is not written in the spirit of carping criticism or fault-finding. We hold no such mental attitude, and indeed could not if we remain true to our conception of Truth. We are mentioning these matters simply that the student may avoid this "I Am God" pitfall which awaits the Candidate just as he has well started on the Path. It would not be such a serious matter if it were merely a question of faulty metaphysics, for that would straighten itself out in time. But it is far more serious than this, for the teaching inevitably leads to the accompanying teaching that all is Illusion or *Maya*, and that Life is but a dream—a false thing—a lie—a nightmare; that the journey along the Path is but an illusion; that everything is "nothing"; that there is no soul; that You are God in disguise, and that He is fooling Himself in making believe that He is You; that Life is but a Divine masquerade or sleight-of-hand performance; that You are God, but that You (God) are fooling Yourself (God) in order to amuse Yourself (God). Is not this horrible? And yet it shows to what lengths the human mind will go before it will part with some pet theory of metaphysics with which it has been hypnotized. Do you think that we have overdrawn the picture? Then read some of the teachings of these schools of the Oriental Philosophy, or listen to some of the more radical of the Western teachers preaching this philosophy. The majority of the latter lack the courage of the Hindu teachers in carrying their theories to a logical conclusion, and, consequently they veil their teachings with metaphysical subtlety. But a few of them are more courageous, and come out into the open and preach their doctrine in full.

Some of the modern Western teachers of this philosophy explain matters by saying that "God is masquerading as different forms of life, including Man, in order that he may gain the experience resulting therefrom, for although He has Infinite and Absolute Wisdom and Knowledge, he lacks the experience that comes only from actually living the life of the lowly forms, and therefore He descend thus in order to gain the needed experience." Can you imagine the Absolute, possessed of all possible Knowledge and Wisdom, feeling the need of such petty "experience," and living the life of the lowly forms (including Man) in order "to gain experience?" To what Depths do these vain theories of Man drive us? Another leading Western teacher, who has absorbed the teaching of certain branches of the Oriental Philosophy, and who possesses the courage of his convictions, boldly announces that "You, yourself, are the *totality* of being, and with your mind alone create, preserve and destroy the universe, which is your own mental product." And again the last mentioned teacher states: "the entire universe is a bagatelle illustration of your own creative power, which you are now exhibiting for your own inspection." "By their fruits shall you know them," is a safe rule to apply to all teachings. The philosophy that teaches that the Universe is an illusion perpetrated by you (God) to amuse, entertain or fool yourself (God), can have but one result, and that is the conclusion that "everything is nothing," and all that is necessary to do is to sit down, fold your hands and enjoy the Divine exhibition of legerdemain that you are performing for your own entertainment, and then, when the show is over, return to your state of conscious Godhood and recall with smiles the pleasant memories of the "conjure show" that you created to fool yourself with during several billions of ages. That is what it amounts to, and the result is that those accepting this philosophy thrust upon them by forceful teachers, and knowing in their hearts that they are *not* God, but absorbing the suggestions of "nothingness," are driven into a state of mental apathy and negativeness, the soul sinking into a stupor from which it may not be roused for a long period of time.

We wish you to avoid confounding our teaching with this just mentioned. We wish to teach you that You are a real Being—*not* God Himself, but a manifestation of Him who is the Absolute. You are a Child of the Absolute, if you prefer the term, possessed of the Divine Heritage, and whose mission it is to unfold qualities which are your inheritances from your Parent. Do not make the great mistake of confounding the Relative with the Absolute. Avoid this pitfall into which so many have fallen. Do not allow yourself to fall into the "Slough of Despond," and wallow in the mud of "nothingness," and to see no reality except in the person of some forceful teacher who takes the place of the Absolute in your mind. But raise your head and assert your Divine Parentage, and your Heritage from the Absolute, and step out boldly on the Path, asserting the "I."

(We must refer the Candidate back to our "Advanced Course," for our teachings regarding the Absolute and the Relative. The last three lessons of that course will throw light upon what we have just said To repeat the teaching at this point would be to use space which is needed for the lesson before us.)

And yet, while the "I" is *not* God, the Absolute, it is infinitely greater than we have imagined it to be before the light dawned upon us. It extends itself far beyond what we had conceived to be its limits. It touches the Universe at all its points, and is in the closest union with all of Life. It is in the closest touch with all that has emanated from the Absolute—all the world of Relativity. And while it faces the Relative Universe, it has its roots in the Absolute, and draws nourishment therefrom, just as does the babe in the womb obtain nourishment from the mother. It is verily a manifestation of God, and God's very essence is in it. Surely this is almost as "high" a statement as the "I Am God" of the teachers just mentioned,—and yet how different. Let us consider the teaching in detail in this lesson, and in portions of others to follow.

Let us begin with a consideration of the instruments of the Ego, and the material with which and through which the Ego works. Let us realize that the physical body of man is identical in substance with all other forms of matter, and that its atoms are continually changing and being replaced, the material being drawn from the great storehouse of matter, and that there is a Oneness of matter underlying all apparent differences of form and substance. And then let us realize that the vital energy or *Prana* that man uses in his life work is but a portion of that great universal energy which permeates everything and everywhere, the portion being used by us at any particular moment being drawn from the universal supply, and again passing out from us into the great ocean of force or energy. And then let us realize that even the mind, which is so close to the real Self that it is often mistaken for it—even that wonderful thing Thought—is but a portion of the Universal Mind, the highest emanation of the Absolute beneath the plane of Spirit, and that the Mind—substance or *Chitta* that we are using this moment, is not ours separately and distinctly, but is simply a portion from the great universal supply, which is constant and unchangeable. Let us then realize that even this thing that we feel pulsing within us—that which is so closely bound up with the Spirit as to be almost inseparable from it—that which we call Life—is but a bit of that Great Life Principle that pervades the Universe, and which cannot be added to, nor subtracted from. When we have realized these things, and have begun to feel our relation (in these particulars) to the One Great Emanation of the Absolute, then we may begin to grasp the idea of the Oneness of Spirit, and the relation of the "I" to every other "I," and the merging of the Self into the one great Self, which is not the extinction of Individuality, as some have supposed, but the enlargement and extension of the Individual Consciousness until it takes in the Whole.

In Lessons X and XI, of the "Advanced Course" we called your attention to the Yogi teachings concerning *Akasa* or Matter, and showed you that all forms of what we know as Matter are but different forms of manifestation of the principle called *Akasa*, or as the Western scientists call it, "Ether." This Ether or *Akasa* is the finest, thinnest and most tenuous form of Matter, in fact it is Matter in its ultimate or fundamental form, the different forms of what we call Matter being but manifestations of this *Akasa* or Ether, the apparent difference resulting from different rates of vibration, etc. We mention this fact here merely to bring clearly before your mind the fact of the Universality of Matter, to the end that you may realize that each and every particle of your physical body is but a portion of this great principle of the Universe, fresh from the great store-house, and just about returning to it again, for the atoms of the body are constantly changing. That which appears as your flesh to-day, may have been part of a plant a few days before, and may be part of some other living thing a few days hence. Constant change is going on, and what is yours to-day was someone's else yesterday, and still another's to-morrow. You do not own one atom of matter *personally,* it is all a part of the common supply, the stream flowing through you and through all Life, on and on forever.

And so it is with the Vital Energy that you are using every moment of your life. You are constantly drawing upon the great Universal supply of *Prana,* then using what is given you, allowing the force to pass on to assume some other form. It is the property of all, and all you can do is to use what you need, and allow it to pass on. There is but one Force or Energy, and that is to be found everywhere at all times.

And even the great principle, Mind-substance, is under the same law. It is hard for us to realize this. We are so apt to think of our mental operations as distinctively our own—something that belongs to us personally—that it is difficult for us to realize that Mind-substance is a Universal principle just as Matter or Energy, and that we are but drawing upon the Universal supply in our mental operations. And more than this, the particular portion of Mind-substance that we are using, although separated from the Mind-substance used by other individuals by a thin wall of the very finest kind of Matter, is really in touch with the other apparently separated minds, and with the Universal Mind of which it forms a part. Just as is the Matter of which our physical bodies are composed really in touch with all Matter; and just as is the Vital Force used by us really in touch with all Energy; so is our Mind-substance really in touch with all Mind-substance. It is as if the Ego in its progress were moving through great oceans of Matter, Energy, or Mind-substance, making use of that of each which it needed and which immediately surrounded it, and leaving each behind as it moved on through the great volume of the ocean. This illustration is clumsy, but it may bring to your consciousness a realization that the Ego is the only thing that is really *Yours*, unchangeable and unaltered, and that all the rest is merely that portion of the Universal supply that you draw to yourself for the wants of the moment. It may also bring more clearly before your mind the great Unity of things—may enable you to see things as a Whole, rather than as separated parts. Remember, *You*—the "I"—are the only Real thing about and around you—all that has permanence—and Matter, Force and even Mind-substance, are but your instruments for use and expression. There are great oceans of each surrounding the "I" as it moves along.

It is well for you also to bear in mind the Universality of Life. All of the Universe is alive, vibrating and pulsating with life and energy and motion. There is nothing dead in the Universe. Life is everywhere, and always accompanied by intelligence. There is no such thing as a dead, unintelligent Universe. *Instead of being atoms of Life floating in a sea of death, we are atoms of Life surrounded by an ocean of Life, pulsating, moving, thinking, living.* Every atom of what we call Matter is alive. It has energy or force with it, and is always accompanied by intelligence and life. Look around us as we will—at the animal world—at the plant world—yes, even at the world of minerals and we see life,

life, life—all alive and having intelligence. When we are able to bring this conception into the realm of actual consciousness—when we are able not only to intellectually accept this fact, but to even go still further and *feel* and be conscious of this Universal Life on all sides, then are we well on the road to attaining the Cosmic Consciousness.

But all these things are but steps leading up to the realization of the Oneness in Spirit, on the part of the Individual. Gradually there dawns upon him the realization that there is a Unity in the manifestation of Spirit from the Absolute—a unity with itself, and a Union with the Absolute. All this manifestation of Spirit on the part of the Absolute—all this begetting of Divine Children—was in the nature of a single act rather than as a series of acts, if we may be permitted to speak of the manifestation as an *act*. Each Ego is a Centre of Consciousness in this great ocean of Spirit—each is a Real Self, apparently separate from the others and from its source, but the separation is only apparent in both cases, for there is the closest bond of union between the Egos of the Universe of Universes—each is knit to the other in the closest bond of union, and each is still attached to the Absolute by spiritual filaments, if we may use the term. In time we shall grow more conscious of this mutual relationship, as the sheaths are outgrown and cast aside, and in the end we will be withdrawn into the Absolute—shall return to the Mansion of the Father.

It is of the highest importance to the developing soul to unfold into a realization of this relationship and unity, *for when this conception is once fully established the soul is enabled to rise above certain of the lower planes, and is free from the operation of certain laws that bind the undeveloped soul.* Therefore the Yogi teachers are constantly leading the Candidates toward this goal. First by this path, and then by that one, giving them different glimpses of the desired point, until finally the student finds a path best fitted for his feet, and he moves along straight to the mark, and throwing aside the confining bonds that have proved so irksome, he cries aloud for joy at his new found Freedom.

The following exercises and Mental Drills are intended to aid the Candidate in his work of growing into a realization of his relationship with the Whole of Life and Being.

MENTAL DRILL.

(1) Read over what we have said in the "Advanced Course" regarding the principle known as Matter. Realize that all Matter is One at the last—that the real underlying substance of Matter is *Akasa* or Ether, and that all the varying forms evident to our senses are but modifications and grosser forms of that underlying principle. Realize that by known chemical processes all forms of Matter known to us, or rather all combinations resulting in "forms," may be resolved into their original elements, and that these elements

are merely *Akasa* in different states of vibration. Let the idea of the Oneness of the visible Universe sink deeply into your mind, until it becomes fixed there. The erroneous conception of diversity in the material world must be replaced by the consciousness of Unity—Oneness, at the last, in spite of the appearance of variety and manifold forms. You must grow to see behind the world of forms of Matter, and see the great principle of Matter (*Akasa* or Ether) back of, within, and under it all. You must grow to *feel* this, as well as to intellectually see it.

(2) Meditate over the last mentioned truths, and then follow the matter still further. Read what we have said in the "Advanced Course" (Lesson XI) about the last analysis of Matter showing it fading away into Force or Energy until the dividing line is lost, and Matter merges into Energy or Force, showing them both to be but the same thing, Matter being a grosser form of Energy or Force. This idea should be impressed upon the understanding, in order that the complete edifice of the Knowing of the Oneness may be complete in all of its parts.

(3) Then read in the "Advanced Lessons" about Energy or Force, in the oneness underlying its various manifestations. Consider how one form of Energy may be transformed into another, and so on around the circle, the one principle producing the entire chain of appearances. Realize that the energy within you by which you move and act, is but one of the forms of this great Principle of Energy with which the Universe is filled, and that you may draw to you the required Energy from the great Universal supply. But above all endeavor to grasp the idea of the Oneness pervading the world of Energy or Force, or Motion. See it in its entirety, rather than in its apparent separateness. These steps may appear somewhat tedious and useless, but take our word for it, they are all helps in fitting the mind to grasp the idea of the Oneness of All. Each step is important, and renders the next higher one more easily attained. In this mental drill, it will be well to mentally picture the Universe in perpetual motion—everything is in motion—all matter is moving and changing its forms, and manifesting the Energy within it. Suns and worlds rush through space, their particles constantly changing and moving. Chemical composition and decomposition is constant and unceasing, everywhere the work of building up and breaking down is going on. New combinations of atoms and worlds are constantly being formed and dissolved. And after considering this Oneness of the principle of Energy, reflect that through all these changes of form the Ego—the Real Self—YOU—stand unchanged and unharmed—Eternal, Invincible, Indestructible, Invulnerable, *Real* and Constant among this changing world of forms and force. You are above it all, and it revolves around and about you—Spirit.

(4) Read what we have said in the "Advanced Course" about Force or Energy, shading into Mind-substance which is its parent. Realize that Mind is back of all this great

exhibition of Energy and Force that you have been considering. Then will you be ready to consider the Oneness of Mind.

(5) Read what we have said in the "Advanced Lessons" about Mind-substance. Realize that there is a great world of Mind-substance, or an Universal Mind, which is at the disposal of the Ego. All Thought is the product of the Ego's use of this Mind-substance, its tool and instrument. Realize that this Ocean of Mind is entire and Whole, and that the Ego may draw freely from it. Realize that *You* have this great ocean of Mind at your command, when you unfold sufficiently to use it. Realize that Mind is back of and underneath all of the world of form and names and action, and that in that sense: "All is Mind," although still higher in the scale than even Mind are *You*, the Real Self, the Ego, the Manifestation of the Absolute.

(6) Realize your identity with and relationship to All of Life. Look around you at Life in all its forms, from the lowest to the highest, all being exhibitions of the great principle of Life in operation along different stages of The Path. Scorn not the humblest forms, but look behind the form and see the reality—Life. Feel yourself a part of the great Universal Life. Let your thought sink to the depths of the ocean, and realize your kinship with the Life back of the forms dwelling there. Do not confound the forms (often hideous from your personal point of view) with the principle behind them. Look at the plant-life, and the animal life, and seek to see behind the veil of form into the real Life behind and underneath the form. Learn to feel your Life throbbing and thrilling with the Life Principle in these other forms, and in the forms of those of your own race. Gaze into the starry skies and see there the numerous suns and worlds, all peopled with life in some of its myriad forms, and feel your kinship to it. If you can grasp this thought and consciousness, you will find yourself at-one-ment with those whirling worlds, and, instead of feeling small and insignificant by comparison, you will be conscious of an expansion of Self, until you feel that in those circling worlds is a part of yourself—that You are there also, while standing upon the Earth—that you are akin to all parts of the Universe—nay, more, that they are as much your home as is the spot upon which you are standing. You will find sweeping upon you a sense of consciousness that the Universe is your home—not merely a part of it, as you had previously thought. You will experience a sense of greatness, and broadness and grandness such as you have never dreamed of. You will begin to realize at least a part of your Divine inheritance, and to know indeed that you are a Child of the Infinite, the very essence of your Divine Parent being in the fibres of your being, At such times of realization one becomes conscious of what lies before the soul in its upward path, and how small the greatest prizes that Earth has to offer are when compared to some of these things before the soul, as seen by the eyes of the Spiritual Mind in moments of clear vision.

You must not dispute with these visions of the greatness of the soul, but must treat them hospitably, for they are your very own, coming to you from the regions of your Spiritual Mind which are unfolding into consciousness.

(7) The highest step in this dawning consciousness of the Oneness of All, is the one in which is realized that there is but One Reality, and at the same time the sense of consciousness that the "I" is in that Reality. It is most difficult to express this thought in words for it is something that must be felt, rather than seen by the Intellect. When the Soul realizes that the Spirit within it is, at the last, the only *real* part of it, and that the Absolute and its manifestation as Spirit is the only *real* thing in the Universe, a great step has been taken. But there is still one higher step to be taken before the full sense of the Oneness and Reality comes to us. That step is the one in which we realize the Identity of the "I" with the great "I" of the Universe. The mystery of the manifestation of the Absolute in the form of the Spirit, is veiled from us—the mind confesses its inability to penetrate behind the veil shielding the Absolute from view, although it will give us a report of its being conscious of the presence of the Absolute just at the edge of the boundary line. But the highest region of the Spiritual Mind, when explored by the advanced souls who are well along the Path, reports that it sees beyond the apparent separation of Spirit from Spirit, and realizes that there is but one Reality of Spirit, and that all the "I"'s are really but different views of that One—Centres of Consciousness upon the surface of the One Great "I," the Centre of which is the Absolute Itself. This certainly penetrates the whole region of the Spiritual Mind, and gives us all the message of Oneness of the Spirit, just as the Intellect satisfies us with its message of the Oneness of Matter, Energy, and Mind. The idea of Oneness permeates all planes of Life.

The sense of Reality of the "I" that is apparent to You in the moments of your clearest mental vision, is really the reflection of the sense of Reality underlying the Whole—it is the consciousness of the Whole, manifesting through your point or Centre of Consciousness. The advanced student or Initiate finds his consciousness gradually enlarging until it realizes its identity with the Whole. He realizes that under all the forms and names of the visible world, there is to be found One Life—One Force—One Substance—One Existence—One Reality—ONE. And, instead of his experiencing any sense of the loss of identity or individuality, he becomes conscious of an enlargement of an expansion of individuality or identity—instead of feeling himself absorbed in the Whole, he feels that he is spreading out and embracing the Whole. This is most hard to express in words, for there are no words to fit the conception, and all that we can hope to do is to start into motion, by means of our words, the vibrations that will find a response in the minds of those who read the words, to the end that they will experience the consciousness which will bring its own understanding. This consciousness cannot be transmitted by words proceeding from the Intellect, but vibrations may be set up that will prepare the mind to receive the message from its own higher planes.

Even in the early stages of this dawning consciousness, one is enabled to identify the *real* part of himself with the *real* part of all the other forms of life that pass before his notice. In every other man—in every animal—in every plant—in every mineral—he sees behind the sheath and form of appearance, an evidence of the presence of the Spirit which is akin to his own Spirit—yea, more than akin, for the two are One. He sees Himself in all forms of life, in all time in all places. He realizes that the Real Self is everywhere present and everlasting, and that the Life within himself is also within all the Universe—in everything, for there is nothing dead in the Universe, and all Life, in all of its varying phases, is simply the One Life, held, used and enjoyed in common by all. Each Ego is a Centre of Consciousness in this great ocean of Life, and while apparently separate and distinct, is yet really in touch with the Whole, and with every apparent part.

It is not our intention, in this lesson, to go into the details of this great mystery of Life, or to recite the comparatively little of the Truth that the most advanced teachers and Masters have handed down. This is not the place for it—it belongs to the subject of Gnani Yoga rather than to Raja Yoga—and we touch upon it here, not for the purpose of trying to explain the scientific side of it to you, but merely in order that your minds may be led to take up the idea and gradually manifest it in conscious realization. There is quite a difference between the scientific, intellectual teaching of Gnani Yoga, whereby the metaphysical and scientific sides of the Yogi teachings are presented to the minds of the students, in a logical, scientific manner, and the methods of Raja Yoga, in which the Candidate is led by degrees to a *consciousness* (outside of mere intellectual belief) of his real nature and powers. We are following the latter plan, for this course is a Course in *Raja* Yoga. We are aiming to present the matter to the mind in such a manner that it may prepare the way for the dawning consciousness, by brushing away the preconceived notions and prejudices, and allowing a clean entrance for the new conception. Much that we have said in this lesson may appear, on the one hand, like useless repetition, and, on the other hand, like an incomplete presentation of the scientific side of the Yogi teachings. But it will be found, in time, that the effect has been that the mind of the student has undergone a change from the absorbing of the idea of the Oneness of Life, and the Expansion of the Self. The Candidate is urged not to be in too much of a hurry. Development must not be forced. Read what we have written, and practice the Mental Drills we have given, even if they may appear trifling and childish to some of you—we know what they will do for you, and you will agree with us in time. Make haste slowly. You will find that the mind will work out the matter, even though you be engaged in your ordinary work, and have forgotten the subject for the time. The greater portion of mental work is done in this way, while you are busy with something else, or even asleep, for the sub-conscious portion of the mind works along the lines pointed out for it, and performs its task.

As we have said, the purpose of this lesson is to bring you in the way of the unfoldment of consciousness, rather than to teach you the details of the scientific side of the Yogi teachings. Development is the keynote of Raja Yoga. And the reason that we wish to develop this sense of the Reality of the "I," and the Expansion of the Self, at this place is that thereby you may assert your Mastery over Matter, Energy and Mind. Before you may mount your throne as King, you must fully realize in consciousness that you *are* the *Reality* in this world of appearances. You must realize that you—the *real* You—are not only existent, and real, but that you are in touch with all else that is real, and that the roots of your being are grounded in the Absolute itself. You must realize that instead of being a separate atom of Reality, isolated and fixed in a narrow space, you are a Centre of Consciousness in the Whole of Reality, and that the Universe of Universes is your home—that your Centre of Consciousness might be moved on to a point trillions of miles from the Earth (which distance would be as nothing in Space) and still you—the awakened soul—would be just as much at home there as here—that even while you are here, your influence extends far out into space. Your real state, which will be revealed to you, gradually, throughout the ages, is so great and grand, that your mind in its present state of development cannot grasp even the faint reflection of that glory.

We wish you to try to form at least a faint idea of your Real State of Being, in order that you may control the lower principles by the force of your awakened Will, which Will depends upon your degree of consciousness of the Real Self.

As man grows in understanding and consciousness of the Real Self, so does his ability to use his Will grow. Will is the attribute of the Real Self. It is well that this great realization of the Real Self brings with it Love for all of Life, and Kindness, for, were it not so, the Will that comes to him who grows into a realization of his real being could be used to the great hurt of those of the race who had not progressed so far (their *relative* hurt, we mean, for in the end, and at the last, no soul is ever really *hurt*). But the dawning power brings with it greater Love and Kindness, and the higher the soul mounts the more is it filled with the higher ideals and the more does it throw from it the lower animal attributes. It is true that some souls growing into a consciousness of their real nature, without an understanding of what it all means, may commit the error of using the awakened Will for selfish ends, as may be seen in the cases of the Black Magicians spoken of in the occult writings, and also in the cases of well known characters in history and in modern life, who manifest an enormous Will which they misuse. All of this class of people of great Will have stumbled or grown blindly into a consciousness (or partial consciousness) of the real nature, but lack the restraining influence of the higher teachings. But such misuse of the Will brings pain and unrest to the user, and he is eventually driven into the right road.

We do not expect our students to grasp fully this idea of the Expansion of Self. Even the highest grasp it only partially. But until you get a glimmering of the consciousness you will not be able to progress far on the path of Raja Yoga. You must understand *what you are*, before you are able to use the power that lies dormant within you. You must realize that you are the Master, before you can claim the powers of the Master, and expect to have your commands obeyed. So bear patiently with us, your Teachers, while we set before you the lessons to be learned—the tasks to be performed. The road is long, and is rough in places—the feet may become tired and bruised, but the reward is great, and there are resting places along the path. Be not discouraged if your progress seem slow, for the soul must unfold naturally as does the flower, without haste, without force.

And be not dismayed nor affrighted if you occasionally catch a glimpse of your higher self. As "M.C." says, in her notes on "Light on the Path" (see "Advanced Course," page 95): "To have seen thy soul in its bloom, is to have obtained a momentary glimpse in thyself of the transfiguration which shall eventually make thee more than man; to recognize, is to achieve the great task of gazing upon the blazing light without dropping the eyes, and not falling back in terror as though before some ghastly phantom. This happens to some, and so, when the victory is all but won, it is lost."

Peace be with thee.

MANTRAM (AFFIRMATION) FOR THE THIRD LESSON.

There is but one ultimate form of Matter; one ultimate form of Energy; one ultimate form of Mind. Matter proceeds from Energy, and Energy from Mind, and all are an emanation of the Absolute, threefold in appearance but One in substance. There is but One Life, and that permeates the Universe, manifesting in various forms, but being, at the last, but One. My body is one with Universal Matter; My energy and vital force is one with the Universal Energy; My Mind is one with the Universal Mind; My Life is one with the Universal Life. The Absolute has expressed and manifested itself in Spirit, which is the real "I" overshadowing and embracing all the apparently separate "I"s. "I" feel my identity with Spirit and realize the Oneness of All Reality. I feel my unity with all Spirit, and my Union (through Spirit) with the Absolute. I realize that "I" am an Expression and Manifestation of the Absolute, and that its very essence is within me. I am filled with Divine Love. I am filled with Divine Power. I am filled with Divine Wisdom. I am conscious of identity in spirit, in substance; and in nature; with the One Reality.

THE FOURTH LESSON.

MENTAL CONTROL.

In our first three lessons of this series, we have endeavored to bring into realization within your mind (1) the consciousness of the "I"; its independence from the body; its immortality; its invincibility and invulnerability; (2) the superiority of the "I" over the mind, as well as over the body; the fact that the mind is not the "I," but is merely an instrument for the expression of the "I"; the fact that the "I" is master of the mind, as well as of the body; that the "I" is behind all thought; that the "I" can set aside for consideration the sensations, emotions, passions, desires, and the rest of the mental phenomena, and still realize that it, the "I," is apart from these mental manifestations, and remains unchanged, real and fully existent; that the "I" can set aside any and all of its mental tools and instruments, as "not I" things, and still consciously realize that after so setting them aside there remains something—itself—the "I" which cannot be set aside or taken from; that the "I" is the master of the mind, and not its slave; (3) that the "I" is a much greater thing than the little personal "I" we have been considering it to be; that the "I" is a part of that great One Reality which pervades all the Universe; that it is connected with all other forms of life by countless ties, mental and spiritual filaments and relations; that the "I" is a Centre of Consciousness in that great One Reality or Spirit, which is behind and back of all Life and Existence, the Centre of which Reality or Existence, is the Absolute or God; that the sense of Reality that is inherent in the "I," is really the reflection of the sense of Reality inherent in the Whole—the Great "I" of the Universe.

The underlying principle of these three lessons is the Reality of the "I," in itself, over and above all Matter, Force, or Mind—positive to all of them, just as they are positive or negative to each other—and negative only to the Centre of the One—the Absolute itself. And this is the position for the Candidate or Initiate to take: "I am positive to Mind, Energy, and Matter, and control them all—I am negative only to the Absolute, which is the Centre of Being, of which Being I Am. And, as I assert my mastery over Mind, Energy, and Matter, and exercise my Will over them, so do I acknowledge my subordination to the Absolute, and gladly open my soul to the inflow of the Divine Will, and partake of its Power, Strength, and Wisdom."

In the present lesson, and those immediately following it, we shall endeavor to assist the Candidate or Initiate in acquiring a mastery of the subordinate manifestations, Matter, Energy, and Mind. In order to acquire and assert this mastery, one must acquaint himself with the nature of the thing to be controlled.

In our "Advanced Course" we have endeavored to explain to you the nature of the Three Great Manifestations, known as *Chitta*, or Mind-Substance; *Prana*, or Energy; and *Akasa*, or the Principle of Matter. We also explained to you that the "I" of man is superior to these three, being what is known as *Atman* or Spirit. Matter, Energy, and Mind, as we have explained, are manifestations of the Absolute, and are relative things. The Yogi philosophy teaches that Matter is the grossest form of manifested substance, being below Energy and Mind, and consequently negative to, and subordinate to both. One stage higher than Matter, is Energy or Force, which is positive to, and has authority over, Matter (Matter being a still grosser form of substance), but which is negative to and subordinate to Mind, which is a still higher form of substance. Next in order comes the highest of the three—Mind—the finest form of substance, and which dominates both Energy and Matter, being positive to both. Mind, however is negative and subordinate to the "I," which is Spirit, and obeys the orders of the latter when firmly and intelligently given. The "I" itself is subordinate only to the Absolute—the Centre of Being—the "I" being positive and dominant over the threefold manifestation of Mind, Energy, and Matter.

The "I," which for the sake of the illustration must be regarded as a separate thing (although it is really only a Centre of Consciousness in the great body of Spirit), finds itself surrounded by the triple-ocean of Mind, Energy and Matter, which ocean extends into Infinity. The body is but a physical form through which flows an unending stream of matter, for, as you know the particles and atoms of the body are constantly changing; being renewed; replaced; thrown off, and supplanted. One's body of a few years ago, or rather the particles composing that body, have passed off and now form new combinations in the world of matter. And one's body of to-day is passing away and being replaced by new particles. And one's body of next year is now occupying some other portion of space, and its particles are now parts of countless other combinations, from which space and combinations they will later come to combine and form the body of next year. There is nothing permanent about the body—even the particles of the bones are being constantly replaced by others. And so it is with the Vital Energy, Force, or Strength of the body (including that of the brain). It is constantly being used up, and expended, a fresh supply taking its place. And even the Mind of the person is changeable, and the Mind-substance or *Chitta*, is being used up and replenished, the new supply coming from the great Ocean of Mind, into which the discarded portion slips, just as is the case with the matter and energy.

While the majority of our students, who are more or less familiar with the current material scientific conceptions, will readily accept the above idea of the ocean of Matter, and Energy, and the fact that there is a continual using up and replenishing of one's store of both, they may have more or less trouble in accepting the idea that Mind is a substance or principle amenable to the same general laws as are the other two manifestations, or attributes of substance. One is so apt to think of his Mind as "himself"—the "I." Notwithstanding the fact that in our Second Lesson of this series we showed you that the "I" is superior to the mental states, and that it can set them aside and regard and consider them as "not-I" things, yet the force of the habit of thought is very strong, and it may take some of you considerable time before you "get into the way" of realizing that your Mind is "something that you use," instead of being You—yourself. And yet, you must persevere in attaining this realization, for in the degree that you realize your dominance over your mind, so will be your control of it, and its amenability to that control. And, as is the degree of that dominance and control, so will be the character, grade and extent of the work that your Mind will do for you. So you see: *Realization brings Control—and Control brings results*. This statement lies at the base of the science of *Raja Yoga*. And many of its first exercises are designed to acquaint the student with that realization, and to develop the realization and control by habit and practice.

The Yogi Philosophy teaches that instead of Mind being the "I." it is the thing through and by means of which the "I" *thinks*, at least so far as is concerned the knowledge concerning the phenomenal or outward Universe—that is the Universe of Name and Form. There is a higher Knowledge locked up in the innermost part of the "I," that far transcends any information that it may receive about or from the outer world, but that is not before us for consideration at this time, and we must concern ourselves with the "thinking" about the world of things.

Mind-substance in Sanscrit is called "*Chitta*," and a wave in the *Chitta* (which wave is the combination of Mind and Energy) is called "*Vritta*," which is akin to what we call a "thought." In other words it is "mind in action," whereas *Chitta* is "mind in repose." *Vritta*, when literally translated means "a whirlpool or eddy in the mind," which is exactly what a thought really is.

But we must call the attention of the student, at this point, to the fact that the word "Mind" is used in two ways by the Yogis and other occultists, and the student is directed to form a clear conception of each meaning, in order to avoid confusion, and that he may more clearly perceive the two aspects of the things which the word is intended to express. In the first place the word "Mind" is used as synonymous with *Chitta*, or Mind-substance, which is the Universal Mind Principle. From this *Chitta*, Mind-substance, or Mind, all the material of the millions of personal minds is obtained. The second meaning of the word "Mind" is that which we mean when we speak of the "mind" of anyone, thereby meaning the mental faculties of that particular person—that which distinguishes his mental personality from that of another. We have taught you that this "mind" in Man, functions on three planes, and have called the respective manifestations (1) the Instinctive Mind; (2) the Intellect; and (3) the Spiritual Mind. (*See "Fourteen Lessons in Yogi Philosophy," etc.*) These three mental planes, taken together, make up the "mind" of the person, or to be more exact they, clustered around the "I" form the "soul" of the individual. The word "soul" is often used as synonymous with "spirit" but those who have followed us will distinguish the difference. The "soul" is the Ego surrounded by its mental principles, while the Spirit is the "soul of the soul"—the "I," or Real Self.

The Science of *Raja Yoga*, to which this series of lessons is devoted, teaches, as its basic principle, the Control of the Mind. It holds that the first step toward Power consists in obtaining a control of one's own mind. It holds that the internal world must be conquered before the outer world is attacked. It holds that the "I" manifests itself in Will, and that that Will may be used to manipulate, guide, govern and direct the mind of its owner, as well as the physical world. It aims to clear away all mental rubbish, and encumbrances—to conduct a "mental house-cleaning," as it were, and to secure a clear, clean, healthy mind. Then it proceeds to control that mind intelligently, and with effect, saving all waste-power, and by means of concentration bringing the Mind in full harmony with the Will, that it may be brought to a focus and its power greatly increased and its efficiency fully secured. Concentration and Will-power are the means by which the Yogis obtain such wonderful results, and by which they manage and direct their vigorous, healthy minds, and master the material world, acting positively upon Energy and Matter. This control extends to all planes of the Mind and the Yogis not only control the Instinctive Mind, holding in subjection its lower qualities and making use of its other parts, but they also develop and enlarge the field of their Intellect and obtain from it wonderful results. Even the Spiritual Mind is mastered, and aided in its unfoldment, and urged to pass down into the field of consciousness some of the wonderful secrets to be found within its area. By means of *Raja Yoga* many of the secrets of existence and Being—many of the Riddles of the Universe—are answered and solved. And by it the latent powers inherent in the constitution of Man are unfolded and brought into action. Those highly advanced in the science are believed to have obtained such a wonderful degree of power and control over the forces of the universe, that they are as gods compared with the ordinary man.

Raja Yoga teaches that not only may power of this kind be secured, but that a wonderful field of Knowledge is opened out through its practice. It holds that when the concentrated mind is focused upon thing or subject, the true nature and inner meaning, of, and concerning, that thing or subject will be brought to view. The concentrated mind passes through the object or subject just as the X-Ray passes through a block of wood, and the thing is seen by the "I" as it *is*—in truth—and not as it had appeared before, imperfectly and erroneously. Not only may the outside world be thus explored, but the mental ray may be turned inward, and the secret places of the mind explored. When it is remembered that the bit of mind that each man possesses, is like a drop of the ocean which contains within its tiny compass all the elements that make up the ocean, and that to know perfectly the drop is to know perfectly the ocean, then we begin to see what such a power really means.

Many in the Western world who have attained great results in the intellectual and scientific fields of endeavor, have developed these powers more or less unconsciously. Many great inventors are practical Yogis, although they do not realize the source of their power. Anyone who is familiar with the personal mental characteristics of Edison, will see that he follows some of the *Raja Yoga* methods, and that Concentration is one of his strongest weapons. And from all reports, Prof. Elmer Gates, of Washington, D.C., whose mind has unfolded many wonderful discoveries and inventions, is also a practical Yogi although he may repudiate the assertion vigorously, and may not have familiarized himself with the principles of this science, which he has "dropped into" unconsciously. Those who have reported upon Prof. Gates' methods, say that he fairly "digs out" the inventions and discoveries from his mind, after going into seclusion and practicing concentration, and what is known as the Mental Vision.

But we have given you enough of theory for one lesson, and must begin to give you directions whereby you may aid yourself in developing these latent powers and unfolding these dormant energies. You will notice that in this series we first tell you something about the theory, and then proceed to give you "something to do." This is the true Yogi method as followed and practiced by their best teachers. Too much theory is tiresome, and sings the mind to sleep, while too much exercise tires one, and does not give the inquiring part of his mind the necessary food. To combine both in suitable proportions is the better plan, and one that we aim to follow.

MENTAL DRILL AND EXERCISES.

Before we can get the mind to do good work for us, we must first "tame" it, and bring it to obedience to the Will of the "I." The mind, as a rule, has been allowed to run wild, and follow its own sweet will and desires, without regard to anything else. Like a spoiled child or badly trained domestic animal, it gets into much trouble, and is of very little pleasure, comfort or use. The minds of many of us are like menageries of wild animals, each pursuing the bent of its own nature, and going its own way. We have the whole menagerie within us—the tiger, the ape, the peacock, the ass, the goose, the sheep the hyena, and all the rest. And we have been letting these animals rule us. Even our Intellect is erratic, unstable, and like the quicksilver to which the ancient occultists compared it, shifting and uncertain. If you will look around you you will see that those men and women in the world who have really accomplished anything worth while have trained their minds to obedience. They have asserted the Will over their own minds, and learned Mastery and Power in that way. The average mind chafes at the restraint of the Will, and is like a frisky monkey that will not be "taught tricks." But taught it must be, if it wants to do good work. And teach it you must if you expect to get any use from it—if you expect to use it, instead of having it use you.

And this is the first thing to be learned in *Raja Yoga*—this control of the mind. Those who had hoped for some royal road to mastery, may be disappointed, but there is only one way and that is to master and control the mind by the Will. Otherwise it will run away when you most need it. And so we shall give you some exercise designed to aid you in this direction.

The first exercise in *Raja Yoga* Is what is called *Pratyahara* or the art of making the mind introspective or turned inward upon itself. It is the first step toward mental control. It aims to turn the mind from going outward, and gradually turning it inward upon itself or inner nature. The object is to gain control of it by the Will. The following exercises will aid in that direction:

EXERCISE I.

(a) Place yourself in a comfortable position, and so far as possible free from outside disturbing influences. Make no violent effort to control the mind, but rather allow it to run along for a while and exhaust its efforts. It will take advantage of the opportunity, and will jump around like an unchained monkey at first, until it gradually slows down and looks to you for orders. It may take some time to tame down at first trial, but each time you try it will come around to you in shorter time. The Yogis spend much time in acquiring this mental peace and calm, and consider themselves well paid for it.

(b) When the mind is well calmed down, and peaceful, fix the thought on the "I Am," as taught in our previous lessons. Picture the "I" as an entity independent of the body; deathless; invulnerable; immortal; real. Then think of it as independent of the body, and able to exist without its fleshly covering. Meditate upon this for a time, and then gradually direct the thought to the realization of the "I" as independent and superior to the mind, and controlling same. Go over the general ideas of the first two lessons, and endeavor to calmly reflect upon them and to see them in the "mind's eye." You will find that your mind is gradually becoming more and more peaceful and calm, and that the distracting thoughts of the outside world are farther and farther removed from you.

(c) Then let the mind pass on to a calm consideration of the Third Lesson, in which we have spoken of the Oneness of All, and the relationship of the "I" to the One Life; Power; Intelligence; Being. You will find that you are acquiring a mental control and calm heretofore unknown to you. The exercises in the first three lessons will have prepared you for this.

(d) The following is the most difficult of the variations or degrees of this exercise, but the ability to perform it will come gradually. The exercise consists in gradually shutting out all thought or impression of the outside world; of the body; and of the thoughts themselves, the student concentrating and meditating upon the word and idea "I AM," the idea being that he shall concentrate upon the idea of mere "being" or "existence," symbolized by the words "I Am." Not "I am *this*," or "I am *that*," or "I *do* this," or "I *think* that," but simply: "I *AM*." This exercise will focus the attention at the very centre of Being within oneself, and will gather in all the mental energies, instead of allowing them to be scattered upon outside things. A feeling of Peace, Strength, and Power will result, for the affirmation, and the thought back of it, is the most powerful and strongest that one may make, for it is a statement of Actual Being, and a turning of the thought inward to that truth. Let the mind first dwell upon the word "I," identifying it with the Self, and then let it pass on to the word "AM," which signifies Reality, and Being. Then combine the two with the meanings thereof, and the result a most powerful focusing of thought inward, and most potent Statement of Being.

It is well to accompany the above exercises with a comfortable and easy physical attitude, so as to prevent the distraction of the attention by the body. In order to do this one should assume an easy attitude and then relax every muscle, and take the tension from every nerve, until a perfect sense of ease, comfort and relaxation is obtained. You should practice this until you have fully acquired it. It will be useful to you in many ways, besides rendering Concentration and Meditation easier. It will act as a "rest cure" for tired body, nerves, and mind.

EXERCISE II.

The second step in *Raja Yoga* is what is known as *Dharana*, or Concentration. This is a most wonderful idea in the direction of focusing the mental forces, and may be cultivated to an almost incredible degree, but all this requires work, time, and patience. But the student will be well repaid for it. Concentration consists in the mind focusing upon a certain subject, or object, and being held there for a time. This, at first thought seems very easy, but a little practice will show how difficult it is to firmly fix the attention and hold it there. It will have a tendency to waver, and move to some other object or subject, and much practice will be needed in order to hold it at the desired point. But practice will accomplish wonders, as one may see by observing people who have acquired this faculty, and who use it in their everyday life. But the following point should be remembered. Many persons have acquired the faculty of concentrating their attention, but have allowed it to become almost involuntary, and they become a slave to it, forgetting themselves and everything else, and often neglecting necessary affairs. This is the ignorant way of concentrating, and those addicted to it become slaves to their habits, instead of masters of their minds. They become day-dreamers, and absent-minded people, instead of Masters. They are to be pitied as much as those who cannot concentrate at all. The secret is in a mastery of the mind. The Yogis can concentrate at will, and completely bury themselves in the subject before them, and extract from it every item of interest, and can then pass the mind from the thing at will, the same control being used in both cases. They do not allow fits of abstraction, or "absent-mindedness" to come upon them, nor are they day-dreamers. On the contrary they are very wide awake individuals; close observers; clear thinkers; correct reasoners. They are masters of their minds, not slaves to their moods. The ignorant concentrator buries himself in the object or subject, and allows it to master and absorb himself, while the trained Yogi thinker asserts the "I," and then directs his mind to concentrate upon the subject or object, keeping it well under control and in view all the time. Do you see the difference? Then heed the lesson.

The following exercises may be found useful in the first steps of Concentration:

(a) Concentrate the attention upon some familiar object—a pencil, for instance. Hold the mind there and consider the pencil to the exclusion of any other object. Consider its size; color; shape; kind of wood. Consider its uses, and purposes; its materials; the process of its manufacture, etc., etc., etc. In short think as many things about the pencil as possible allowing the mind to pursue any associated by-paths, such as a consideration of the graphite of which the "lead" is made; the forest from which came the wood used in making the pencil; the history of pencils, and other implements used for writing, etc. In short exhaust the subject of "Pencils." In considering a subject under concentration, the following plan of synopsis will be found useful. Think of the thing in question from the following view-points:

(1) The thing itself.

(2) The place from whence it came.

(3) Its purpose or use.

(4) Its associations.

(5) Its probable end.

Do not let the apparently trivial nature of the inquiry discourage you, for the simplest form of mental training is useful, and will help to develop your Will and Concentration. It is akin to the process of developing a physical muscle by some simple exercise, and in both cases one loses sight of the unimportance of the exercise itself, in view of the end to be gained.

(b) Concentrate the attention upon some part of the body—the hand for instance, and fixing your entire attention upon it, shut off or inhibit all sensation from the other parts of the body. A little practice will enable you to do this. In addition to the mental training, this exercise will stimulate the part of the body concentrated upon, for reasons that will appear in future lessons. Change the parts of the body concentrated upon, and thus give the mind a variety of exercises, and the body the effect of a general stimulation.

(c) These exercises may be extended indefinitely upon familiar objects about you. Remember always, that the thing in itself is of no importance, the whole idea being to train the mind to obey the Will, so that when you really wish to use the mental forces upon some important object, you may find them well trained and obedient. Do not be tempted to slight this part of the work because it is "dry" and uninteresting, for it leads up to things that are most interesting, and opens a door to a fascinating subject.

(d) Practice focusing the attention upon some abstract subject—that is upon some subject of interest that may offer a field for mental exploration. Think about the subject in all its phases and branches, following up one by-path, and then another, until you feel that you know all about the subject that your mind has acquired. You will be surprised to find how much more you know about any one thing or subject than you had believed possible. In hidden corners of your mind you will find some useful or interesting information about the thing in question, and when you are through you will feel well posted upon it, and upon the things connected with it. This exercise will not only help, to develop your intellectual powers, but will strengthen your memory, and broaden your mind, and give you more confidence in yourself. And, in addition, you will have taken a valuable exercise in Concentration or *Dharana*.

The Importance of Concentration.

Concentration is a focusing of the mind. And this focusing of the mind requires a focusing, or bringing to a center, of the Will. The mind is concentrated because the Will is focused upon the object. The mind flows into the mould made by the Will. The above exercises are designed not only to accustom the mind to the obedience and direction of the Will, but also tend to accustom the Will to command. We speak of strengthening the Will, when what we really mean is training the mind to obey, and accustoming the Will to command. Our Will is strong enough, but we do not realize it. The Will takes root in the very center of our being—in the "I," but our imperfectly developed mind does not recognize this tact. We are like young elephants that do not recognize their own strength, but allow themselves to be mastered by puny drivers, whom they could brush aside with a movement. The Will is back of all action—all doing—mental and physical.

We shall have much to say touching the Will, in these lessons and the student should give the matter his careful attention. Let him look around him, and he will see that the great difference between the men who have stepped forward from the ranks, and those who remain huddled up in the crowd, consists in Determination and Will. As Buxton has well said: "The longer I live, the more certain I am that the great difference between men, the feeble and the powerful; the great and the insignificant; is Energy and Invincible Determination." And he might have added that the thing behind that "energy and invincible determination" was Will.

The writers and thinkers of all ages have recognized the wonderful and transcendent importance of the Will. Tennyson sings: "O living Will thou shalt endure when all that seems shall suffer shock." Oliver Wendell Holmes says: "The seat of the Will seems to vary with the organ through which it is manifested; to transport itself to different parts of the brain, as we may wish to recall a picture, a phrase, a melody; to throw its force on the muscles or the intellectual processes. Like the general-in-chief, its place is everywhere in the field of action. It is the least like an instrument of any of our faculties; the farthest removed from our conceptions of mechanism and matter, as we commonly define them." Holmes was correct in his idea, but faulty in his details. The Will does not change its seat, which is always in the center of the Ego, but the Will forces the mind to all parts, and in all directions, and it directs the *Prana* or vital force likewise. The Will is indeed the general-in-chief, but it does not rush to the various points of action, but sends its messengers and couriers there to carry out its orders. Buxton has said: "The Will will do anything that can be done in this world. And no talents, no circumstances, no opportunities will make a two-legged creature a Man without it." Ik Marvel truly says: "Resolve is what makes a man manifest; not puny resolve, not crude determinations, not errant purpose—but that strong and indefatigable Will which treads down difficulties and danger, as a boy treads down the heaving frost-lands of winter; which kindles his eye and brain with a proud pulse-beat toward the unattainable. Will makes men giants."

The great obstacle to the proper use of the Will, in the case of the majority of people, is the lack of ability to focus the attention. The Yogis clearly understand this point, and many of the *Raja Yoga* exercises which are given to the students by the teachers, are designed to overcome this difficulty. Attention is the outward evidence of the Will. As a French writer has said: "The attention is subject to the superior authority of the Ego. I yield it, or I withhold it, as I please. I direct it in turn to several points. I concentrate it upon each point as long as my Will can stand the effort." Prof. James has said: "The essential achievement of the Will, when it is most voluntary, is to attend to a difficult object, and hold it fast before the mind. Effort of Attention is the essential phenomenon of the Will." And Prof. Halleck says: "The first step toward the development of Will lies in the exercise of Attention. Ideas grow in distinctness and motor-power as we attend to them. If we take two ideas of the same intensity and center the attention upon one, we shall notice how much it grows in power." Prof. Sully says: "Attention may be roughly defined as the active self-direction of the mind to any object which presents itself at the moment." The word "Attention" is derived from two Latin words, *ad tendere*, meaning "to stretch towards," and this is just what the Yogis know it to be. By means of their psychic or clairvoyant sight, they see the thought of the attentive person stretched out toward the object attended to, like a sharp wedge, the point of which is focused upon the object under consideration, the entire force of the thought being concentrated at that point. This is true not only when the person is considering an object, but when he is earnestly impressing his ideas upon another, or upon some task to be accomplished. Attention means reaching the mind out to and focusing it upon something.

The trained Will exhibits itself in a tenacious Attention, and this Attention is one of the signs of the trained Will. The student must not hastily conclude that this kind of Attention is a common faculty among men. On the contrary it is quite rare, and is seen only among those of "strong" mentality. Anyone may fasten his Attention upon some passing, *pleasing* thing, but it takes a trained will to fasten it upon some unattractive thing, and hold it there. Of course the trained occultist is able to throw interest into the most unattractive thing upon which it becomes advisable to focus his Attention, but this, in itself, comes with the trained Will, and is not the possession of the average man. Voluntary Attention is rare, and is found only among strong characters. But it may be cultivated and grown, until he who has scarcely a shade of it to-day, in time may become a giant. It is all a matter of practice, exercise, and Will.

It is difficult to say too much in favor of the development of the faculty of tenacious Attention. One possessing this developed faculty is able to accomplish far more than even a much "brighter" man who lacks it. And the best way to train the Attention, under the direction of the Will, is to practice upon *uninteresting* objects, and ideas, holding them before the mind until they begin to assume an Interest. This is difficult at first, but the task soon begins to take on a pleasant aspect, for one finds that his Will-power and Attention are growing, and he feels himself acquiring a Force and Power that were lacking before—he realizes that he is growing Stronger. Charles Dickens said that the secret of his success consisted in his developing a faculty of throwing his entire Attention into whatever he happened to be doing at the moment and then being able to turn that same degree of Attention to the next thing coming before him for consideration. He was like a man behind a great searchlight, which was successively turned upon point after point, illuminating each in turn. The "I" is the man behind the light, and the Will is the reflector, the light being the Attention.

This discussion of Will and Attention may seem somewhat "dry" to the student, but that is all the more reason that he should attend to it. It is the secret that lies at the basis of the Science of *Raja Yoga*, and the Yogi Masters have attained a degree of Concentrated Will and Attention that would be inconceivable to the average "man on the street." By reason of this, they are able to direct the mind here and there, outward or inward, with an enormous force. They are able to focus the mind upon a small thing with remarkable intensity, just as the rays of the sun may be focused through a "sun-glass" and caused to ignite linen, or, on the other hand, they are able to send forth the mind with intense energy, illuminating whatever it rests upon, just as happens in the case of the strong electric searchlight, with which many of us are familiar. By all means start in to cultivate the Attention and Will. Practice on the unpleasant tasks—do the things that you have before you, and from which you have been shrinking because they were unpleasant. Throw interest into them, and the difficulty will vanish, and you will come out of it much stronger, and filled with a new sense of Power.

MANTRAM (AFFIRMATION).

"I" have a Will—it is my inalienable property and right. I determine to cultivate and develop it by practice and exercise. My mind is obedient to my Will. I assert my Will over my Mind. I am Master of my mind and body. I *assert* my Mastery. My Will is Dynamic—full of Force and Energy, and Power. I feel my strength. I am Strong. I am Forceful. I am Vital. I am Center of Consciousness, Energy, Strength, and Power, and I claim my birthright.

THE FIFTH LESSON.

THE CULTIVATION OF ATTENTION.

In our last lesson we called your attention to the fact that the Yogis devote considerable time and practice to the acquirement of Concentration. And we also had something to say regarding the relation of Attention to the subject of Concentration. In this lesson we shall have more to say on the subject of Attention, for it is one of the important things relating to the practice of *Raja Yoga*, and the Yogis insist upon their students practicing systematically to develop and cultivate the faculty. Attention lies at the base of Will-power, and the cultivation of one makes easy the exercise of the other.

To explain why we lay so much importance to the cultivation of Attention, would necessitate our anticipating future lessons of this series, which we do not deem advisable at this time. And so we must ask our students to take our word for it, that all that we have to say regarding the importance of the cultivation of Attention, is occasioned by the relation of that subject to the use of the mind in certain directions as will appear fully later on.

In order to let you know that we are not advancing some peculiar theory of the Yogis, which may not be in harmony with modern Western Science, we give you in this article a number of quotations, from Western writers and thinkers, touching upon this important faculty of the mind, so that you may see that the West and East agree upon this main point, however different may be their explanations of the fact, or their use of the power gained by the cultivation of Attention.

As we said in our last lesson, the word Attention is derived from two Latin words "*ad tendere*," meaning "to stretch toward," which is really what Attention is. The "I" wills that the mind be focused on some particular object or thing, and the mind obeys and "stretches toward" that object or thing, focusing its entire energy upon it, observing every detail, dissecting, analyzing, consciously and sub-consciously, drawing to itself every possible bit of information regarding it, both from within and from without. We cannot lay too much stress upon the acquirement of this great faculty, or rather, the development of it, for it is necessary for the intelligent study of *Raja Yoga*.

In order to bring out the importance of the subject, suppose we start in by actually giving our Attention to the subject of Attention, and see how much more there is in it than we had thought. We shall be well repaid for the amount of time and trouble expended upon it.

Attention has been defined as a focusing of consciousness, or, if one prefers the form of expression, as "detention in consciousness." In the first case, we may liken it to the action of the sun-glass through which the sun's rays are concentrated upon an object, the result being that the heat is gathered together at a small given point, the intensity of the same being raised many degrees until the heat is sufficient to burn a piece of wood, or evaporate water. If the rays were not focused, the same rays and heat would have been scattered over a large surface, and the effect and power lessened. And so it is with the mind. If it is allowed to scatter itself over the entire field of a subject, it will exert but little power and the results will be weak. But if it is passed through the sun-glass of attention, and focused first over one part, and then over another, and so on, the matter may be mastered in detail, and a result accomplished that will seem little less than marvelous to those who do not know the secret.

Thompson has said: "The experiences most permanently impressed upon consciousness, are those upon which the greatest amount of attention has been fixed."

Another writer upon the subject has said that "Attention is so essentially necessary to understanding, that without some degree of it the ideas and perceptions that pass through the mind seem to leave no trace behind them."

Hamilton has said: "An act of attention, that is, an act of concentration, seems thus necessary to every exertion of consciousness, as a certain contraction of the pupil is requisite to every exertion of vision. Attention then is to consciousness what the contraction of the pupil is to sight, or, to the eye of the mind what the microscope or telescope is to the bodily eye. It constitutes the better half of all intellectual power."

And *Brodie* adds, quite forcibly: "It is Attention much more than any difference in the abstract power of reasoning, which constitutes the vast difference which exists between minds of different individuals."

Butler gives us this important testimony: "The most important intellectual habit I know of is the habit of attending exclusively to the matter in hand. It is commonly said that genius cannot be infused by education, yet this power of concentrated attention, which belongs as a part of his gift to every great discoverer, is unquestionably capable of almost indefinite augmentation by resolute practice."

And, concluding this review of opinions, and endorsements of that which the Yogis have so much to say, and to which they attach so much importance, let us listen to the words of *Beattie*, who says: "The force wherewith anything strikes the mind, is generally in proportion to the degree of attention bestowed upon it. Moreover, the great art of memory is attention, and inattentive people always have bad memories."

There are two general kinds of Attention. The first is the Attention directed within the mind upon mental objects and concepts. The other is the Attention directed outward upon objects external to ourselves. The same general rules and laws apply to both equally.

Likewise there may be drawn another distinction and division of attention into two classes, *viz.*, Attenion attracted by some impression coming into consciousness without any conscious effort of the Will—this is called Involuntary Attention, for the Attention and Interest is caught by the attractiveness or novelty of the object. Attention directed to some object by an effort of the Will, is called Voluntary Attention. Involuntary Attention is quite common, and requires no special training. In fact, the lower animals, and young children seem to have a greater share of it than do adult men. A great percentage of men and women never get beyond this stage to any marked degree. On the other hand, Voluntary Attention requires effort, will, and determination—a certain mental training, that is beyond the majority of people, for they will not "take the trouble" to direct their attention in this way. Voluntary Attention is the mark of the student and other thoughtful men. They focus their minds on objects that do not yield immediate interest or pleasure, in order that they may learn and accomplish. The careless person will not thus fasten his Attention, at least not more than a moment or so, for his Involuntary Attention is soon attracted by some passing object of no matter how trifling a nature, and the Voluntary

Attention disappears and is forgotten. Voluntary Attention is developed by practice and perseverance, and is well worth the trouble, for nothing in the mental world is accomplished without its use.

The Attention does not readily fasten itself to uninteresting objects, and, unless interest can be created it requires a considerable degree of Voluntary Attention in order that the mind may be fastened upon such an object. And, more than this, even if the ordinary attention is attracted it will soon waver, unless there is some interesting change in the aspect of the object, that will give the attention a fresh hold of interest, or unless some new quality, characteristic or property manifests itself in the object. This fact occurs because the mind mechanism has not been trained to bear prolonged Voluntary Attention, and, in fact, the physical brain is not accustomed to the task, although it may be so trained by patient practice.

It has been noticed by investigators that the Attention may be rested and freshened, either by withdrawing the Voluntary Attention from the object, and allowing the Attention to manifest along Involuntary lines toward passing objects, etc.; or, on the other hand, by directing the Voluntary Attention into a new field of observation—toward some new object. Sometimes one plan will seem to give the best results, and again the other will seem preferable.

We have called your attention to the fact that Interest develops Attention, and holds it fixed, while an uninteresting object or subject requires a much greater effort and application. This fact is apparent to anyone. A common illustration may be found in the matter of reading a book. Nearly everyone will give his undivided attention to some bright, thrilling story, while but few are able to use sufficient Voluntary Attention to master the pages of some scientific work. But, right here, we wish to call your attention to the other side of the case, which is another example of the fact that Truth is composed of paradoxes.

Just as Interest develops Attention, so it is a truth that Attention develops Interest. If one will take the trouble to give a little Voluntary Attention to an object, he will soon find that a little perseverance will bring to light points of Interest in the object. Things before unseen and unsuspected, are quickly brought to light. And many new phases, and aspects of the subject or object are seen, each one of which, in turn, becomes an object of Interest. This is a fact not so generally known, and one that it will be well for you to remember, and to use in practice. *Look* for the interesting features of an uninteresting thing, and they will appear to your view, and before long the uninteresting object will have changed into a thing having many-sided interests.

Voluntary Attention is one of the signs of a developed Will. That is, of a mind that has been well trained by the Will, for the Will is always strong, and it is the mind that has to be trained, not the Will. And on the other hand, one of the best ways to train the mind by the Will, is by practice in Voluntary Attention. So you see how the rule works both ways. Some Western psychologists have even advanced theories that the Voluntary Attention is the *only* power of the Will, and that that power is sufficient, for if the Attention be firmly fixed, and held upon an object the mind will "do the rest." We do not agree with this school of philosophers, but merely mention the fact as an illustration of the importance attributed by psychologists to this matter of Voluntary Attention.

A man of a strongly developed Attention often accomplishes far more than some much brighter man who lacks it. Voluntary Attention and Application is a very good substitute for Genius, and often accomplishes far more in the long run.

Voluntary Attention is the fixing of the mind earnestly and intently upon some particular object, at the same time shutting out from consciousness other objects pressing for entrance. *Hamilton* has defined it as "consciousness voluntarily applied under its law of limitations to some determinate object." The same writer goes on to state that "the greater the number of objects to which our consciousness is simultaneously extended, the smaller is the intensity with which it is able to consider each, and consequently the less vivid and distinct will be the information it contains of the several objects. When our interest in any particular object is excited, and when we wish to obtain all the knowledge concerning it in our power, it behooves us to limit our consideration to that object to the exclusion of others."

The human mind has the power of attending to only one object at a time, although it is able to pass from one object to another with a marvelous degree of speed, so rapidly, in fact, that some have held that it could grasp several things at once. But the best authorities, Eastern and Western, hold to the "single idea" theory as being correct. On this point we may quote a few authorities.

Jouffroy says that "It is established by experience that we cannot give our attention to two different objects at the same time." And *Holland* states that "Two thoughts, however closely related to one another, cannot be presumed to exist at the same time." And *Lewes* has told us that "The nature of our organism prevents our having more than one aspect of an object at each instant presented to consciousness." *Whateley* says: "The best philosophers are agreed that the mind cannot actually attend to more than one thing at a time, but, when it appears to be doing so it is really shifting with prodigious rapidity backward and forward from one to the other."

By giving a concentrated Voluntary Attention to an object, we not only are able to see and think about it with the greatest possible degree of clearness, but the mind has a tendency, under such circumstances, to bring into the field of consciousness all the different ideas associated in our memory with that object or subject, and to build around the object or subject a mass of associated facts and information. And at the same time the Attention given the subject makes more vivid and clear all that we learn about the thing at the time, and, in fact, all that we may afterwards learn about it. It seems to cut a channel, through which knowledge flows.

Attention magnifies and increases the powers of perception, and greatly aids the exercise of the perceptive faculties. By "paying attention" to something seen or heard, one is enabled to observe the details of the thing seen or heard, and where the inattentive mind acquires say three impressions the attentive mind absorbs three times three, or perhaps three times "three times three," or twenty-seven. And, as we have just said, Attention brings into play the powers of association, and gives us the "loose end" of an almost infinite chain of associated facts, stored away in our memory, forming new combinations of facts which we had never grouped together before, and bring out into the field of consciousness all the many scraps of information regarding the thing to which we are giving attention. The proof of this is within the experience of everyone. Where is the one who does not remember sitting down to some writing, painting, reading, etc., with interest and attention, and finding, much to his surprise, what a flow of facts regarding the matter in hand was passing through his mind. Attention seems to focus all the knowledge of a thing that you possess, and by bringing it to a point enables you to combine, associate, classify, etc., and thus create new knowledge. *Gibbon* tells us that after he gave a brief glance and consideration to a new subject, he suspended further work upon it, and allowed his mind (under concentrated attention) to bring forth all his associated knowledge regarding the subject, after which he renewed the task with increased power and efficiency.

The more one's attention is fixed upon a subject under consideration, the deeper is the impression which the subject leaves upon the mind. And the easier will it be for him to afterwards pursue the same train of thought and work.

Attention is a prerequisite of good memory, and in fact there can be no memory at all unless some degree of attention is given. The degree of memory depends upon the degree of attention and interest. And when it is considered that the work of today is made efficient by the memory of things learned yesterday, the day before yesterday, and so on, it is seen that the degree of attention given today regulates the quality of the work of tomorrow.

Some authorities have described Genius as the result of great powers of attention, or, at least, that the two seem to run together. Some writer has said that "possibly the best definition of genius is the power of concentrating upon some one given subject until its possibilities are exhausted and absorbed." *Simpson* has said that "The power and habit of thinking closely and continuously upon the subject at hand, to the exclusion, for the time, of all other subjects, is one of the principal, if, indeed, not the principal, means of success." *Sir Isaac Newton* has told us his plan of absorbing information and knowledge. He has stated that he would keep the subject under consideration before him continually, and then would wait till the first dawning of perception gradually brightened into a clear light, little by little. A mental sunrise, in fact.

That sage observer, *Dr. Abercrombie*, has written that he considered that he knew of no more important rule for rising to eminence in any profession or occupation than the Ability to do one thing at a time, avoiding all distracting and diverting objects or subjects, and keeping the leading matter continually before the mind. And others have added that such a course will enable one to observe relations between the subject and other things that will not be apparent to the careless observer or student.

The degree of Attention cultivated by a man is the degree of his capacity for intellectual work. As we have said, the "great" men of all walks of life have developed this faculty to a wonderful degree, and many of them seem to get results "intuitively," whereas, in truth, they obtain them by reason of their concentrated power of Attention, which enables them to see right into the center of a subject or proposition—and all around it, back and front, and all sides, in a space of time incredible to the man who has not cultivated this mighty power. Men who have devoted much attention to some special line of work or research, are able to act almost as if they possessed "second sight," providing the subject is within their favorite field of endeavor. Attention quickens every one of the faculties—the reasoning faculties—the senses—the deriding qualities—the analytical faculties, and so on, each being given a "fine edge" by their use under a concentrated Attention.

And, on the other hand, there is no surer indication of a weak mind than the deficiency in Attention. This weakness may arise from illness or physical weakness reacting upon the brain, in which case the trouble is but temporary. Or it may arise from a lack of mental development. Imbeciles and idiots have little or no Attention. The great French psychologist, *Luys*, speaking of this fact, says "Imbeciles and idiots see badly, hear badly, feel badly, and their sensorium is, in consequence, in a similar condition of sensitive poverty. Its impressionability for the things of the external world is at a minimum, its sensibility weak, and consequently, it is difficult to provoke the physiological condition necessary for the absorption of the external impression."

In old age the Attention is the first faculty to show signs of decay. Some authorities have held that the Memory was the first faculty to be affected by the approach of old age, but this is incorrect, for it is a matter of common experience that the aged manifest a wonderfully clear memory of events occurring in the far past. The reason that their memory of recent events is so poor is because their failing powers of Attention has prevented them from receiving strong, clear mental impressions, and as is the impression so is the memory. Their early impressions having been clear and strong, are easily recalled, while their later ones, being weak, are recalled with difficulty. If the Memory were at fault, it would be difficult for them to recall any impression, recent or far distant in time.

But we must stop quoting examples and authorities, and urging upon you the importance of the faculty of Attention. If you do not now realize it, it is because you have not given the subject the Attention that you should have exercised, and further repetition would not remedy matters.

Admitting the importance of Attention, from the psychological point of view, not to speak of the occult side of the subject, is it not a matter of importance for you to start in to cultivate that faculty? We think so. And the only way to cultivate any mental or physical part or faculty is to Exercise it. Exercise "uses up" a muscle, or mental faculty, but the organism makes haste to rush to the scene additional material—cell-stuff, nerve force, etc., to repair the waste, and it always sends a little more than is needed. And this "little more," continually accruing and increasing, is what increases the muscles and brain centers. And improved and strengthened brain centers give the mind better instruments with which to work.

One of the first things to do in the cultivation of Attention is to learn to think of, and do, one thing at a time. Acquiring the "knack" or habit of attending closely to the things before us, and then passing on to the next and treating it in the same way, is most conducive to success, and its practice is the best exercise for the cultivation of the faculty of Attention. And on the contrary, there is nothing more harmful from the point of view of successful performance—and nothing that will do more to destroy the power of giving Attention—than the habit of trying to do one thing while thinking of another. The thinking part of the mind, and the acting part should work together, not in opposition.

Dr. Beattie, speaking of this subject, tells us "It is a matter of no small importance that we acquire the habit of doing only one thing at a time; by which I mean that while attending to any one object, our thoughts ought not to wander to another." And *Granville* adds, "A frequent cause of failure in the faculty of Attention is striving to think of more than one thing at a time." And *Kay* quotes, approvingly, a writer who says: "She did things easily, because she attended to them in the doing. When she made bread, she thought of the bread, and not of the fashion of her next dress, or of her partner at the last dance." *Lord Chesterfield said,* "There is time enough for everything in the course of the day, if you do but one thing at a time; but there is not time enough in the year if you try to do two things at a time."

To attain the best results one should practice concentrating upon the task before him, shutting out, so far as possible, every other idea or thought. One should even forget self—personality—in such cases, as there is nothing more destructive of good thinking than to allow morbid self-consciousness to intrude. One does best when he "forgets himself" in his work, and sinks his personality in the creative work. The "earnest" man or woman is the one who sinks personality in the desired result, or performance of the task undertaken. The actor, or preacher, or orator, or writer, must lose sight of himself to get the best results. Keep the Attention fixed on the thing before you, and let the self take care of itself.

In connection with the above, we may relate an anecdote of *Whateley* that may be interesting in connection with the consideration of this subject of "losing one's self" in the task. He was asked for a recipe for "bashfulness," and replied that the person was bashful simply because he was thinking of himself and the impression he was making. His recipe was that the young man should think of others—of the pleasure he could give them—and in that way he would forget all about himself. The prescription is said to have effected the cure. The same authority has written, "Let both the extemporary speaker, and the reader of his own compositions, study to avoid as far as possible all thoughts of self, earnestly fixing the mind on the matter of what is delivered; and they will feel less that embarrassment which arises from the thought of what opinion the hearers will form of them."

The same writer, *Whateley*, seems to have made quite a study of Attention and has given us some interesting information on its details. The following may be read with interest, and if properly understood may be employed to advantage. He says, "It is a fact, and a very curious one. that many people find that they can best attend to any serious matter when they are occupied with something else which requires a little, and but a little, attention, such as working with the needle, cutting open paper leaves, or, for want of some such employment, fiddling anyhow with the fingers." He does not give the reason for this, and at first sight it might seem like a contradiction of the "one thing at a time" idea. But a closer examination will show us that the minor work (the cutting leaves, etc.) is in the nature of an involuntary or automatic movement, inasmuch as it requires little or no voluntary attention, and seems to "do itself." It does not take off the Attention from the main subject, but perhaps acts to catch the "waste Attention" that often tries to divide the Attention from some voluntary act to another. The habit mind may be doing one thing, while the Attention is fixed on another. For instance, one may be writing with his attention firmly fixed upon the thought he wishes to express, while at the time his hand is doing the writing, apparently with no attention being given it. But, let a boy, or person unaccustomed to writing, try to express his thoughts in this way, and you will find that he is hampered in the flow of his thoughts by the fact that he has to give much attention to the mechanical act of writing. In the same way, the beginner on the typewriter finds it difficult to compose to the machine, while the experienced typist finds the mechanical movements no hindrance whatever to the flow of thought and focusing of Attention; in fact, many find that they can compose much better while using the typewriter than they can by dictating to a stenographer. We think you will see the principle. And now for a little Mental Drill in Attention, that you may be started on the road to cultivate this important faculty.

MENTAL DRILL IN ATTENTION.

Exercise I. Begin by taking some familiar object and placing it before you, try to get as many impressions regarding it as is possible for you. Study its shape, its color, its size, and the thousand and one little peculiarities about it that present themselves to your attention. In doing this, reduce the thing to its simplest parts—analyze it as far as is possible—dissect it, mentally, and study its parts in detail. The more simple and small the part to be considered, the more clearly will the impression be received, and the more vividly will it be recalled. Reduce the thing to the smallest possible proportions, and then examine each portion, and mastering that, then pass on to the next part, and so on, until you have covered the entire field. Then, when you have exhausted the object, take a pencil and paper and put down as nearly as possible all the things or details of the object examined. When you have done this, compare the written description with the object itself, and see how many things you have failed to note.

The next day take up the same object, and after re-examining it, write down the details and you will find that you will have stored away a greater number of impressions regarding it, and, moreover, you will have discovered many new details during your second examination. This exercise strengthens the memory as well as the Attention, for the two are closely connected, the memory depending largely upon the clearness and strength of the impressions received, while the impressions depend upon the amount of attention given to the thing observed. Do not tire yourself with this exercise, for a tired Attention is a poor Attention. Better try it by degrees, increasing the task a little each time you try it. Make a game of it if you like, and you will find it quite interesting to notice the steady but gradual improvement.

It will be interesting to practice this in connection with some friend, varying the exercise by both examining the object, and writing down their impressions, separately, and then comparing results. This adds interest to the task, and you will be surprised to see how rapidly both of you increase in your powers of observation, which powers, of course, result from Attention.

Exercise II. This exercise is but a variation of the first one. It consists in entering a room, and taking a hasty glance around, and then walking out, and afterward writing down the number of things that you have observed, with a description of each. You will be surprised to observe how many things you have missed at first sight, and how you will improve in observation by a little practice. This exercise, also, may be improved by the assistance of a friend, as related in our last exercise. It is astonishing how many details one may observe and remember, after a little practice. It is related of Houdin, the French conjurer, that he improved and developed his faculty of Attention and Memory by playing this game with a young relative. They would pass by a shop window, taking a hasty, attentive glance at its contents. Then they would go around the corner and compare notes. At first they could remember only a few prominent articles—that is, their Attention could grasp only a few. But as they developed by practice, they found that they could observe and remember a vast number of things and objects in the window. And, at last, it is related that Houdin could pass rapidly before any large shop window, bestowing upon it but one hasty glance, and then tell the names of, and closely describe, nearly every object in plain sight in the window. The feat was accomplished by the fact that the cultivated Attention enabled Houdin to fasten upon his mind a vivid mental image of the window and its contents, and then he was able to describe the articles one by one from the picture in his mind.

Houdin taught his son to develop Attention by a simple exercise which may be interesting and of value to you. He would lay down a domino before the boy—a five-four, for example. He would require the boy to tell him the combined number at once, without allowing him to stop to count the spots, one by one. "Nine" the boy would answer after a moment's hesitation. Then another domino, a three-four, would be added. "That makes sixteen," cried the boy. Two dominoes at a time was the second day's task. The next day, three was the standard. The next day, four, and so on, until the boy was able to handle twelve dominoes—that is to say, give instantaneously the total number of spots on twelve dominoes, after a single glance. This was Attention, in earnest, and shows what practice will do to develop a faculty. The result was shown by the wonderful powers of observation, memory and attention, together with instantaneous mental action, that the boy developed. Not only was he able to add dominoes instantaneously, but he had powers of observation, etc., that seemed little short of miraculous. And yet it is related that he had poor attention, and deficient memory to begin with.

If this seems incredible, let us remember how old whist players note and remember every card in the pack, and can tell whether they have been played or not, and all the circumstances attending upon them. The same is true of chess players, who observe every move and can relate the whole game in detail long after it has been played. And remember, also, how one woman may pass another woman on the street, and without seeming to give her more than a careless glance, may be able to relate in detail every feature of the other woman's apparel, including its color, texture, style of fashioning, probable price of the material, etc., etc. And a mere man would have noticed scarcely anything about it—because he would not have given it any attention. But how soon would that man learn to equal his sister in attention and observation of women's wearing apparel, if his business success depended upon it, or if his speculative instinct was called into play by a wager with some friend as to who could remember the most about a woman's clothing, seen in a passing glance? You see it is all a matter of Interest and Attention.

But we forget that the Attention may be developed and cultivated, and we complain that we "cannot remember things," or that we do not seem to be able to "take notice." A little practice will do wonders in this direction.

Now, while the above exercises will develop your memory and powers of observation, still that is not the main reason that we have given them to you. We have an ulterior object, that will appear in time. We aim to develop your Will-power, and we know that Attention stands at the gate of Will-power. In order to be able to use your Will, you must be able to focus the Attention forcibly and distinctly. And these childish exercises will help you to develop the mental muscles of the Attention. If you could but realize the childish games the young Yogi students are required to play, in order to develop the mental faculties, you would change your minds about the Yogi Adepts whom you have been thinking about as mere dreamers, far removed from the practical. These men, and their students, are intensely practical. They have gained the mastery of the Mind, and its faculties, and are able to use them as sharp edged tools, while the untrained man finds that he has but a dull, unsharpened blade that will do nothing but hack and hew roughly, instead of being able to produce the finished product.

The Yogi believes in giving the "I" good tools with which to work, and he spends much time in tempering and sharpening these tools. Oh, no, the Yogi are not idle dreamers. Their grasp of "practical things" would surprise many a practical, matter-of-fact Western business man, if he could but observe it.

And so, we ask you to practice "observing things." The two exercises we have given are but indications of the general line. We could give you thousands, but you can prepare them yourselves as well as could we. The little Hindu boy is taught Attention by being asked to note and remember the number, color, character and other details of a number of colored stones, jewelry, etc., shown for an instant in an open palm, the hand being closed the moment after. He is taught to note and describe passing travelers, and their equipages—houses he sees on his journeys—and thousands of other everyday objects. The results are almost marvelous. In this way he is prepared as a *chela* or student, and he brings to his *guru* or teacher a brain well developed—a mind thoroughly trained to obey the Will of the "I"—and with faculties quickened to perceive instantly that which others would fail to see in a fortnight. It is true that he does not turn these faculties to "business" or other so-called "practical" pursuits, but prefers to devote them to abstract studies and pursuits outside of that which the Western man considers to be the end and aim of life. But remember that the two civilizations are quite different—following different ideals—having different economic conditions—living in different worlds, as it were. But that is all a matter of taste and ideals—the faculty for the "practical life" of the West is possessed by the *chela*, if he saw fit to use it. But all Hindu youths are not *chelas*, remember—nor are all Western youths "captains of industry," or Edisons.

MANTRAM (AFFIRMATION).

I am using my Attention to develop my mental faculties, so as to give the "I" a perfect instrument with which to work. The mind is *My* instrument and I am bringing it to a state of capacity for perfect work.

MANTRAM (OR AFFIRMATION).

There is but One Life—One Life Underlying. This Life is manifesting through ME, and through every other shape, form, and thing. I am resting on the bosom of the Great Ocean of Life, and it is supporting me, and will carry me safely, though the waves rise and fall—though the storms rage and the tempests roar. I am safe on the Ocean of Life, and rejoice as I feel the sway of its motion. Nothing can harm me—though changes may come and go, I am Safe. I am One with the All Life, and its Power, Knowledge, and Peace are behind, underneath, and within Me. O! One Life! express Thyself through me—carry me now on the crest of the wave, now deep down in the trough of the ocean—supported always by Thee—all is good to me, as I feel Thy life moving in and through me. I am Alive, through thy life, and I open myself to thy full manifestation and inflow.

THE SIXTH LESSON.

CULTIVATION OF PERCEPTION.

Man gains his knowledge of the outside world through his senses. And, consequently, many of us are in the habit of thinking of these senses as if *they* did the sensing, instead of being merely carriers of the vibrations coming from the outside world, which are then presented to the Mind for examination. We shall speak of this at greater length a little later on in this lesson. Just now we wish to impress upon you the fact that it is the Mind that perceives, not the senses. And, consequently, a development of Perception is really a development of the Mind.

The Yogis put their students through a very arduous course of practice and exercises designed to develop their powers of perception. To many this would appear to be merely a development of the Senses, which might appear odd in view of the fact that the Yogis are constantly preaching the folly of being governed and ruled by the senses. But there is nothing paradoxical about all this, for the Yogis, while preaching the folly of sense life, and manifesting the teaching in their lives, nevertheless believe in any and all exercises calculated to "sharpen" the Mind, and develop it to a keen state and condition.

They see a great difference between having a sharpened perception, on the one hand, and being a slave to the senses on the other. For instance, what would be thought of a man who objected to acquiring a keen eyesight, for fear it would lead him away from higher things, by reason of his becoming attached to the beautiful things he might see. To realize the folly of this idea, one may look at its logical conclusion, which would be that one would then be much better off if all their senses were destroyed. The absurdity, not to say wickedness, of such an idea will be apparent to everyone, after a minute's consideration.

The secret of the Yogi theory and teachings regarding the development of the Mental powers, lies in the word "*Mastery*." The Yoga student accomplishes and attains this mastery in two ways. The first way is by subordinating all the feelings, sense-impressions, etc., to the Mastery of the "I," or Will, the Mastery being obtained in this way by the assertion of the dominancy of the "I" over the faculties and emotions, etc. The second step, or way, lies in the Yogi, once having asserted the mastery, beginning to develop and perfect the Mental instrument, so as to get better work and returns from it. In this way he increases his kingdom and is Master over a much larger territory.

In order for one to gain knowledge, it is necessary to use to the best advantage the mental instruments and tools that he finds at his disposal. And again, one must develop and improve such tools—put a keen edge upon them, etc. Not only does one gain a great benefit from a development of the faculties of perception, but he also acquires an additional benefit from the training of the whole mind arising from the mental discipline and training resulting from the former exercises, etc. In our previous lessons we have pointed out some of the means by which these faculties might be greatly improved, and their efficiency increased. In this lesson we shall point out certain directions in which the Perceptive faculties may be trained. We trust that the simplicity of the idea may not cause any of our students to lose interest in the work. If they only knew just what such development would lead to they would gladly follow our suggestions in the matter. Every one of the ideas and exercises given by us are intended to lead up to the strengthening of the Mind, and the attainment of powers and the unfoldment of faculties. There is no royal road to Raja Yoga, but the student will be well repaid for the work of climbing the hill of Attainment.

In view of the above, let us examine the question of The Senses. Through the doors of the senses Man receives all his information regarding the outside world. If he keeps these doors but half open, or crowded up with obstacles and rubbish, he may expect to receive but few messages from outside. But if he keeps his doorways clear, and clean, he will obtain the best that is passing his way.

If one were born without sense-organs—no matter how good a Mind he might have—he would be compelled to live his life in a dreamy plant-life stage of existence, with little or no consciousness. The Mind would be like a seed in the earth, that for some reason was prevented from growing.

One may object that the highest ideas do not come to us through the senses, but the reply is that the things obtained through the senses are the "raw material" upon which the mind works, and fashions the beautiful things that it is able to produce in its highest stages. Just as is the body dependent for growth upon the nourishment taken into it, so is the mind dependent for growth upon the impressions received from the Universe—and these impressions come largely through the senses. It may be objected to that we know many things that we have not received through our senses. But, does the objector include the impressions that came through his senses in some previous existence, and which have been impressed upon his instinctive mind, or soul-memory? It is true that there are higher senses than those usually recognized, but Nature insists upon one learning the lessons of the lower grades before attempting those of the higher.

Do not forget that all that we know we have "worked for." There is nothing that comes to the idler, or shirker. What we know is merely the result of "stored-up accumulations of previous experience," as Lewes has so well said.

So it will be seen that the Yogi idea that one should develop all parts of the Mind is strictly correct, if one will take the trouble to examine into the matter. A man sees and knows but very little of what is going on about him. His limitations are great. His powers of vision report only a few vibrations of light, while below and above the scale lie an infinity of vibrations unknown to him. The same is true of the powers of hearing, for only a comparatively small portion of the sound-waves reach the Mind of Man—even some of the animals hear more than he does.

If a man had only one sense he would obtain but a one-sense idea of the outside world. If another sense is added his knowledge is doubled. And so on. The best proof of the relation between increased sense perception and development is had in the study of the evolution of animal forms. In the early stages of life the organism has only the sense of feeling—and very dim at that—and a faint sense of taste. Then developed smell, hearing and sight, each marking a distinct advance in the scale of life, for a new world has been opened out to the advancing forms of life. And, when man develops new senses—and this is before the race—he will be a much wiser and greater being.

Carpenter, many years ago, voiced a thought that will be familiar to those who are acquainted with the Yogi teachings regarding the unfoldment of new senses. He said: "It does not seem at all improbable that there are properties of matter of which none of our senses can take immediate cognizance, and which other beings might be formed to perceive in the same manner as we are sensible to light, sound, etc."

And Isaac Taylor said: "It may be that within the field observed by the visible and ponderable universe there is existing and moving another element fraught with another species of life—corporeal, indeed, and various in its orders, but not open to cognizance of those who are confined to the conditions of animal organization. Is it to be thought that the eye of man is the measure of the Creator's power?—and that He created nothing but that which he has exposed to our present senses? The contrary seems much more than barely possible; ought we not to think it almost certain?"

Another writer. Prof. Masson, has said: "If a new sense or two were added to the present normal number, in man, that which is now the phenomenal world for all of us might, for all that we know, burst into something amazingly different and wider, in consequence of the additional revelations of these new senses."

But not only is this true, but Man may increase his powers of knowledge and experience if he will but develop the senses he has to a higher degree of efficiency, instead of allowing them to remain comparatively atrophied. And toward this end, this lesson is written.

The Mind obtains its impressions of objects of the outside world by means of the brain and sense organs. The sensory organs are the instruments of the Mind, as is also the brain and the entire nervous system. By means of the nerves, and the brain, the Mind makes use of the sensory organs in order that it may obtain information regarding external objects.

The senses are usually said to consist of five different forms, *viz.*, sight, hearing, smell, touch, and taste.

The Yogis teach that there are higher senses, undeveloped, or comparatively so, in the majority of the race, but toward the unfoldment of which the race is tending. But we shall not touch upon these latent senses in this lesson, as they belong to another phase of the subject. In addition to the five senses above enumerated, some physiologists and psychologists have held that there were several others in evidence. For instance, the sense by which the inner organs revealed their presence and condition, The muscular system reports to the mind through some sense that is not that of "touch," although closely allied to it. And the feelings of hunger, thirst, etc., seem to come to us through an unnamed sense.

Bernstein has distinguished between the five senses and the one just referred to as follows: "The characteristic distinction between these common sensations and the sensations of the senses is that by the latter we gain knowledge of the occurrences and objects which belong to the external world (and which sensations we refer to external objects), whilst by the former we only feel conditions of our own body."

A sensation is the internal, mental conception, resulting from an external object or fact exciting the sense organs and nerves, and the brain, thus making the mind "aware" of the external object or fact. As Bain has said, it is the "mental impression, feeling, or conscious state, resulting from the action of external things on some part of the body, called on that account, sensitive."

Each channel of sense impressions has an organ, or organs, peculiarly adapted for the excitation of its substance by the particular kind of vibrations through which it receives impressions. The eye is most cunningly and carefully designed to receive the light-waves; and sound-waves produce no effect upon it. And, likewise, the delicate mechanism of the ear responds only to sound-waves; light-waves failing to register upon it. Each set of sensations is entirely different, and the organs and nerves designed to register each particular set are peculiarly adapted to their own special work. The organs of sense, including their special nervous systems, may be compared to a delicate instrument that the mind has fashioned for itself, that it may investigate, examine and obtain reports from the outside world.

We have become so accustomed to the workings of the senses that we take them as a "matter of course," and fail to recognize them as the delicate and wonderful instruments that they are—designed and perfected by the mind for its own use. If we will think of the soul as designing, manufacturing and using these instruments, we may begin to understand their true relations to our lives, and, accordingly treat them with more respect and consideration.

We are in the habit of thinking that we are aware of all the sensations received by our mind. But this is very far from being correct. The unconscious regions of the mind are incomparably larger than the small conscious area that we generally think of when we say "my mind." In future lessons we shall proceed to consider this wonderful area, and examine what is to be found there. Taine has well said, "There is going on within us a subterranean process of infinite extent; its products alone are known to us, and are only known to us in the mass. As to elements, and their elements, consciousness does not attain to them. They are to sensations what secondary molecules and primitive molecules are to bodies. We get a glance here and there at obscure and infinite worlds extending beneath our distinct sensations. These are compounds and wholes. For their elements to be perceptible to consciousness, it is necessary for them to be added together, and so to acquire a certain bulk and to occupy a certain time, for if the group does not attain this bulk, and does not last this time, we observe no changes in our state. Nevertheless, though it escapes us, there is one."

But we must postpone our consideration of this more than interesting phase of the subject, until some future lesson, when we shall take a trip into the regions of Mind, under and above Consciousness. And a most wonderful trip many of us will find it, too.

For the present, we must pay our attention to the channels by which the material for knowledge and thought enter our minds. For these sense impressions, coming to us from without, are indeed "material" upon which the mind works in order to manufacture the product called "Thought."

This material we obtain through the channels of the senses, and then store in that wonderful storehouse, the Memory, from whence we bring out material from time to time, which we proceed to weave into the fabric of Thought. The skill of the worker depends upon his training, and his ability to select and combine the proper materials. And the acquiring of good materials to be stored up is an important part of the work.

A mind without stored-up material of impressions and experiences would be like a factory without material. The machinery would have nothing upon which to work, and the shop would be idle. As Helmholtz has said, "Apprehension by the senses supplies directly or indirectly, the material of all human knowledge, or at least the stimulus necessary to develop every inborn faculty of the mind." And Herbert Spencer, has this to say of this phase of the subject, "It is almost a truism to say that in proportion to the numerousness of the objects that can be distinguished, and in proportion to the variety of coexistences and sequences that can be severally responded to, must be the number and rapidity and variety of the changes within the organism—must be the amount of vitality."

A little reflection upon this subject will show us that the greater degree of exercise and training given the senses, the greater the degree of mental power and capability. As we store our mental storehouse with the materials to be manufactured into thought, so is the quality and quantity of the fabric produced.

It therefore behooves us to awaken from our "lazy" condition of mind, and to proceed to develop our organs of sense, and their attendant mechanism, as by doing so we increase our capacity for thought and knowledge.

Before passing to the exercises, however, it may be well to give a hasty passing glance at the several senses, and their peculiarities.

The sense of Touch is the simplest and primal sense. Long before the lower forms of life had developed the higher senses, they had evidenced the sense of Touch or Feeling. Without this sense they would have been unable to have found their food, or to receive and respond to outside impressions. In the early forms of life it was exercised equally by all parts of the body, although in the higher forms this sense has become somewhat localized, as certain parts of the body are far more sensitive than are others. The skin is the seat of the sense of Touch, and its nerves are distributed over the entire area of the skin. The hand, and particularly the fingers, and their tips, are the principal organs of this sense.

The acuteness of Touch varies materially in different parts of the body. Experiments have shown that a pair of compasses would register impressions as a very slight distance apart when applied to the tip of the tongue. The distance at which the two points could be distinguished from one point, on the tip of the tongue, was called "one line." Using this "line" as a standard, it was found that the palmar surface of the third finger registered 2 lines; the surface of the lips 4 lines, and the skin of the back, and on the middle of the arm or thigh, as high as 60 lines The degree of sensitiveness to Touch varies greatly with different individuals, some having a very fine sense of touch in their fingers, while others manifested a very much lower degree.

In the same way, there is a great difference in the response of the fingers to weight—a great difference in the ability to distinguish the difference of the weight of objects. It has been found that some people can distinguish differences in weight down to very small fractions of an ounce. Fine distinctions in the differences in temperature have also been noticed.

The sense of touch, and its development has meant much for Man. It is the one sense in which Man surpasses the animals in the matter of degree and acuteness. The animal may have a keener smell, taste, hearing and sight, but its sense of Touch is far beneath that of

Man. Anaxagoras is quoted as saying that "if the animals had hands and fingers, they would be like men."

In developing the sense of Touch, the student must remember that Attention is the key to success. The greater the amount of Attention the greater the degree of development possible in the case of any sense. When the Attention is concentrated upon any particular sense, the latter becomes quickened and more acute, and repeated exercise, under the stimulus of Attention, will work wonders in the case of any particular sense. And on the other hand, the sense of touch may be almost, or completely inhibited, by firmly fixing the Attention upon something else. As an extreme proof of this latter fact, the student is asked to remember the fact that men have been known to suffer excruciating torture, apparently without feeling, owing to the mind being intently riveted upon some idea or thought. As Wyld has said, "The martyr borne above sensuous impressions, is not only able to endure tortures, but is able to endure and quench them. The pinching and cutting of the flesh only added energy to the death song of the American Indian, and even the slave under the lash is sustained by the indignant sense of his wrongs."

In the cases of persons engaged in occupations requiring a fine degree of Touch, the development is marvelous. The engraver passes his hand over the plate, and is able to distinguish the slightest imperfection. And the handler of cloth and fabrics is able to distinguish the finest differences, simply by the sense of touch. Wool sorters also exercise a wonderfully high degree of fineness of touch. And the blind are able to make up for the loss of sight by their greatly increased sense of Touch, cases being recorded where the blind have been able to distinguish *color* by the different "feel" of the material.

The sense of Taste is closely allied to that of Touch—in fact some authorities have considered Taste as a very highly developed sense of Touch in certain surfaces of the body, the tongue notably. It will be remembered that the tongue has the finest sense of Touch, and it also has the sense of Taste developed to perfection. In Taste and Touch the object must be brought in direct contact with the organ of sense, which is not the case in Smell, Hearing, or Sight. And, be it remembered, that the latter senses have special nerves, while Taste is compelled to fall back upon the ordinary nerves of Touch. It is true that Taste is confined to a very small part of the surface of the body, while Touch is general. But this only indicates a special development of the special area. The sense of Taste also depends to a great extent upon the presence of fluids, and only substances that are soluble make their presence known through the organs and sense of Taste.

Physiologists report that the sense of Taste in some persons is so acute that one part of strychnine in one million parts of water has been distinguished. There are certain occupations, such as that of wine-tasters, tea-tasters, etc., the followers of which manifest a degree of fineness of Taste almost incredible.

The sense of Smell is closely connected with the sense of Taste, and often acts in connection therewith, as the tiny particles of the substance in the mouth arise to the organs of Smell, by means of the opening or means of communication situated in the back part of the mouth. Besides which the nose usually detects the odor of substances before they enter the mouth. The sense of Smell operates by reason of the tiny particles or the object being carried to the mucous membrane of the interior of the nose, by means of the air. The membrane, being moist, seizes and holds these particles for a moment, and the fine nervous organism reports differences and qualities and the Mind is thus informed of the nature of the object.

The sense of Smell is very highly developed among animals, who are compelled to rely upon it to a considerable extent. And many occupations among men require the development of this sense, for instance, the tobacconist, the wine dealer, the perfumers, the chemist, etc. It is related that in the cases of certain blind people, it has been observed that they could distinguish persons in this manner.

The sense of Hearing is a more complex one than in the case of Taste, Touch and Smell. In the latter three the objects to be sensed must be brought in close contact with the sense-organs, while in Hearing the object may be far removed, the impressions being carried by the vibrations of the air, which are caught up and reported upon by the nervous organism of the sense of Hearing. The internal mechanism of the ear is most wonderfully intricate and complex, and excites to wonder the person examining it. It cannot be described here for want of space, but the student is advised to inquire into it if he has access to any library containing books on the subject. It is a wonderful illustration of the work of the mind in building up for itself instruments with which to work—to acquire knowledge.

The ear records vibrations in the air from 20 or 32 per second, the rate of the lowest audible note, to those of 38,000 per second, the rate of the highest audible note. There is a great difference in individuals in regard to the fineness of the sense of Hearing. But all may develop this sense by the application of Attention. The animals and savages have wonderfully acute senses of Hearing developed only along the lines of distinctness, however—on the other hand musicians have developed the sense along different lines.

The sense of Sight is generally conceded to be the highest and most complex of all the senses of Man. It deals with a far larger number of objects—at longer distances—and gives a far greater variety of reports to the mind than any of its associate senses. It is the sense of Touch magnified many times. As Wilson says of it, "Our sight may be considered as a more delicate and diffusive kind of touch that spreads itself over an infinite number of bodies; comprehends the largest figures, and brings into our reach some of the most remote parts of the universe."

The sense of Sight receives its impressions from the outside world by means of waves that travel from body to body—from sun to earth, and from lamp to eye. These waves of light arise from vibrations in substance, of an almost incredible degree of rapidity. The lowest light vibration is about 450,000,000,000,000 per second, while the highest is about 750,000,000,000,000 per second. These figures deal only with the vibrations recognizable by the eye as light. Above and below these figures of the scale are countless other degrees invisible to the eye, although some of them may be recorded by instruments. The different sensations of color, depend upon the rate of the vibrations, red being the limit of the lowest, and violet the limit of the highest visible vibrations—orange, yellow, green, blue, and indigo being the intermediate rates or colors.

The cultivation of the sense of Sight, under the aid of Attention is most important to ail persons. By being able to clearly see and distinguish the parts of an object, a degree of knowledge regarding it is obtained that one may not acquire without the said exercise of the faculty. We have spoken of this under the subject of Attention, in a previous lesson, to which lesson we again refer the student. The fixing of the eye upon an object has the power of concentrating the thoughts and preventing them from wandering. The eye has other properties and qualities that will be dwelt upon in future lessons. It has other uses than seeing. The influence of the eye is a marvelous thing, and may be cultivated and developed.

We trust that what we have said will bring the student to a realization of the importance of developing the powers of Perception. The senses have been developed by the mind during a long period of evolution and effort that surely would not have been given unless the object in view was worth it all. The "I" insists upon obtaining knowledge of the Universe, and much of this knowledge may be obtained only through the senses. The Yogi student must be "wide awake" and possessed of developed senses and powers of Perception. The senses of Sight and Hearing, the two latest in the scale of Evolutionary growth and unfoldment, must receive a particular degree of attention. The student must make himself "aware" of what is going on about and around him, so that he may "catch" the best vibrations.

It would surprise many Westerners if they could come in contact with a highly developed Yogi, and witness the marvelously finely developed senses he possesses. He is able to distinguish the finest differences in things, and his mind is so trained that, in thought, he may draw conclusions from what he has perceived, in a manner that seems almost "second-sight" to the uninitiated. *In fact, a certain degree of second-sight is possible to one who develops his sense of Sight, under the urge of Attention.* A new world is opened out to such a person. One must learn to master the senses, not only in the direction of being independent of and superior to their urgings, but also in the matter of developing them to a high degree. The development of the physical senses, also has much to do with the development of the "Astral Senses," of which we have spoken in our "Fourteen Lessons," and of which we may have more to say in the present series. The idea of *Raja Yoga* is to render the student the possessor of a highly developed Mind, with highly developed instruments with which the mind may work.

In our future lessons we shall give the student many illustrations, directions, and exercises calculated to develop the different faculties of the mind—not only the ordinary faculties of everyday use, but others hidden behind these familiar faculties and senses. Commencing with the next lesson, we shall present a system of exercises, drills, etc., the purpose of which will be the above mentioned development of the faculties of the Mind.

In this lesson we shall not attempt to give specific exercises, but will content ourselves with calling the attention of the student to a few general rules underlying the development of Perception.

GENERAL RULES OF PERCEPTION.

The first thing to remember in acquiring the art of Perception is that one should not attempt to perceive the whole of a complex thing or object at the same time, or at once. One should consider the object in detail, and then, by grouping the details, he will find that he has considered the whole. Let us take the face of a person as a familiar object. If one tries to perceive a face as a whole, he will find that he will meet with a certain degree of failure, the impression being indistinct and cloudy, it following, also, that the memory of that face will correspond with the original perception.

But let the observer consider the face in detail, first the eyes, then the nose, then the mouth, then the chin, then the hair, then the outline of the face, the complexion, etc., and he will find that he will have acquired a clear and distinct impression or perception of the whole face.

The same rule may be applied to any subject or object. Let us take another familiar illustration. You wish to observe a building. If you simply get a general perception of the building as a whole, you will be able to remember very little about it, except its general outlines, shape, size, color, etc. And a description will prove to be very disappointing. But if you have noted, *in detail*, the material used, the shape of the doors, chimney, roof, porches, decorations, trimmings, ornamentation, size and number of the window-panes etc., etc., the shape and angles of the roof, etc., you will have an *intelligent* idea of the building, in the place of a mere general outline or impression of such as might be acquired by an animal in passing.

We will conclude this lesson with an anecdote of the methods of that famous naturalist Agassiz, in his training of his pupils. His pupils became renowned for their close powers of observation and perception, and their consequent ability to "think" about the things they had seen. Many of them rose to eminent positions, and claimed that this was largely by reason of their careful training.

The tale runs that a new student presented himself to Agassiz one day, asking to be set to work. The naturalist took a fish from a jar in which it had been preserved, and laying it before the young student bade him observe it carefully, and be ready to report upon what he had noticed about the fish. The student was then left alone with the fish. There was nothing especially interesting about that fish—it was like many other fishes that he had seen before. He noticed that it had fins and scales, and a mouth and eyes, yes, and a tail. In a half hour he felt certain that he had observed all about that fish that there was to be perceived. But the naturalist remained away.

The time rolled on, and the youth, having nothing else to do, began to grow restless and weary. He started out to hunt up the teacher, but he failed to find him, and so had to return and gaze again at that wearisome fish. Several hours had passed, and he knew but little more about the fish than he did in the first place.

He went out to lunch and when he returned it was still a case of watching the fish. He felt disgusted and discouraged, and wished he had never come to Agassiz, whom, it seemed, was a stupid old man after all,—one away behind the times. Then, in order to kill time, he began to count the scales. This completed he counted the spines of the fins. Then he began to draw a picture of the fish. In drawing the picture he noticed that the fish had no eyelids. He thus made the discovery that as his teacher had expressed it often, in lectures, "a pencil is the best of eyes." Shortly after the teacher returned, and after ascertaining what the youth had observed, he left rather disappointed, telling the boy to keep on looking and maybe he would see something.

This put the boy on his mettle, and he began to work with his pencil, putting down little details that had escaped him before, but which now seemed very plain to him. He began to catch the secret of observation. Little by little he brought to light new objects of interest about the fish. But this did not suffice his teacher, who kept him at work on the same fish for three whole days. At the end of that time the student really knew something about the fish, and, better than all, had acquired the "knack" and habit of careful observation and perception in detail.

Years after, the student, then attained to eminence, is reported as saying: "That was the best zoological lesson I ever had—a lesson whose influence has extended to the details of every subsequent study; a legacy that the professor left to me, as he left to many others, of inestimable value, which we could not buy, and with which we cannot part."

Apart from the value to the student of the particular information obtained, was the quickening of the perceptive faculties that enabled him to observe the important points in a subject or object, and, consequently to deduce important information from that which was observed. The Mind is hungry for knowledge, and it has by years of weary evolution and effort built up a series of sense systems in order to yield it that knowledge and it is still building. The men and women in the world who have arrived at the point of success have availed themselves of these wonderful channels of information, and by directing them under the guidance of Will and Attention, have attained wonderful results. These things are of importance, and we beg of our students not to pass by this portion of the subject as uninteresting. Cultivate a spirit of wide-awakeness and perception, and the "knowing" that will come to you will surprise you.

No only do you develop the existing senses by such practice and use, *but you help in the unfoldment of the latent powers and senses that are striving for unfoldment*. By using and exercising the faculties that we have, we help to unfold those for the coming of which we have been dreaming.

MANTRAM (AFFIRMATION).

I am a Soul, possessed of channels of communication with the outer world. I will use these channels, and thereby acquire the information and knowledge necessary for my mental development. I will exercise and develop my organs of sense, knowing that in so doing I shall cause to unfold the higher senses, of which they are but forerunners and symbols. I will be "*wide-awake*" and open to the inflow of knowledge and information. The Universe is my Home—I will explore it.

THE SEVENTH LESSON.

THE UNFOLDMENT OF CONSCIOUSNESS.

We have thought it well to make a slight change in the arrangement of these lessons—that is, in the order in which they should appear. We had contemplated making this Seventh Lesson a series of Mental Drills, intended to develop certain of the mental faculties, but we have decided to postpone the same until a later lesson, believing that by so doing a more logical sequence or order of arrangement will be preserved. In this lesson we will tell you of the unfoldment of consciousness in Man, and in the next lesson, and probably in the one following it, we shall present to you a clear statement regarding the states of mind, below and over consciousness—a most wonderful region, we assure you, and one that has been greatly misunderstood and misinterpreted. This will lead up to the subject of the cultivation of the various faculties—both conscious and outside of consciousness, and the series will be concluded by three lessons going right to the heart of this part of the subject, and giving certain rules and instruction calculated to develop Man's wonderful "thought-machine" that will be of the greatest interest and importance to all of our students. When the lessons are concluded you will see that the present arrangement is most logical and proper.

In this lesson we take up the subject of "The Unfoldment of Consciousness"—a most interesting subject. Many of us have been in the habit of identifying "consciousness" with mind, but as we proceed with this series of lessons we will see that that which is called "consciousness" is but a small portion of the mind of the individual, and even that small part is constantly changing its states, and unfolding new states undreamed of.

"Consciousness" is a word we use very often in considering the science of the Mind. Let us see what it means. Webster defines it as one's "knowledge of sensations and mental operations, or of what passes in one's own mind." Halleck defines it as "that undefinable characteristic of mental states which causes one to be aware of them." But, as Halleck states, "Consciousness is incapable of definition. To define anything we are obliged to describe it in terms of something else. And there is nothing else in the world like consciousness, hence we can define it only in terms of itself, and that is very much like trying to lift one's self by one's own boot straps. Consciousness is one of the greatest mysteries that confronts us."

Before we can understand what Consciousness really is, we must know just what "Mind" really is—and that knowledge is lacking, notwithstanding the many injenious theories evolved in order to explain the mystery. The metaphysicians do not throw much light on the subject, and as for materialistic science, listen to what Huxley says: "How it comes about that anything so remarkable as a state of consciousness comes about by the result of irritating nervous tissue, is just as unaccountable as the appearance of the genie when Aladdin rubbed his lamp."

To many persons the words "consciousness" and "mental process," or "thought" are regarded as synonymous. And, in fact, psychologists so held until quite recently. But now it is generally accepted as a fact that mental processes are not limited to the field of consciousness, and it is now generally taught that the field of sub-consciousness (that is, "under" conscious) mentation, is of a much greater extent than that of conscious mentation.

Not only is it true that the mind can hold in consciousness but one fact at any one instant, and that, consequently, only a very small fraction of our knowledge can be in consciousness at any one moment, but it is also true that the consciousness plays but a very small part in the totality of mental processes, or mentation. The mind is not conscious of the greater portion of its own activities—Maudsley says that only ten per cent comes into the field of consciousness. Taine has stated it in these words: "Of the world which makes up our being, we only perceive the highest points—the lighted up peaks of a continent whose lower levels remain in the shade."

But it is not our intention to speak of this great subconscious region of the mind at this point, for we shall have much to do with it later on. It is mentioned here in order to show that the enlargement or development of consciousness is not so much a matter of "growth" as it is an "unfoldment"—not a new creation or enlargement from outside, but rather an unfoldment outward from within.

From the very beginning of Life—among the Particles of Inorganic Substance, may be found traces of something like Sensation, and response thereto. Writers have not cared to give to this phenomenon the name of "sensation," or "sensibility," as the terms savored too much of "senses," and "sense-organs." But Modern Science has not hesitated to bestow the names so long withheld. The most advanced scientific writers do not hesitate to state that in reaction, chemical response, etc., may be seen indications of rudimentary sensation. Haeckel says: "I cannot imagine the simplest chemical and physical process without attributing the movement of the material particles to unconscious sensation. The idea of Chemical Affinity consists in the fact that the various chemical elements perceive the qualitative differences in other elements and experience 'pleasure' or 'revulsion' at contacts with them, and execute their specific movements on this ground." He also speaks of the sensitiveness of "plasm," or the substance of "living bodies," as being "only a superior degree of the general irritability of substance."

Chemical reaction, between atoms, is spoken of by chemists as a "sensitive" reaction. Sensitiveness is found even in the Particles of Inorganic Substance, and may be regarded as the first glimmerings of thought. Science recognizes this when it speaks of the unconscious sensation of the Particles as *athesis* or "feeling," and the unconscious Will that responds thereto, as *tropesis*, or "inclination." Haeckel says of this that "Sensation perceives the different qualities of the stimuli, and feeling the quantity," and also, "We may ascribe the feeling of pleasure and pain (in the contact with qualitatively differing atoms) to all atoms, and so explain the elective affinity in chemistry (attraction of loving atoms, inclination; repulsion of hating atoms, disinclination)."

It is impossible to form a clear or intelligent idea of the phenomenon of chemical affinity, etc., unless we attribute to the Atoms something akin to Sensation. It is likewise impossible to understand the actions of the Molecules, unless we think of them as possessing something akin to Sensation. The Law of Attraction is based upon Mental States in Substance. The response of Inorganic Substance to Electricity and Magnetism is also another evidence of Sensation and the response thereto.

In the movements and operations of crystal-life we obtain evidences of still a little higher forms of Sensation and response thereto. The action of crystallization is very near akin to that of some low forms of plasmic action. In fact, the "missing link" between plant life and the crystals is claimed to have been found in some recent discoveries of Science, the connection being found in certain crystals in the interior of plants composed of carbon combinations, and resembling the inorganic crystals in many ways.

Crystals grow along certain lines and forms up to a certain size. Then they begin to form "baby-crystals" on their surfaces, which then take on the growth—the processes being almost analogous to cell-life. Processes akin to fermentation have been detected among chemicals. In many ways it may be seen that the beginning of Mental Life must be looked for among the Minerals and Particles—the latter, be it remembered, composing not only inorganic, but also Organic Substance.

As we advance in the scale of life, we are met with constantly increasing unfoldment of mentation, the simple giving place to the complex manifestations. Passing by the simple vital processes of the monera, or single-celled "things," we notice the higher forms of cell life, with growing sensibility or sensation. Then we come to the cell-groups, in which the individual cells manifest sensation of a kind, coupled with a community-sensation. Food is distinguished, selected and captured, and movements exercised in pursuit of the same. The living thing is beginning to manifest more complex mental states. Then the stage of the lower plants is reached, and we notice the varied phenomena of that region, evidencing an increased sensitiveness, although there are practically no signs of special organs of sense. Then we pass on to the higher plant life, in which begin to manifest certain "sensitive-cells," or groups of such cells, which are rudimentary sense organs. Then the forms of animal life, and considered with rising degrees of sensations and growing sense apparatus, or sense organs, gradually unfolding into something like nervous systems.

Among the lower animal forms there are varying degrees of mentation with accompanying nerve centers and sense-organs, but little or no signs of consciousness, gradually ascending until we have dawning consciousness in the reptile kingdom, etc., and fuller consciousness and a degree of intelligent thought in the still higher forms, gradually increasing until we reach the plane of the highest mammals, such as the horse, dog, elephant, ape, etc., which animals have complex nervous systems, brains and well developed consciousness. We need not further consider the forms of mentation in the forms of life below the Conscious stage, for that would carry us far from our subject.

Among the higher forms of animal life, after a "dawn period" or semi-consciousness, we come to forms of life among the lower animals possessing a well developed degree of mental action and Consciousness, the latter being called by psychologists "Simple Consciousness," but which term we consider too indefinite, and which we will term "Physical Consciousness," which will give a fair idea of the thing itself. We use the word "Physical" in the double sense of "External," and "Relating to the material structure of a living being," both of which definitions are found in the dictionaries. And that is just what Physical Consciousness really is—an "awareness" in the mind, or a "consciousness" of the "external" world as evidenced by the senses; and of the "body" of the animal or person. The animal or person thinking on the plane of Physical Consciousness (all the higher animals do, and many men seem unable to rise much higher) identifies itself with the physical body, and is conscious only of thoughts of that body and the outside world. It "knows," but not being conscious of mental operations, or of the existence of its mind, it does not "know that it knows." This form of consciousness, while infinitely above the mentation of the nonconscious plane of "sansation," is like a different world of thought from the consciousness of the highly developed intellectual man of our age and race.

It is difficult for a man to form an idea of the Physical Consciousness of the lower animals and savages, particularly as he finds it difficult to understand his own consciousness except by the act of being conscious. But observation and reason have given us a fair degree of understanding of what this Physical Consciousness of the animal is like—or at least in what respect it differs from our own consciousness. Let us take a favorite illustration. A horse standing out in the cold sleet and rain undoubtedly *feels* the discomfort, and possibly pain, for we know by observation that animals feel both. But he is not able to analyze his mental states and wonder when his master will come out to him—think how cruel it is to keep him out of the warm stable—wonder whether he will be taken out in the cold again tomorrow—feel envious of other horses who are indoors—wonder why he is compelled to be out cold nights, etc., etc.,—in short, he does not think as would a reasoning man under such circumstances. He is aware of the discomfort, just as would be the man—and he would run home if he could just as would the man. But he is not able to pity himself, nor to think about his personality as would the man, nor does he wonder whether such a life is worth living, after all. He "knows," but is not able to think of himself as knowing—he does not "know that he knows," as we do. He experiences the physical pain and discomfort, but is spared the mental discomfort and concern arising from the physical, which man so often experiences.

The animal cannot shift its consciousness from the sensations of the outer world to the inner states of being. It is not able to "know itself." The difference may be clumsily illustrated by the example of a man feeling, seeing or hearing something that gives him a pleasurable sensation, or the reverse. He is conscious of the feeling or sensation, and that it is pleasurable or otherwise. That is Physical Consciousness, and the animal may share it with him. But it stops right there with the animal. But the man may begin to wonder *why* the sensation is pleasurable and to associate it with other things and persons; or speculate *why* he dislikes it, what will follow, and so on—that is Mental Consciousness, because he recognizes an inward self, and is turning his attention *inward.* He may see another man and experience a feeling or sensation of attraction or aversion—like or dislike. This is Physical Consciousness, and an animal also may experience the sensation. But the man goes further than the animal, and wonders just what there is about the man he likes or detests, and may compare himself to the man and wonder whether the latter feels as he does, and so on—this is Mental Consciousness.

In animals the mental gaze is freely directed outward, and never returns upon itself. In man the mental gaze may be directed inward, or may return inward after its outward journey. The animal "knows"—the man not only "knows," but he "knows that he knows," and is able to investigate that "knowing" and speculate about it. We call this higher consciousness Mental Consciousness. The operation of Physical Consciousness we call Instinct—the operation of Mental Consciousness we call Reason.

The Man who has Mental Consciousness not only "feels" or "senses" things, but he has words or mental concepts of these feelings and sensations and may think of himself as experiencing them, separating himself, the sensation or feeling, and the thing felt or sensed. The man is able to think: "I feel; I hear; I see; I smell; I taste; I desire; I do," etc., etc. The very words indicate Mental Consciousness recognizing mental states and giving them names, and also recognizing something called "I" that experiences the sensations. This latter fact has caused psychologists to speak of this stage as "Self-consciousness," but we reserve this idea of the "I" consciousness for a higher stage.

The animal experiences something that gives it the impressions or feeling that we call "pain," "hurt," "pleasant," "sweet," "bitter," etc., all being forms of sensation, but it is unable to think of them in words. The pain seems to be a part of itself, although possibly associated with some person or thing that caused it. The study of the unfoldment of consciousness in a young baby will give one a far better idea of the grades and distinctions than can be obtained from reading mere words.

Mental Consciousness is a growth. As Halleck says, "Many persons never have more than a misty idea of such a mental attitude. They always take themselves for granted, and never turn the gaze inward." It has been doubted whether the savages have developed Self-consciousness, and even many men of our own race seem to be but little above the animals in intellect and consciousness. They do not seem able to "know themselves" even slightly. To them the "I" seems to be a purely physical thing—a body having desires and feeling but little more. They are able to feel an act, but scarcely more. They are not able to set aside any physical "not—I," being utterly unable to think of themselves as anything else but a Body. The "I" and the Body are one with them, and they seem incapable of distinguishing between them.

Then comes another stage in which mental-consciousness proper sets in. The man begins to realize that he has "a mind." He is able to "know himself" as a mental being, and to turn the gaze inward a little. This period of development may be noticed in young children. For a time they speak of themselves as a third person, until finally they begin to say "I." Then a little later comes the ability to know their own mental states as such—they know that they have a mind, and are able to distinguish between it and the body. It is related that some children experience a feeling of terror when they pass into this stage. They exhibit signs of bashfulness and what is commonly termed "self-consciousness" in that sense. Some tell us in after years that when they became aware of themselves as an entity they were overcome with alarm, as if by a sense of loneliness and apartness from the Universe. Young people often feel this way for several years. There seems to be a distinct feeling that the Universe is antagonistic to and set apart from them.

And, although this feeling of separateness and apartness grows less acute as the man grows older, yet it is always present to a greater or less degree until a still higher stage—the Ego-consciousness is reached, when it disappears as we shall see. And this mental-conscious stage is a hard one for many. They are entangled in a mass of mental states which the man thinks is "himself," and the struggle between the real "I" and its confining sheaths is painful. And it becomes still more painful as the end is neared, for as man advances in mental-consciousness and knowledge he feels more keenly and suffers accordingly. Man eats the fruit of the Tree of Knowledge and begins to suffer, and is driven out of the Garden of Eden of the child and primitive races, who live like the birds of the air and concern themselves not about mental states and problems. But there is deliverance ahead in the shape of a higher consciousness, although but few realize it and still fewer have gained it. Perhaps this lesson may point out the way for you.

With the birth of mental-consciousness comes the knowledge that there is a mind in others. Man is able to speculate and reason about the mental states of other men, because he recognizes these states within himself. As man advances in the Mental Consciousness he begins to develop a constantly increasing degree and grade of Intellect, and accordingly he attaches the greatest importance to that part of his nature. Some men worship Intellect as a God, ignoring its limitations which other thinkers have pointed out. Such people are apt to reason that because the human intellect (in its present state of development) reports that such a thing *must* be, or *cannot* possibly be, that the matter is forever settled. They ignore the fact that it is possible that Man's Intellect, in its present state of unfoldment, may be able to take cognizance of only a very small part of the Universal Fact, and that there may be regions upon regions of Reality and Fact of which he cannot even dream, so far are they removed from his experience. The unfoldment of a new sense would open out a new world and might bring to light facts that would completely revolutionize our entire world of conceptions by reason of the new information it would give us.

But, nevertheless, from this Mental Consciousness has come the wonderful work of Intellect, as shown in the achievements of Man up to this time, and while we must recognize its limitations, we gladly join in singing its praises. Reason is the tool with which Man is digging into the mine of Facts, bringing to light new treasures every day. This stage of Mental Consciousness is bringing to Man knowledge of himself—knowledge of the Universe—that is well worth the price he pays for it. For Man *does* pay a price for entrance into this stage—and he pays an increasing price as he advances in its territory, for the higher he advances the more keenly he feels and suffers, as well as enjoys. Capacity for pain is the price Man pays for Attainment, up to a certain stage. His pain passes from the Physical to the Mental consciousness, and he becomes aware of problems that he never dreamt existed, and the lack of an intelligent answer produces mental suffering. And the mental suffering that comes to him from unsatisfied longings, disappointment, the pain of others whom he loves, etc., is far worse than any physical suffering.

The animal lives its animal life and is contented, for it knows no better. If it has enough to eat—a place to sleep—a mate—it is happy. And some men are likewise. But others find themselves involved in a world of mental discomfort. New wants arise, and the lack of satisfaction brings pain. Civilization becomes more and more complex, and brings its new pains as well as new pleasures. Man attaches himself to "things," and each day creates for himself artificial wants, which he must labor to meet. His Intellect may not lead him upward, but instead may merely enable him to invent new and subtle means and ways of gratifying his senses to a degree impossible to the animals. Some men make a religion of the gratification of their sensuality—their appetites—and become beasts magnified by the power of Intellect. Others become vain, conceited and puffed up with a sense of the importance of their Personality (the false "I"). Others become morbidly introspective, and spend their time analyzing and dissecting their moods, motives, feelings, etc. Others exhaust their capacity for pleasure and happiness, but looking outside for it instead of within, and become *blase*, bored, *ennuied* and an affliction to themselves We mention these things not in a spirit of Pessimism but merely to show that even this great Mental Consciousness has a reverse and ugly side as well as the bright face that has been ascribed to it.

As man reaches the higher stages of this Mental Consciousness, and the next higher stage begins to dawn upon him, he is apt to feel more keenly than ever the insufficiency of Life as it appears to him. He is unable to understand Himself—his origin, destiny, purpose and nature—and he chafes against the bars of the cage of Intellect in which he is confined. He asks himself the question, "Whence come I—Whither go I—What is the object of my Existence?" He becomes dissatisfied with the answers the world has to give him to these questions, and he cries aloud in despair—and but the answer of his own voice comes back to him from the impassable walls with which he is surrounded. He does not realize that his answer must come from Within—but so it is.

Psychology stops when it reaches the limits of Mental Consciousness, or as it calls it "Self-Consciousness," and denies that there is anything beyond—any unexplored regions of the Mind. It laughs at the reports that come from those who have penetrated farther within the recesses of their being, and dismisses the reports as mere "dreams," "fantasies," "illusions," "ecstatic imaginings," "abnormal states," etc., etc. But, nevertheless, there are schools of thought that teach of these higher states, and there are men of all ages and races that have entered them and have reported concerning them. And we feel justified in asking you to take them into consideration.

There are two planes of Consciousness, of which we feel it proper to speak, for we have obtained more or less information regarding them. There are still higher planes, but they belong to higher phases of life than are dealt with here.

The first of these planes or states of Consciousness, above the "Self-Consciousness" of the psychologists (which we have called "Mental Consciousness") may be called "Ego-consciousness," for it brings an "awareness" of the Reality of the Ego. This "awareness" is far above the Self-consciousness of the man who is able to distinguish "I" from "You," and to give it a name. And far above the consciousness that enables a man, as he rises in the scale, to distinguish the "I" from faculty after faculty of the mind, which he is able to recognize as "not—I," until he finds left a mental something that he cannot set aside, which he calls "I"—although this stage alone is very much higher than that of the average of the race, and is a high degree of Attainment itself. It is akin to this last stage, and yet still fuller and more complete. In the dawning of Ego Consciousness the "I" recognizes itself still more clearly and, more than this, is fully imbued with a sense and "awareness" of its own *Reality*, unknown to it before. This awareness is not a mere matter of reasoning—it is a "consciousness," just as is Physical Consciousness and Mental Consciousness something different from an "intellectual conviction." It is a Knowing, not a Thinking or Believing. The "I" *knows* that it is Real—that it has its roots in the Supreme Reality underlying all the Universe, and partakes of its Essence. It does not know what this Reality is, but it knows that it is Real, and something different from anything in the world of name, form, number, time, space, cause and effect—something Transcendental and surpassing all human experience. And knowing this, it knows that it cannot be destroyed or hurt; cannot die, but is immortal; and that there is Something which is the very essence of Good behind of, underneath and even *in* itself. And in this certainty and consciousness is there Peace, Understanding and Power. When it fully bursts upon one, Doubt, Fear, Unrest and Dissatisfaction drop from him like wornout garments and he finds himself clothed in the Faith that Knows; Fearlessness; Restfulness; Satisfaction. Then he is able to say understandingly and with meaning "I AM."

This Ego Consciousness is coming to many as a dawning knowledge—the light is just rising from behind the hills. To others it has come gradually and slowly, but fully, and they now live in the full light of the consciousness. Others it has burst upon like a flash, or vision—like a light falling from the clear sky, almost blinding them at first, but leaving them changed men and women, possessed of that something that cannot be understood by or described to those who have not experienced it. This last stage is called "Illumination" in one of its forms.

The man of the Ego Consciousness may not understand the Riddle of the Universe or be able to give an answer to the great Questions of Life—but he has ceased to worry about them—they now disturb him not. He may use his intellect upon them as before, but never with the feeling that in their intellectual solution rests his happiness or peace of mind. He knows that he stands on solid rock, and though the storms of the world of matter and force may beat upon him, he will not be hurt. This and other things he knows. He cannot prove these things to others, for they are not demonstrable by argument—he himself did not get them in that way. And so he says but little about it—but lives his life as if he knew them not, so far as outward appearances go. But inwardly he is a changed man—his life is different from that of his brothers, for while their souls are wrapped in slumber or are tossing in troubled dreams, his Soul has awakened and is gazing upon the world with bright and fearless eyes. There are, of course, different stages or degrees of this Consciousness, just as there are in the lower planes of consciousness. Some have it to a slight degree, while others have it fully. Perhaps this lesson will tell some of its readers just what is the thing that has "happened" to them and which they hesitate to speak of to their closest friend or life companion. To others it may open the way to a fuller realization. We sincerely trust so, for one does not begin to Live until he knows the "I" as Reality.

There is a stage still higher than this last mentioned but it has come to but very few of the race. Reports of it come from all times, races, countries. It has been called "Cosmic Consciousness," and is described as an awareness of the Oneness of Life—that is, a consciousness that the Universe is filled with One Life—an actual perception and "awareness" that the Universe is full of Life, Motion and Mind, and that there is no such thing as Blind Force, or Dead Matter, but that All is alive, vibrating and intelligent. That is, of course, that the *Real Universe*, which is the Essence or background of the Universe of Matter, Energy and Mind, is as they describe. In fact, the description of those who have had glimpses of this state would indicate that they see the Universe as All Mind—that All is Mind at the last. This form of consciousness has been experienced by men here and there—only a few—in moments of "Illumination," the period lasting but a very short space of time, then fading away, leaving but a memory. In the moment of the "Illumination" there came to those experiencing it a sense of "intouch-ness" with Universal Knowledge and Life, impossible to describe, accompanied by a Joy beyond understanding.

Regarding this last, "Cosmic Consciousness," we would state that it means more than an intellectual conviction, belief or realization of the facts as stated, for an actual *vision* and *consciousness* of these things came in the moment of Illumination. Some others report that they have a deep abiding sense of the reality of the facts described by the report of the Illumined, but have not experienced the "vision" or ecstasy referred to. These last people seem to have with them always the same mental state as that possessed by those who had the "vision" and passed out of it, carrying with them the remembrance and feeling, but not the actual consciousness attained at the moment. They agree upon the essential particulars of the reports. Dr. Maurice Bucke, now passed out of this plane of life, wrote a book entitled "Cosmic Consciousness," in which he describes a number of these cases, including his own, Walt Whitman's and others, and in which he holds that this stage of consciousness is before the race and will gradually come to it in the future. He holds that the manifestation of it which has come to some few of the race, as above stated, is but the first beams of the sun which are flashing upon us and which are but prophecies of the appearance of the great body of light itself.

We shall not here consider at length the reports of certain great religious personages of the past, who have left records that in moments of great spiritual exaltation they became conscious of "being in the presence of the Absolute," or perhaps within the radius of "the light of Its countenance." We have great respect for these reports, and have every reason for believing many of them authentic, notwithstanding the conflicting reports that have been handed down to us by those experiencing them. These reports are conflicting because of the fact that the minds of those who had these glimpses of consciousness were not prepared or trained to fully understand the nature of the phenomena. They found themselves in the spiritual presence of Something of awful grandeur and spiritual rank, and were completely dazed and bewildered at the sight. They did not understand the nature of the Absolute, and when they had sufficiently recovered they reported that they had been in the "presence of God"—the word "God" meaning their particular conception of Deity—that is, the one appearing as Deity in their own particular religious creed or school. They saw nothing to cause them to identify this Something with their particular conception of Deity, except that they thought that "it *must* be God," and knowing no other God except their own particular conception, they naturally identifying the Something with "God" as they conceived Him to be. And their reports naturally were along these lines.

Thus the reports of all religions are filled with accounts of the so-called miraculous occurrences. The Catholic saint reports that he "saw of light of God's countenance," and the non-Catholic reports likewise regarding God as he knows him. The Mohammedan reports that he caught a glimpse of the face of Allah, and the Buddhist tells us that he saw Buddha under the tree. The Brahman has seen the face of Brahma, and the various Hindu sects have men who give similar reports regarding their own particular deities. The Persians have given similar reports, and even the ancient Egyptians have left records of similar occurrences. These conflicting reports have led to the belief, on the part of those who did not understand the nature of the phenomena, that these things were "all imagination" and fancy, if indeed not rank falsehood and imposture. But the Yogis know better than this. They know that underneath all these varying reports there is a common ground of truth, which will be apparent to anyone investigating the matter. They know that all of these reports (except a few based upon fraudulent imitation of the real phenomenon) are based upon truth and are but the bewildered reports of the various observers. They know that these people were temporarily lifted above the ordinary plane of consciousness and were made aware of the existence of a Being or Beings higher than mortal. It does not follow that they saw "God" or the Absolute, for there are many Beings of high spiritual growth and development that would appear to the ordinary mortal as a very God. The Catholic doctrine of Angels and Arch-angels is corroborated by those among the Yogis who have been "behind the Veil," and they give us reports of the "Devas" and other advanced Beings. So the Yogi accepts these reports of the various mystics, saints and inspired ones, and accounts for them all by laws perfectly natural to the students of the Yogi Philosophy, but which appear as supernatural to those who have not studied along these lines.

But we cannot speak further of this phase of the subject in this lesson, for a full discussion of it would lead us far away from the phase of the general subject before us. But we wish to be understood as saying that there are certain centers in the mental being of Man from which may come light regarding the existence of the Absolute and higher order of Beings. In fact, from these centers come to man that part of his mental "feelings" that he calls "the religious instinct or intuition." Man does not arrive at that underlying consciousness of "Something Beyond" by means of his Intellect—it is the glimmer of light coming from the higher centers of the Self. He notices these gleams of light, but not understanding them, he proceeds to erect elaborate theological and creedal structures to account for them, the work of the Intellect, however, always lacking that "feeling" that the intuition itself possesses. True religion, no matter under what name it may masquerade, comes from the "heart" and is not comforted or satisfied with these

Intellectual explanations, and hence comes that unrest and craving for satisfaction which comes to Man when the light begins to break through.

But we must postpone a further discussion of this part of the subject for the present. We shall consider it again in a future lesson in connection with other matters. As we have said, our next two lessons will take upon the inquiry regarding the regions outside of the consciousness of the ordinary man. You will find it a most fascinating and instructive inquiry and one that will open up new fields of thought for many of you.

MANTRAM (AFFIRMATION.)

I Am a Being far greater and grander than I have as yet conceived. I am unfolding gradually but surely into higher planes of consciousness. I am moving Forward and Upward constantly. My goal is the Realization of the True Self, and I welcome each stage of Unfoldment that leads me toward my aim. I am a manifestation of REALITY. I *AM.*

THE EIGHTH LESSON.

THE HIGHLANDS AND LOWLANDS OF MIND.

The Self of each of us has a vehicle of expression which we call the Mind, but which vehicle is much larger and far more complex than we are apt to realize. As a writer has said "Our Self is greater than we know; it has peaks above, and lowlands below the plateau of our conscious experience." That which we know as the "conscious mind" is not the Soul. The Soul is not a part of that which we know in consciousness, but, on the contrary, that which we know in consciousness is but a small part of the Soul—the conscious vehicle of a greater Self, or "I."

The Yogis have always taught that the mind has many planes of manifestation and action—and that many of its planes operated above and below the plane of consciousness. Western science is beginning to realize this fact, and its theories regarding same may be found in any of the later works on psychology. But this is a matter of recent development in Western science. Until very recently the text books held that Consciousness and Mind were synonymous, and that the Mind was conscious of all of its activities, changes and modifications.

Liebnitz was one of the first Western philosophers to advance the idea that there were planes of mental activity outside of the plane of consciousness, and since his time the leading thinkers have slowly but surely moved forward to his position.

At the present time it is generally conceded that at least ninety per cent of our mental operations take place in the out-of-conscious realm. Prof. Elmer Gates, the well known scientist, has said: "At least ninety per cent of our mental life is sub-conscious. If you will analyze your mental operations you will find that conscious thinking is never a continuous line of consciousness, but a series of conscious data with great intervals of subconscious. We sit and try to solve a problem, and fail. We walk around, try again, and fail. Suddenly an idea dawns that leads to the solution of the problem. The subconscious processes were at work. We do not volitionally create our own thinking. It takes place in us. We are more or less passive recipients. We cannot change the nature of a thought, or of a truth, but we can, as it were, *guide the ship by a moving of the helm*. Our mentation is largely the result of the great Cosmic Whole upon us."

Sir William Hamilton says that the sphere of our consciousness is only a small circle in the center of a far wider sphere of action and thought, of which we are conscious through its effects.

Taine says: "Outside of a little luminous circle, lies a large ring of twilight, and beyond this an indefinite night; but the events of this twilight and this night are as real as those within the luminous circle."

Sir Oliver Lodge, the eminent English scientist, speaking of the planes of the mind, says: "Imagine an iceberg glorying in its crisp solidity, and sparkling pinnacles, resenting attention paid to its submerged self, or supporting region, or to the saline liquid out of which it arose, and into which in due course it will some day return. Or, reversing the metaphor, we might liken our present state to that of the hulls of ships submerged in a dim ocean among strange monsters, propelled in a blind manner through space; proud perhaps of accumulating many barnacles as decoration; only recognizing our destination by bumping against the dock-wall; and with no cognizance of the deck and cabins above us, or the spars and sails—no thought of the sextant, and the compass, and the captain—no perception of the lookout on the mast—of the distant horizon. With no vision of objects far ahead—dangers to be avoided—destinations to be reached—other ships to be spoken to by means other than by bodily contact—a region of sunshine and cloud, of space, or perception, and of intelligence utterly inaccessible to parts below the waterline."

We ask our students to read carefully the above expression of Sir Oliver Lodge, for it gives one of the clearest and most accurate figures of the actual state of affairs concerning the mental planes that we have seen in Western writings.

And other Western writers have noted and spoken of these out-of-conscious realms. Lewes has said: "It is very certain that in every conscious volition—every act that is so characterized—the larger part of it is quite unconscious. It is equally certain that in every perception there are unconscious processes of reproduction and inference. There is a middle distance of sub-consciousness, and a background of unconsciousness."

Taine has told us that: "Mental events imperceptible to consciousness are far more numerous than the others, and of the world that makes up our being we only perceive the highest points—the lighted-up peaks of a continent whose lower levels remain in the shade. Beneath ordinary sensations are their components, that is to say, the elementary sensations, which must be combined into groups to reach our consciousness."

Maudsley says: "Examine closely and without bias the ordinary mental operations of daily life, and you will find that consciousness has not one-tenth part of the function therein which it is commonly assumed to have. In every conscious state there are at work conscious, sub-conscious, and infra-conscious energies, the last as indispensable as the first."

Oliver Wendall Holmes said: "There are thoughts that never emerge into consciousness, which yet make their influence felt among the perceptible mental currents, just as the unseen planets sway the movements of those that are watched and mapped by the astronomer."

Many other writers have given us examples and instances of the operation of the out-of-consciousness planes of thought. One has written that when the solution of a problem he had long vainly dealt with, flashed across his mind, he trembled as if in the presence of another being who had communicated a secret to him. All of us have tried to remember a name or similar thing without success, and have then dismissed the matter from our minds, only to have the missing name or thought suddenly presented to our conscious mind a few minutes, or hours, afterwards. Something in our mind was at work hunting up the missing word, and when it found it it presented it to us.

A writer has mentioned what he called "unconscious rumination," which happened to him when he read books presenting new points of view essentially opposed to his previous opinions. After days, weeks, or months, he found that to his great astonishment the old opinions were entirely rearranged, and new ones lodged there. Many examples of this unconscious mental digestion and assimilation are mentioned in the books on the subject written during the past few years.

It is related of Sir W. R. Hamilton that he discovered quarternions one day while walking with his wife in the observatory at Dublin. He relates that he suddenly felt "the galvanic circle of thought" close, and the sparks that fell from it was the fundamental mathematical relations of his problem, which is now an important law in mathematics.

Dr. Thompson has written: "At times I have had a feeling of the uselessness of all voluntary effort, and also that the matter was working itself clear in my mind. It has many times seemed to me that I was really a passive instrument in the hands of a person not myself. In view of having to wait for the results of these unconscious processes, I have proved the habit of getting together material in advance, and then leaving the mass to digest itself till I am ready to write about it. I delayed for a month the writing of my book 'System of Psychology,' but continued reading the authorities. I would not try to think about the book. I would watch with interest the people passing the windows. One evening when reading the paper, the substance of the missing part of the book flashed upon my mind, and I began to write. This is only a sample of many such experiences."

Berthelot, the founder of Synthetic Chemistry has said that the experiments leading to his wonderful discoveries have never been the result of carefully followed trains of thought—of pure reasoning processes—but have come of themselves, so to speak, from the clear sky.

Mozart has written: "I cannot really say that I can account for my compositions. My ideas flow, and I cannot say whence or how they come. I do not hear in my imagination the parts successively, but I hear them, as it were, all at once. The rest is merely an attempt to reproduce what I have heard."

Dr. Thompson, above mentioned, has also said: "In writing this work I have been unable to arrange my knowledge of a subject for days and weeks, until I experienced a clearing up of my mind, when I took my pen and unhesitatingly wrote the result. I have best accomplished this by leading the (conscious) mind as far away as possible from the subject upon which I was writing."

Prof. Barrett says: "The mysteriousness of our being is not confined to subtle physiological processes which we have in common with all animal life. There are higher and more capacious powers wrapped up in our human personality than are expressed even by what we know of consciousness, will, or reason. There are supernormal and transcendental powers of which, at present, we only catch occasional glimpses; and behind and beyond the supernormal there are fathomless abysses, the Divine ground of the soul; the ultimate reality of which our consciousness is but the reflection or faint perception. Into such lofty themes I do not propose to enter, they must be forever beyond the scope of human inquiry; nor is it possible within the limits of this paper to give any adequate conception of those mysterious regions of our complex personality, which are open to, and beginning to be disclosed by, scientific investigation."

Rev. Dr. Andrew Murray has written: "Deeper down than where the soul with its consciousness can enter there is spirit matter linking man with God; and deeper down than the mind and feelings or will—in the unseen depths of the hidden life—there dwells the Spirit of God." This testimony is remarkable, coming from that source, for it corroborates and reiterates the Yogi teachings of the Indwelling Spirit Schofield has written: "Our conscious mind as compared with the unconscious mind, has been likened to the visible spectrum of the sun's rays, as compared to the invisible part which stretches indefinitely on either side. We know now that the chief part of heat comes from the ultra-red rays that show no light; and the main part of the chemical changes in the vegetable world are the results of the ultra-violet rays at the other end of the spectrum, which are equally invisible to the eye, and are recognized only by their potent effects. Indeed as these invisible rays extend indefinitely on both sides of the visible spectrum, so we may say that the mind includes not only the visible or conscious part, and what we have termed the sub-conscious, that which lies below the red line, but the supraconscious mind that lies at the other end—all those regions of higher soul and spirit life, of which we are only at times vaguely conscious, but which always exist, and link us on to eternal verities, on the one side, as surely as the sub-conscious mind links us to the body on the other."

We know that our students will appreciate the above testimony of Dr. Schofield, for it is directly in the line of our teachings in the Yogi Philosophy regarding the Planes of the Mind (see "Fourteen Lessons").

We feel justified in quoting further from Dr. Schofield, for he voices in the strongest manner that which the Yogi Philosophy teaches as fundamental truths regarding the mind. Dr. Schofield is an English writer on Psychology, and so far as we know has no tendency toward occultism, his views having been arrived at by careful scientific study and investigation along the lines of Western psychology, which renders his testimony all the more valuable, showing as it does, how the human mind will instinctively find its way to the Truth, even if it has to blaze a new trail through the woods, departing from the beaten tracks of other minds around it, which lack the courage or enterprise to strike out for themselves.

Dr. Schofield writes: "The mind, indeed, reaches all the way, and while on the one hand it is inspired by the Almighty, on the other it energizes the body, all whose purposive life it originates. We may call the supra-conscious mind the sphere of the spirit life, the sub-conscious the sphere of the body life, and the conscious mind the middle region where both meet."

Continuing, Dr. Schofield says: "The Spirit of God is said to dwell in believers, and yet, as we have seen, His presence is not the subject of direct consciousness. We would include, therefore, in the supra-conscious, all such spiritual ideas, together with conscience—the voice of God, as Max Muller calls it—which is surely a half-conscious faculty. Moreover, the supra-conscious, like the sub-conscious, is, as we have said, best apprehended when the conscious mind is not active. Visions, meditations, prayers, and even dreams have been undoubtedly occasions of spiritual revelations, and many instances may be adduced as illustrations of the workings of the Spirit apart from the action of reason or mind. The truth apparently is that the mind as a whole is an unconscious state, by that its middle registers, excluding the highest spiritual and lowest physical manifestations, are fitfully illuminated in varying degree by consciousness; and that it is to this illuminated part of the dial that the word "mind," which rightly appertains to the whole, has been limited."

Oliver Wendell Holmes has said: "The automatic flow of thought is often singularly favored by the fact of listening to a weak continuous discourse, with just enough ideas in it to keep the (conscious) mind busy. The induced current of thought is often rapid and brilliant in inverse ratio to the force of the inducing current."

Wundt says: "The unconscious logical processes are carried on with a certainty and regularity which would be impossible where there exists the possibility of error. Our mind is so happily designed that it prepares for us the most important foundations of cognition, whilst we have not the slightest apprehension of the *modus operandi*. This unconscious soul, like a benevolent stranger, works and makes provisions for our benefit, pouring only the mature fruits into our laps."

A writer in an English magazine interestingly writes: "Intimations reach our consciousness from unconsciousness, that the mind is ready to work, is fresh, is full of ideas." "The grounds of our judgment are often knowledge so remote from consciousness that we cannot bring them to view." "That the human mind includes an unconscious part; that unconscious events occurring in that part are proximate causes of consciousness; that the greater part of human intuitional action is an effect of an unconscious cause; the truth of these propositions is so deducible from ordinary mental events, and is so near the surface that the failure of deduction to forestall induction in the discerning of it may well excite wonder." "Our behavior is influenced by unconscious assumptions respecting our own social and intellectual rank, and that of the one we are addressing. In company we unconsciously assume a bearing quite different from that of the home circle. After being raised to a higher rank the whole behavior subtly and unconsciously changes in accordance with it." And Schofield adds to the last sentence: "This is also the case in a minor degree with different styles and qualities of dress and different environments. Quite unconsciously we change our behavior, carriage, and style, to suit the circumstance."

Jensen writes: "When we reflect on anything with the whole force of the mind, we may fall into a state of entire unconsciousness, in which we not only forget the outer world, but also know nothing at all of ourselves and the thoughts passing within us after a time.

We then suddenly awake as from a dream, and usually at the same moment the result of our meditations appears as distinctly in consciousness without our knowing how we reached it."

Bascom says: "It is inexplicable how premises which lie below consciousness can sustain conclusions in consciousness; how the mind can wittingly take up a mental movement at an advanced stage, having missed its primary steps."

Hamilton and other writers have compared the mind's action to that of a row of billiard balls, of which one is struck and the impetus transmitted throughout the entire row, the result being that only the last ball actually moves, the others remaining in their places. The last ball represents the conscious thought—the other stages in the unconscious mentation. Lewes, speaking of this illustration, says: "Something like this, Hamilton says, seems often to occur in a train of thought, one idea immediately suggesting another into consciousness—this suggestion passing through one or more ideas which do not themselves rise into consciousness. This point, that we are not conscious of the formation of groups, but only of a formed group, may throw light on the existence of unconscious judgments, unconscious reasonings, and unconscious registrations of experience."

Many writers have related the process by which the unconscious mentation emerges gradually into the field of consciousness, and the discomfort attending the process. A few examples may prove interesting and instructive.

Maudsley says: "It is surprising how uncomfortable a person may be made by the obscure idea of something which he ought to have said or done, and which he cannot for the life of him remember. There is an effort of the lost idea to get into consciousness, which is relieved directly the idea bursts into consciousness."

Oliver Wendell Holmes said: "There are thoughts that never emerge into consciousness, and which yet make their influence felt among the perceptive mental currents, just as the unseen planets sway the movements of the known ones." The same writer also remarks: "I was told of a business man in Boston who had given up thinking of an important question as too much for him. But he continued so uneasy in his brain that he feared he was threatened with palsy. After some hours the natural solution of the question came to him, worked out, as he believed, in that troubled interval."

Dr. Schofield mentions several instances of this phase of the workings of the unconscious planes of the mind. We mention a couple that seem interesting and to the point:

"Last year," says Dr. Schofield, "I was driving to Phillmore Gardens to give some letters to a friend. On the way, a vague uneasiness sprang up, and a voice seemed to say, 'I doubt if you have those letters.' Conscious reason rebuked it, and said, 'Of course you have; you took them out of the drawer specially.' The vague feeling was not satisfied, but could not reply. On arrival I found the letters were in none of my pockets. On returning I found them on the hall table, where they had been placed a moment putting on my gloves."

"The other day I had to go to see a patient in Folkestone, in Shakespeare Terrace. I got there very late, and did not stay but drove down to the Pavilion for the night, it being dark and rainy. Next morning at eleven I walked up to find the house, knowing the general direction, though never having walked there before. I went up the main road, and, after passing a certain turning, began to feel a vague uneasiness coming into consciousness, that I had passed the terrace. On asking the way, I found it was so; and the turning was where the uneasiness began. The night before was pitch dark, and very wet, and anything seen from a close carriage was quite unconsciously impressed on my mind."

Prof. Kirchener says: "Our consciousness can only grasp one quite clear idea at once. All other ideas are for the time somewhat obscure. They are really existing, but only potentially for consciousness, *i.e.,* they hover, as it were, on our horizon, or beneath the threshold of consciousness. The fact that former ideas suddenly return to consciousness is simply explained by the fact that they have continued psychic existence: and attention is sometimes voluntarily or involuntarily turned away from the present, and the appearance of former ideas is thus made possible."

Oliver Wendell Holmes says: "Our different ideas are stepping-stones; how we get from one to another we do not know; something carries us. We (our conscious selves) do not take the step. The creating and informing spirit, which is *within* us and not *of* us, is recognized everywhere in real life. It comes to us as a voice that will be heard; it tells us what we must believe; it frames our sentences and we wonder at this visitor who chooses our brain as his dwelling place."

Galton says: "I have desired to show how whole states of mental operation that have lapsed out of ordinary consciousness, admit of being dragged into light."

Montgomery says: "We are constantly aware that feelings emerge unsolicited by any previous mental state, directly from the dark womb of unconsciousness. Indeed all our most vivid feelings are thus mystically derived. Suddenly a new irrelevant, unwilled, unlooked-for presence intrudes itself into consciousness. Some inscrutable power causes it to rise and enter the mental presence as a sensorial constituent. If this vivid dependence on unconscious forces has to be conjectured with regard to the most vivid mental occurrences, how much more must such a sustaining foundation be postulated for those faint revivals of previous sensations that so largely assist in making up our complex mental presence!"

Sir Benjamin Brodie says: "It has often happened to me to have accumulated a store of facts, but to have been able to proceed no further. Then after an interval of time, I have found the obscurity and confusion to have cleared away: the facts to have settled in their right places, though I have not been sensible of having made any effort for that purpose."

Wundt says: "The traditional opinion that consciousness is the entire field of the internal life cannot be accepted. In consciousness, psychic acts are very distinct from one another, and observation itself necessarily conducts to unity in psychology. But the agent of this unity is outside of consciousness, which knows only the result of the work done in the unknown laboratory beneath it. Suddenly a new thought springs into being. Ultimate analysis of psychic processes shows that the unconscious is the theater of the most important mental phenomena. The conscious is always conditional upon the unconscious."

Creighton says: "Our conscious life is the sum of these entrances and exits. Behind the scenes, as we infer, there lies a vast reserve which we call 'the unconscious,' finding a name for it by the simple device of prefixing the negative article. The basis of all that lies behind the scene is the mere negative of consciousness."

Maudsley says: "The process of reasoning adds nothing to knowledge (in the reasoner). It only displays what was there before, and brings to conscious possession what before was unconscious." And again: "Mind can do its work without knowing it. Consciousness is the light that lightens the process, not the agent that accomplishes it."

Walstein says: "It is through the sub-conscious self that Shakespeare must have perceived, without effort, great truths which are hidden from the conscious mind of the student; that Phidias painted marble and bronze; that Raphael painted Madonnas, and Beethoven composed symphonies."

Ribot says: "The mind receives from experience certain data, and elaborates them unconsciously by laws peculiar to itself, and the result merges into consciousness."

Newman says: "When the unaccustomed causes surprise, we do not perceive the thing and then feel the surprise; but surprise comes first, and then we search out the cause; so the theory must have acted on the unconscious mind to create the feeling, before being perceived in consciousness."

A writer in an English magazine says: "Of what transcendent importance is the fact that the unconscious part of the mind bears to the conscious part such a relation as the magic lantern bears to the luminous disc which it projects; that the greater part of the intentional action, the whole practical life of the vast majority of men, is an effect of events as remote from consciousness as the motion of the planets."

Dr. Schofield says: "It is quite true that the range of the unconscious mind must necessarily remain indefinite; none can say how high or low it may reach.... As to how far the unconscious powers of life that, as has been said, can make eggs and feathers out of Indian corn, and milk and beef and mutton out of grass, are to be considered within or beyond the lowest limits of unconscious mind, we do not therefore here press. It is enough to establish the fact of its existence; to point out its more important features; and to show that in all respects it is as worthy of being called mind as that which works in consciousness. We therefore return to our first definition of Mind, as 'the sum of psychic action in us, whether conscious or unconscious.'"

Hartmann calls our attention to a very important fact when he says: "The unconscious does not fall ill, the unconscious does not grow weary, but all conscious mental activity becomes fatigued."

Kant says: "To have ideas and yet not be conscious of them—therein seems to lie a contradiction. However, we may still be immediately aware of holding an idea, though we are not directly conscious of it."

Maudsley says: "It may seem paradoxical to assert not merely that ideas may exist in the mind without any consciousness of them, but that an idea, or a train of associated ideas, may be quickened into action and actuate movements without itself being attended to. When an idea disappears from consciousness it does not necessarily disappear entirely; it may remain latent below the horizon of consciousness. Moreover it may produce an effect upon movement, or upon other ideas, when thus active below the horizon of consciousness."

Liebnitz says: "It does not follow that because we do not perceive thought that it does not exist. It is a great source of error to believe that there is no perception in the mind but that of which it is conscious."

Oliver Wendell Holmes says: "The more we examine the mechanism of thought the more we shall see that anterior unconscious action of the mind that enters largely into all of its processes. People who talk most do not always think most. I question whether persons who think most—that is who have most conscious thought pass through their mind—necessarily do most mental work. Every new idea planted in a real thinker's mind grows when he is least conscious of it."

Maudsley says: "It would go hard with mankind indeed, if they must act wittingly before they acted at all. Men, without knowing why, follow a course for which good reasons exist. Nay, more. The practical instincts of mankind often work beneficially in actual contradiction to their professed doctrines."

The same writer says: "The best thoughts of an author are the unwilled thoughts which surprise himself; and the poet, under the influence of creative activity, is, so far as consciousness is concerned, being dictated to."

A writer in an English magazine says: "When waiting on a pier for a steamer, I went on to the first, which was the wrong one. I came back and waited, losing my boat, which was at another part of the pier, on account of the unconscious assumption I had made, that this was the only place to wait for the steamer. I saw a man enter a room, and leave by another door. Shortly after, I saw another man exactly like him do the same. It was the same man; but I said it must be his twin brother, in the unconscious assumption that there was no exit for the first man but by the way he came (that by returning)."

Maudsley says: "The firmest resolve or purpose sometimes vanishes issueless when it comes to the brink of an act, while the true will, which determines perhaps a different act, springs up suddenly out of the depths of the unconscious nature, surprising and overcoming the conscious."

Schofield says: "Our unconscious influence is the projection of our unconscious mind and personality unconsciously over others. This acts unconsciously on their unconscious centers, producing effects in character and conduct, recognized in consciousness. For instance, the entrance of a good man into a room where foul language is used, will unconsciously modify and purify the tone of the whole room. Our minds cast shadows of which we are as unconscious as those cast by our bodies, but which affect for good or evil all who unconsciously pass within their range. This is a matter of daily experience, and is common to all, though more noticeable with strong personalities."

Now we have given much time and space to the expressions of opinion of various Western writers regarding this subject of there being a plane or planes of the mind outside of the field of consciousness. We have given space to this valuable testimony, not alone because of its intrinsic value and merit, but because we wished to impress upon the minds of our students that these out-of-conscious planes of mind are now being recognized by the best authorities in the Western world, although it has been only a few years back when the idea was laughed at as ridiculous, and as a mere "dream of the Oriental teachers." Each writer quoted has brought out some interesting and valuable point of the subject, and the student will find that his own experiences corroborate the points cited by the several writers. In this way we think the matter will be made plainer, and will become fixed in the mind of those who are studying this course of lessons.

But we must caution our students from hastily adopting the several theories of Western writers, advanced during the past few years, regarding these out-of-conscious states. The trouble has been that the Western writers dazzled by the view of the subconscious planes of mentation that suddenly burst upon the Western thought, hastily adopted certain theories, which they felt would account for all the phenomena known as "psychic," and which they thought would fully account for all the problems of the subject. These writers while doing a most valuable work, which has helped thousands to form new ideas regarding the nature and workings of the mind, nevertheless did not sufficiently explore the nature of the problem before them. A little study of the Oriental philosophies might have saved them and their readers much confusion.

For instance, the majority of these writers hastily assumed that because there *was* an out-of-conscious plane of mentation, therefore all the workings of the mind might be grouped under the head of "conscious" and "sub-conscious," and that all the out-of-conscious phenomena might be grouped under the head of "subconscious mind," "subjective mind," etc., ignoring the fact that this class of mental phenomena embraced not only the highest but the lowest forms of mentation In their newly found "mind" (which they called "subjective" or "sub-conscious"), they placed the lowest traits and animal passions; insane impulses; delusions; bigotry; animal-like intelligence, etc., etc., as well as the inspiration of the poet and musician, and the high spiritual longings and feelings that one recognizes as having come from the higher regions of the soul.

This mistake was a natural one, and at first reading the Western world was taken by storm, and accepted the new ideas and theories as Truth. But when reflection came, and analysis was applied there arose a feeling of disappointment and dissatisfaction, and people began to feel that there was something lacking. They intuitively recognized that their higher inspirations and intuitions came from a different part of the mind than the lower emotions, passions, and other sub-conscious feelings, and instincts.

A glance at the Oriental philosophies will give one the key to the problem at once. The Oriental teachers have always held that the conscious mentation was but a small fraction of the entire volume of thought, but they have always taught that just as there was a field of mentation *below* consciousness, so was there a field of mentation *above* consciousness as much higher than Intellect as the other was lower than it. The mere mention of this fact will prove a revelation to those who have not heard it before, and who have become entangled with the several "dual-mind" theories of the recent Western writers. The more one has read on this subject the more he will appreciate the superiority of the Oriental theory over that of the Western writers. It is like the chemical which at once clears the clouded liquid in the test-tube.

In our next lesson we shall go into this subject of the above-conscious planes, and the below-conscious planes, bringing out the distinction clearly, and adding to what we have said on the subject in previous books.

And all this is leading us toward the point where we may give you instruction regarding the training and cultivation—the retraining and guidance of these out-of-conscious faculties. By retraining the lower planes of mentation to their proper work, and by stimulating the higher ones, man may "make himself over." mentally, and may acquire powers of which he but dreams now. This is why we are leading you up to the understanding of this subject, step by step. We advise you to acquaint yourself with each phase of the matter, that you may be able to apply the teachings and instructions to follow in later lessons of the course.

MANTRAM (AFFIRMATION).

I recognize that my Self is greater than it seems—that above and below consciousness are planes of mind—that just as there are lower planes of mind which belong to my past experience in ages past and over which I must now assert my Mastery—so are there planes of mind into which I am unfolding gradually, which will bring me wisdom, power, and joy. I Am Myself, in the midst of this mental world—I am the Master of my Mind—I assert my control of its lower phases, and I demand of its higher all that it has in store for me.

THE NINTH LESSON.

THE MENTAL PLANES.

In our last lesson we told you something about the operation of the mind outside of the field of consciousness. In this lesson we will attempt to classify these out-of-consciousness planes, by directing your attention to the several mental planes above and below the plane of consciousness. As we stated in the last lesson, over 90 per cent of our mental operations are conducted outside of the field of consciousness, so that the consideration of the planes is seen to be an important subject.

Man is a Centre of Consciousness in the great One Life of the Universe. His soul has climbed a great many steps before it reached its present position and stage of unfoldment.

And it will pass through many more steps until it is entirely free and delivered from the necessity of its swaddling clothes.

In his mental being man contains traces of all that has gone before—all the experiences of himself and the great race movement of which he is a part. And, likewise, his mind contains faculties and mental planes which have not as yet unfolded into consciousness, and of the existence of which he is but imperfectly aware. All of these mental possessions, however, are useful and valuable to him—even the lowest. The lowest may be used to advantage, under proper mastery, and are only dangerous to the man who allows them to master him instead of serving him as they should, considering his present stage of development.

In this consideration of the several mental planes we shall not confine ourselves to the technical occult terms given to these several planes, but will place them in general groups and describe the features and characteristics of each, rather than branch off into long explanations of the growth and reason of the several planes, which would take us far away from the practical consideration of the subject.

Beginning at the lowest point of the scale we see that man has a body. The body is composed of minute cells of protoplasm. These cells are built up of countless molecules, atoms and particles of matter—precisely the same matter that composes the rocks, trees, air, etc., around him. The Yogi philosophy tells us that even the atoms of matter have life and an elementary manifestation of mind, which causes them to group together according to the law of attraction, forming different elements, combinations, etc. This law of attraction is a mental operation, and is the first evidence of mental choice, action and response. Below this is Prana or Force, which, strictly speaking, is also a manifestation of mind, although for convenience we designate it as a separate manifestation of the Absolute.

And therefore we find that this law of attraction between the atoms and particles of matter is a mental action, and that it belongs to man's mental kingdom, because he has a body and this mental action is continually going on in his body. So therefore this is the lowest mental plane to be considered in the make-up of the man. This plane is, of course, far sunken beneath the plane of consciousness, and is scarcely identified with the personality of the man at all, but rather belongs to the life of the whole, manifest in the rock as well as in the man.

But after these atoms have been grouped by the law of attraction and have formed molecules of matter, they are taken possession of by a higher mental activity and built up into cells by the mental action of the plant. The life impulse of the plant begins by drawing to it certain particles of inorganic matter—chemical elements—and then building them into a single cell. Oh, mystery of the cell! The intellect of man is unable to duplicate this wonderful process. The Mind Principle on the Vegetative Plane, however, knows exactly how to go to work to select and draw to itself just the elements needed to build up the single cell. Then taking up its abode in that cell—using it as a basis of operations, it proceeds to duplicate its previous performance, and so cell after cell is added, by the simple reproductive process of division and subdivision—the primitive and elemental sex process—until the mighty plant is built up. From the humblest vegetable organism up to the greatest oak the process is the same.

And it does not stop there. The body of man is also built up in just this way, and he has this vegetative mind also within him, below the plane of consciousness, of course. To many this thought of a vegetative mind may be somewhat startling. But let us remember that every part of our body has been built up from the vegetable cell. The unborn child starts with the coalition of two cells. These cells begin to build up the new body for the occupancy of the child—that is, the mind principle in the cells directs the work, of course—drawing upon the body of the mother for nourishment and supplies. The nourishment in the mother's blood, which supplies the material for the building up of the child's body, is obtained by the mother eating and assimilating the vegetable cells of plants, directly or indirectly. If she eats fruit, nuts, vegetables, etc., she obtains the nourishment of the plant life directly—if she eats meat she obtains it indirectly, for the animal from which the meat was taken built up the meat from vegetables. There is no two ways about this—all nourishment of the animal and human kingdom is obtained from the vegetable kingdom, directly or indirectly.

And the cell action in the child is identical with the cell action in the plant. Cells constantly reproducing themselves and building themselves up into bodily organs, parts, etc., under the direction and guidance of the mind principle. The child grows in this way until the hour of birth. It is born, and then the process is but slightly changed. The child begins to take nourishment either from the mother's milk or from the milk of the cow, or other forms of food. And as it grows larger it partakes of many different varieties of food. But always it obtains building material from the cell life of the plants.

And this great building up process is intelligent, purposeful, to a wonderful degree. Man with his boasted intellect cannot explain the real "thingness" of the process. A leading scientist who placed the egg of a small lizard under microscopical examination and then watched it slowly develop has said that it seemed as if some hand was tracing the outlines of the tiny vertebrae, and then building up around it. Think for a moment of the development of the germ within the egg of the humming-bird, or the ant, or the gnat, or the eagle. Every second a change may be noticed. The germ cell draws to itself nourishment from the other part of the egg, and then it grows and reproduces another cell. Then both cells divide—then subdivide until there are millions and millions and millions of cells. And all the while the building up process continues, and the bird or insect assumes shape and form, until at last the work is accomplished and the young bird emerges from the egg.

And the work thus commenced continues until the death of the animal. For there is a constant using-up and breaking-down of cell and tissue, which the organism must replace. And so the vegetative mind of the plant, or insect, or animal, or man, is constantly at work building up new cells from the food, throwing out worn-out and used-up material from the system. Not only this, but it attends to the circulation of the blood in order that the materials for the building up may be carried to all parts of the system. It attends to the digestion and assimilation of the food—the wonderful work of the organs of the body. It attends to the healing of wounds, the fight against disease, the care of the physical body. And all this out of the plane of consciousness—in the infant man the animal world, the vegetable kingdom—ever at work, untiring, intelligent, wonderful. And this plane of mind is in man as well as in the plant, and it does its work without aid from the conscious part of man, although man may interfere with it by adverse conscious thought, which seems to paralyze its efforts. Mental Healing is merely the restoring of normal conditions, so that this part of the body may do its work without the hindrance of adverse conscious thought.

On this plane of the mind is found all of the vital functions and operations. The work is done out-of-consciousness, and the consciousness is aware of this part of the mind only when it makes demands upon the conscious for food, etc. On this plane also resides the elementary instinct that tends toward reproduction and sexual activity. The demand of this part of the mind is always "increase and multiply," and according to the stage of growth of the individual is the mandate carried out, as we shall see presently. The elementary impulses and desires that we find rising into the field of consciousness come from this plane of the mind. Hunger, thirst and the reproductive desires are its messages to the higher parts of the mind. And these messages are natural and free from the abuses and prostitution often observed attached to them by the intellect of man in connection with his unrestrained animal impulses. Gluttony and unnatural lust arise not from the primitive demand of this plane of the mind—for the lower animals even are free from them to a great extent—but it is reserved for man to so prostitute these primitive natural tendencies, in order to gratify unnatural and artificial appetites, which serve to frustrate nature rather than to aid her.

As Life advanced in the scale and animal forms appeared on the scene new planes of mind were unfolded, in accordance to the necessity of the living forms. The animal was compelled to hunt for his food—to prey upon other forms, and to avoid being preyed upon by others. He was compelled to struggle for the unfoldment of latent powers of his mind that would give him means to play his part in the scheme of life. He was compelled to do certain things in order to live and reproduce his kind. And he demanded not in vain. For there came to him slowly an unfolding knowledge of the things necessary for the requirements of his life. We call this Instinct. But, pray remember, by Instinct we do not mean the still higher something that is really rudimentary Intellect that we notice in the higher animals. We are speaking now of the unreasoning instinct observed in the lower animals, and to a certain degree in man. This Instinctive plane of mentality causes the bird to build its nest before its eggs are laid, which instructs the animal mother how to care for its young when born, and after birth; which teaches the bee to construct its cell and to store up its honey. These and countless other things in animal life, and in the higher form of plant life, are manifestations of Instinct—that great plane of the mind. In fact, the greater part of the life of the animal is instinctive although the higher forms of animals have developed something like rudimentary Intellect or Reason, which enables them to meet new conditions where Intellect alone fails them.

And man has this plane of mind within him, below consciousness. In fact the lower forms of human life manifest but little Intellect, and live almost altogether according to their Instinctive impulses and desires.

Every man has this Instinctive mental region within him and from it are constantly arising impulses and desires to perplex and annoy him, as well as to serve him occasionally. The whole secret consists in whether the man has Mastery of his lower self or not.

From this plane of the mind arise the hereditary impulses coming down from generations of ancestors, reaching back to the cavemen, and still further back into the animal kingdom. A queer storehouse is this. Animal instincts—passions, appetites, desires, feelings, sensations, emotions, etc., are there. Hate, envy, jealousy, revenge, the lust of the animal seeking the gratification of his sexual impulses, etc., etc., are there, and are constantly intruding upon our attention until we have asserted our mastery. And often the failure to assert this mastery comes from an ignorance of the nature of the desire, etc. We have been taught that these thoughts were "bad" without being told *why*, and we have feared them and thought them the promptings of an impure nature, or a depraved mind, etc. This is all wrong. These things are not "bad" of themselves—they came to us honestly—they are our heritage from the past. They belong to the animal part of our nature, and were necessary to the animal in his stage of development. We have the whole menagerie within us, but that does not mean that we should turn the beasts loose upon ourselves or others. It was necessary for the animal to be fierce, full of fight, passionate, regardless of the rights of others, etc., but we have outgrown that stage of development, and it is ignoble for us to return to it, or to allow it to master us.

This lesson is not intended as a discourse upon Ethics or morals. We do not intend going into a discussion of the details of "Right and Wrong," for we have touched upon that phase of the subject in other works. But we feel justified in calling your attention to the fact that the human mind intuitively recognizes the "Rightness" of the living up to that which comes to us from the highest parts of the mind—the highest product of our unfoldment. And it likewise intuitively recognizes the "Wrongness" of the falling back into that which belongs to the lower stages of our mentality—to the animal part of us, that is our heritage from the past and that which has gone before.

While we may be puzzled about many details of morals and ethics and may not be able to "explain" why we consider certain things right or wrong, we still intuitively feel that the highest "Right" of which we are capable is the acting out of that which is coming to us from the highest pole of our mental being, and that the lowest "Wrong" consists in doing that which carries us back to the life of the lower animals, in so far as mentality is concerned. Not because there is anything absolutely "Wrong" in the mental processes and consequent of the animals in themselves—they are all right and perfectly natural in the animals—but we intuitively recognize that for us to fall back to the animal stage is a "going backward" in the scale of evolution. We intuitively shrink at an exhibition of brutality and animality on the part of a man or woman. We may not know just why, but a little reflection will show us that it is a sinking in the evolutionary scale, against which the spiritual part of us revolts and protests.

But this must not be construed to mean that the advanced soul looks upon the animal world with disgust or horror. On the contrary, there is nowhere to be found a higher respect for animal life and being than among the Yogi and other advanced souls. They delight in watching the animals filling their places in life—playing out their parts in the divine scheme of life. Their animal passions and desires are actions viewed sympathetically and lovingly by the advanced soul, and nothing "Wrong" or disgusting is seen there. And even the coarseness and brutality of the savage races are so regarded by these advanced souls. They see everything as natural according to the grade and degree of development of these people.

It is only when these advanced souls view the degeneracies of "civilized" life that they feel sorrow and pain. For here they see instances of devolution instead of evolution—degeneration instead of regeneration and advancement. And not only do they know this to be the fact, but the degenerate specimens of mankind themselves feel and know it. Compare the expression of the animal or savage going through their natural life actions and performances. See how free and natural are their expressions, how utterly apart are evidences of wrong doing. They have not as yet found out the fatal secret of Good and Evil—they have not as yet eaten the forbidden fruit. But, on the contrary, look into the faces of the degenerates and fallen souls of our civilized life. See the furtive glance and the self-consciousness of "Wrong" evident in every face. And this consciousness of "Wrong" bears heavily upon these people—it is heavier than the punishments heaped upon them That nameless something called "conscience" may be smothered for a while, but sooner or later it comes to light and demands the pound of flesh from its victim.

And yet you will say that it seems hard to think that the same thing can be Right in one person and Wrong in another. This seems like a hard saying and a dangerous doctrine, but it is the Truth. And man instinctively recognizes it. He does not expect the same sense of moral responsibility in a young child, or in a savage, that he does in a mature, developed, civilized man. He may restrain the child and the savage, for self-protection and the welfare of all, but he realizes the distinction, or at least should do so. And not only is this true, but as man advances in the scale he casts off many ideas of "Wrong" that he once held, having outgrown the old ideas and having grown into new conceptions. And the tendency is always upward and onward. The tendency is constantly from Force and Restraint toward Love and Freedom. The ideal condition would be one in which there were no laws and no necessity for them—a condition in which men had ceased to do wrong because they had outgrown the desire rather than from fear or restraint or force. And while this condition as yet seems afar off, there is constantly going on an unfoldment of higher planes and faculties of the mind, which when once fully manifest in the race will work a complete revolution in ethics and laws and government—and for the better, of course. In the meantime Mankind moves along, doing the best it can, making a steady though slow progress.

There is another plane of the mind which is often called the "Instinct," but which is but a part of the plane of the Intellect, although its operations are largely below the field of consciousness. We allude to what may be called the "Habit Mind," in order to distinguish it from the Instinctive Plane. The difference is this: The Instinctive plane of mind is made up of the ordinary operations of the mind below the plane of the Intellect, and yet above the plane of the Vegetative mind—and also of the acquired experiences of the race, which have been transmitted by heredity, etc. But the "Habit Mind" contains only that which has been placed there by the person himself and which he has acquired by experience, habit, and observation, repeated so often until the mind knows it so well that it is carried below the field of consciousness and becomes "second nature," and akin to Instinct.

The text books upon psychology are filled with illustrations and examples of the habit phase or plane of the mental operations, and we do not think it necessary to repeat instances of the same kind here. Everyone is familiar with the fact that tasks which at first are learned only by considerable work and time soon become fixed in some part of the mind until their repetition calls for little or no exercise of conscious mental operation. In fact, some writers have claimed that no one really "learns" how to perform a task until he can perform it almost automatically. The pupil who in the early stages of piano playing finds it most difficult to control and manage his fingers, after a time is able to forget all about his fingering and devote his entire attention to the pages of his music, and after this he is able to apparently let his fingers play the entire piece of music by themselves without a thought on his part. The best performers have told us that in the moments of their highest efforts they are aware that the out-of-conscious portion of their mind is doing the work for them, and they are practically standing aside and witnessing the work being done. So true is this that in some cases it is related that if the performer's conscious mind attempts to take up the work the quality is impaired and the musician and the audience notice the difference.

The same thing is true in the case of the woman learning to operate the sewing machine. It is quite difficult at first, but gradually it grows to "run itself." Those who have mastered the typewriter have had the same experience. At first each letter had to be picked out with care and effort. After a gradual improvement the operator is enabled to devote her entire attention to the "copy" and let the fingers pick out the keys for themselves. Many operators learn rapid typewriting by so training the habit mind that it picks out the letter-keys by reason of their position, the letters being covered over in order to force the mind to adapt itself to the new requirements. A similar state of affairs exists wherever men or women have to use tools of any kind. The tool soon is recognized by the mind and used as if it were a part of the body, and no more conscious thought is devoted to the manipulation than we devote to the operation of walking, which, by the way, is learned by the child only by the expenditure of time and labor. It is astonishing how many things we do "automatically" in this way. Writers have called our attention to the fact that the average man cannot consciously inform you how he puts on his coat in the morning—which arm goes in first, how the coat is held, etc. But the habit mind knows—knows very well. Let the student stand up and put on his coat in the regular way, following the leadings of the habit mind. Then, after removing it, let him attempt to put it on by inserting the other arm first, for instance. He will be surprised to find out how awkward it will be for him, and how completely he has been depending upon the habit mind. And tomorrow morning let him find out which shoe the habit mind has been putting on him first and then try to reverse the order and notice how flurried and disturbed the habit mind will become, and how frantically it will signal to the conscious mind: "Something wrong up there!" Or try to button on your collar, reversing the order in which the tabs are placed over the button—right before left, or left before right, as the case may be, and notice the involuntary protest. Or, try to reverse the customary habit in walking and attempt to swing your right arm with the movement of your right leg, and so on, and you will find it will require the exercise of great will power. Or, try to "change hands" and use your knife and fork. But we must stop giving examples and illustrations. Their number is countless.

Not only does the habit mind attend to physical actions, etc., but it also takes a hand in our mental operations. We soon acquire the habit of ceasing to consciously consider certain things, and the habit mind takes the matter for granted, and thereafter we will think automatically on those particular questions, unless we are shaken out of the habit by a rude jolt from the mind of someone else, or from the presentation of some conflicting idea occasioned by our own experience or reasoning processes. And the habit mind hates to be disturbed and compelled to revise its ideas. It fights against it, and rebels, and the result is that many of us are slaves to old outgrown ideas that we realize are false and untrue, but which we find that we "cannot exactly get rid of." In our future lessons we will give methods to get rid of these old outgrown ideas.

There are other planes of mind which have to do with the phenomena known as "psychic," by which is meant the phases of psychic phenomena known as clairvoyance, psychometry, telepathy, etc., but we shall not consider them in this lesson, for they belong to another part of the general subject. We have spoken of them in a general way in our "Fourteen Lessons in Yogi Philosophy, etc."

And now we come to the plane of mind known to us as Intellect or the Reasoning Faculties. Webster defines the word Intellect as follows: The part or faculty of the human soul by which it knows, as distinguished from the power to feel and to will; the thinking faculty; the understanding. The same authority defines the word Reason as follows: "The faculty or capacity of the human mind by which it is distinguished from the intelligence of the inferior animals." We shall not attempt to go into a consideration of the conscious Intellect, for to do so we would be compelled to take up the space of the remaining lessons of the course, and besides, the student may find extended information on this subject in any of the text books on psychology. Instead we will consider other faculties and planes of mind which the said text books pass by rapidly, or perhaps deny. And one of these planes is that of Unconscious Reasoning, or Intellect. To many this term will seem paradoxical, but students of the unconscious will understand just what is meant.

Reasoning is not necessarily conscious in its operations, in fact, a greater part of the reasoning processes are performed below or above the conscious field. In our last lesson we have given a number of examples proving this fact, but a few more remarks may not be out of place, nor without interest to the student.

In our last lesson you will see many instances stated in which the sub-conscious field of the Intellect worked out problems, and then after a time handed to the conscious reason the solution of the matter. This has occurred to many of us, if not indeed to all of us. Who has not endeavored to solve a problem or question of some sort and after "giving it up" has had it suddenly answered and flashed into consciousness when least expected. The experience is common to the race. While the majority of us have noticed these things, we have regarded them as exceptional and out of the general rule. Not so, however, with students of the mental planes. The latter have recognized these planes of reason, and have availed themselves of their knowledge by setting these unconscious faculties to work for them. In our next lesson we will give directions to our students regarding this accomplishment, which may prove of the greatest importance to those who will take the trouble to practice the directions given. It is a plan that is known to the majority of men who have "done things" in the world, the majority of them, however, having discovered the plan for themselves as the result of a need or demand upon the inner powers of mind.

The plane of mind immediately above that of Intellect is that known as Intuition. Intuition is defined by Webster as follows: "Direct apprehension or cognition; immediate knowledge, as in perception or consciousness, involving no reasoning process; quick or ready insight or apprehension." It is difficult to explain just what is meant by Intuition, except to those who have experienced it—and these people do not need the explanation. Intuition is just as real a mental faculty as is Intellect—or, to be more exact, is just as much a collection of mental faculties. Intuition is above the field of consciousness, and its messages are passed downward, though its processes are hidden. The race is gradually unfolding into the plane of Intuition, and the race will some day pass into full consciousness on that plane. In the meantime it gets but flashes and glimpses from the hidden region. Many of the best things we have come from that region. Art, music, the love of the beautiful and good poetry, the higher form of love, spiritual insight to a certain degree, intuitive perception of truth, etc., etc., come from this region. These things are not reasoned out by the intellect, but seem to spring full born from some unknown region of the mind.

In this wonderful region dwells Genius. Many, if not all of the great writers, poets, musicians, artists and other examples of genius have felt that their power came to them from some higher source. Many have thought that it emanated from some being kindly to them, who would inspire them with power and wisdom. Some transcendent power seemed to have been called into operation, and the worker would feel that his product or creation was not his handiwork, but that of some outside intelligence. The Greeks recognized this something in man, and called it man's "Daemon." Plutarch in his discourse on the daemon that guided Socrates speaks of the vision of Timarchus, who, in the case of Trophonius, saw spirits which were partly attached to human bodies, and partly over and above them, shining luminously over their heads. He was informed by the oracle that the part of the spirit which was immersed in the body was called the "soul," but that the outer and unimmersed portion was called the "daemon." The oracle also informed him that every man had his daemon, whom he is bound to obey; those who implicitly follow that guidance are the prophetic souls, the favorites of the gods. Goethe also spoke of the daemon as a power higher than the will, and which inspired certain natures with miraculous energy.

We may smile at these conceptions, but they are really very close to the truth. The higher regions of the mind, while belonging to the individual, and a part of himself, are so far above his ordinary consciousness that to all intents and purposes messages from them are as orders from another and higher soul. But still the voice is that of the "I," speaking through its sheaths as best it is able.

This power belongs to every one of us, although it manifests only in the degree that we are able to respond to it. It grows by faith and confidence, and closes itself up, and withdraws into its recesses when we doubt it and would question its veracity and reality. What we call "originality" comes from this region. The Intuitive faculties pass on to the conscious mind some perception of truth higher than the Intellect has been able to work out for itself, and lo! it is called the work of genius.

The advanced occultist knows that in the higher regions of the mind are locked up intuitive perceptions of all truth, and that he who can gain access to these regions will know everything intuitively, and as a matter of clear sight, without reasoning or explanation. The race has not as yet reached the heights of Intuition—it is just beginning to climb the foothills. But it is moving in the right direction. It will be well for us if we will open ourselves to the higher inner guidance, and be willing to be "led by the Spirit." This is a far different thing from being led by outside intelligence, which may, or may not, be qualified to lead. But the Spirit within each of us has our interests at heart and is desirous of our best good, and is not only ready but willing to take us by the hand and lead us on. The Higher Self is doing the best it can for our development and welfare, but is hampered by the confining sheaths. And alas, many of us glory in these sheaths and consider them the highest part of ourselves. Do not be afraid to let the light of the Spirit pierce through these confining sheaths and dissolve them. The Intuition, however, is not the Spirit, but is one of its channels of communication to us. There are other and still higher planes of mind, but the Intuition is the one next in the line of unfoldment, and we should open ourselves to its influence and welcome its unfoldment.

Above the plane of Intuition is that of the Cosmic Knowing, upon which we will find the consciousness of the Oneness of All. We have spoken of this plane in our lesson on the Unfoldment of Consciousness. When one is able to "conscious" on this plane—this exalted plane of mind—he is able to see fully, plainly and completely that there is One Great Life underlying all the countless forms and shapes of manifestation. He is able to see that separateness is only "the working fiction of the Universe." He is able to see that each Ego is but a Centre of Consciousness in the great Ocean of Life—all in pursuance of the Divine Plan, and that he is moving forward toward higher and higher planes of manifestation, power and individuality, in order to take a greater and grander part in the Universal work and plans.

The Cosmic Knowing in its fulness has come to but few of the race, but many have had glimpses, more or less clear, of its transcendent wonder, and others are on the borderland of this plane. The race is unfolding gradually, slowly but surely, and those who have had this wonderful experience are preparing others for a like experience. The seed is being sown, and the harvest will come later. This and other phases of the higher forms of consciousness are before the race. The individuals who read this lesson are perhaps nearer to it than they think; their interest in the lessons is an indication of that hunger of the soul which is a prophecy of the satisfaction of the cry for spiritual bread. The Law of Life heeds these cries for aid and nourishment and responds accordingly, but along the lines of the highest wisdom and according to the *real requirements* of the individual.

Let us close this lesson with a quotation from "Light on the Path," which bears directly upon the concluding thought. Read it carefully and let it sink down deep into your inner consciousness, and you will feel the thrill of joy that comes to him who is nearing the goal.

"Look for the flower to bloom in the silence that follows the storm; not till then.

"It shall grow, it will shoot up, it will make branches and leaves, and form buds while the storm lasts. But not until the entire personality of the man is dissolved and melted—not until it is held by the divine fragment which has created it, as a mere subject for grave experiment and experience—not until the whole nature has yielded and become subject unto its higher self, can the bloom open. Then will come a calm such as comes in a tropical country after the heavy rain, when nature works so swiftly that one may see her action. Such a calm will come to the harassed spirit. And in the deep silence the mysterious event will occur which will prove that the way has been found. Call it by whatever name you will. It is a voice that speaks where there is none to speak, it is a messenger that comes—a messenger without form or substance—or it is the flower of the soul that has opened. It cannot be described by any metaphor. But it can be felt after, looked for, and desired, even among the raging of the storm. The silence may last a moment of time, or it may last a thousand years. But it will end. Yet you will carry its strength with you. Again and again the battle must be fought and won. It is only for an interval that nature can be still."

* * * * *

The concluding three lessons of this series will be devoted to a practical course of instruction in the development of the hidden planes of the mind, or rather, in the development of the power of the individual to master the same and make use of them in his life. He will be taught to master the lower principles, not only in the surmounting of them, but in the transmitting of the elemental forces toward his higher ends. Power may be obtained from this part of the mind, under the direction of the Will. And the student will be told how to set the unconscious Intellect to work for him. And he will be told how to develop and train the Will. We have now passed the line between the theoretical and the practical phases of the subject, and from now on it will be a case of train, develop, cultivate and apply. Knowing what lies back of it all, the student is now prepared to receive the instructions which he might have misused before. Peace be with thee all.

MANTRAM (AFFIRMATION).

I AM THE MASTER OF MY SOUL.

THE TENTH LESSON.

SUB-CONSCIOUSING.

In the Ninth Lesson we called your attention to the fact that Reasoning was not necessarily conscious in its operations, and that, in fact, a large part of the rational processes of the mind are performed below or above the field of consciousness. And in the Eighth Lesson we gave you a number of examples illustrating this fact. We also gave you a number of cases in which the sub-conscious field of the Intellect worked out problems, and then after a time passed on to the conscious field of the Intellect the solution of the matter. In this lesson we purpose instructing you in the methods by which this part of the Intellect may be set to work for you. Many have stumbled upon bits of this truth for themselves, and, in fact, the majority of successful men and men who have attained eminence in any walk of life have made more or less use of this truth, although they seldom understand the reason of it.

Very few Western writers have recognized the work of this plane of the mind. They have given us full and ingenious theories and examples of the workings of the Instinctive Mind, and in some cases they have touched upon the workings and operations of the Intuitional planes, but in nearly every case they have treated the Intellect as something entirely confined to the Conscious plane of mentation. In this they have missed some of the most interesting and valuable manifestations of sub-conscious mentation.

In this lesson we will take up this particular phase of mentation, and trust to be able to point out the way to use it to the best advantage, giving some simple instructions that have been given by the Hindu teachers to their students for centuries past, such instructions of course, being modified by us to conform to the requirements and necessities of the Western student of today.

We have taken the liberty of bestowing a new title upon this phase of mentation—we have thought it well to call it "Sub-consciousing." The word "Sub," of course means "under; below;" and the word "Consciousing" is a favorite term employed by Prof. Elmer Gates, and means receiving impressions from the mind. In a general way, "Sub-consciousing," as used in this lesson, may be understood to mean "using the subconscious mind, under orders of the conscious mind."

By referring to our Eighth Lesson, we see mention made of the case of the man who indulged in "unconscious rumination," which happened to him when he read books presenting new points of view essentially opposed to his previous opinion. You will note that after days, weeks, or months, he found that to his great astonishment the old opinions were entirely rearranged, and new ones lodged there.

On the same page you will see mentioned the case of Sir William Hamilton, who discovered an important law of mathematics while walking with his wife. In this case he had been previously thinking of the missing link in his chain of reasoning, and the problem was worked out for him by the sub-conscious plane of his Intellect.

On the same page, and the one following, is found the case of Dr. Thompson, who gives an interesting account of the workings of this part of his mind, which caused him at times to experience a feeling of the uselessness of all voluntary effort, coupled with a feeling that the matter was working itself clear in his mind. He tells us that at times he seemed to be merely a passive instrument in the hands of some person other than himself, who compelled him to wait until the work was performed for him by some hidden region of the mind. When the subconscious part of the mind had completed its work, it would flash the message to his conscious mind, and he would begin to write.

On page 178 mention is also made of the great French chemist Berthelot, who relates that some of his best conceptions have flashed upon him as from the clear sky. In fact, the Eighth Lesson is largely made up of examples of this kind, and we ask the student to re-read the same, in order to refresh his mind with the truth of the workings of the sub-conscious mentality.

But you will notice in nearly all the cases mentioned, that those who related instances of the help of the sub-conscious mind had merely stumbled upon the fact that there was a part of the mind below consciousness that could and would work out problems for one, if it could somehow be set in operation. And these people trusted to luck to start that part of the mind in operation. Or rather, they would saturate their conscious mind with a mass of material, like stuffing the stomach with food, and then bid the subconscious mind assort, separate, arrange and digest the mental food, just as does the stomach and digestive apparatus digest the natural food—outside of the realm of consciousness or volition. In none of the cases mentioned was the subconscious mind *directed* specially to perform its wonderful work. It was simply hoped that it might digest the mental material with which it had been stuffed—in pure self defense. But there is a much better way, and we intend to tell you about it. The Hindu Yogis, or rather those who instruct their pupils in *"Raja Yoga,"* give their students directions whereby they may *direct* their sub-conscious minds to perform mental tasks for them, just as one may direct another to perform a task. They teach them the methods whereby, after having accumulated the necessary materials, they may bid the sub-conscious mentality to sort it out, rearrange, analyze, and build up from it some bit of desired knowledge. More than this, they instruct their pupils to direct and order the sub-conscious mentality to search out and report to them certain information to be found only within the mind itself—some question of philosophy or metaphysics. And when such art has been acquired, the student or Yogi rests assured that the desired result will be forthcoming in due time, and consequently dismisses the matter from his conscious mind, and busies himself with other matters, knowing that day and night, incessantly, the sub-consciousing process is going on, and that the sub-conscious mind is actively at work collecting the information, or working out the problem.

You will see at once the great superiority of this method over the old "hit-or-miss," "hope-it-will-work" plan pursued by those who have stumbled upon bits of the truth.

The Yogi teacher begins by impressing upon his students the fact that the mind is capable of extending outward toward an object, material or mental, and by examining it by methods inherent in itself, extracting knowledge regarding the object named. This is not a startling truth, because it is so common, everyone employing it more or less every day. But the process by which the knowledge is extracted is most wonderful, and really is performed below the plane of consciousness, the work of the conscious mind being chiefly concerned in *holding the Attention* upon the object. We have spoken of the importance of Attention in previous lessons, which it will be well for you to re-read, at this time.

When the student is fully impressed with the details of the process of Attention, and the subsequent unfoldment of knowledge, the Yogi proceeds to inform him that there are other means of obtaining knowledge about an object, by the employment of which the Attention may be firmly directed toward the object and then afterwards held there *unconsciously*—that is, a portion of the Attention, or a sub-conscious phase of mentation, which will hold the sub-conscious mind firmly upon the work until accomplished, leaving the conscious Attention and mentality free to employ itself with other things.

The Yogis teach the students that this new form of Attention is far more intense and powerful than is the conscious Attention, for it cannot be disturbed or shaken, or distracted from its object, and that it will work away at its task for days, months, years, or a lifetime if necessary, according to the difficulty of the task, and in fact carries its work over from one life to another, unless recalled by the Will. They teach the student that in everyone's life there is going on a greater or less degree of this sub-conscious work, carried on in obedience to a strong desire for knowledge manifested in some former life, and bearing fruit only in the present existence. Many important discoveries have been made in obedience to this law. But it is not of this phase of the matter that we wish to speak in this lesson.

The Yogi theory is that the sub-conscious intellectual faculty may be set to work under the direction of orders given by the Will. All of you know how the sub-conscious mentality will take up an order of the Will, or a strong wish, that the person be awakened at a certain hour in order to catch a train. Or, in the same way how the remembrance of a certain engagement at, say, four o'clock, will flash into the mind when the hands of the clock approach the stated hour. Nearly every one can recall instances of this sort in his own experience.

But the Yogis go much further than this. They claim that any and all faculties of the mind may be "set going," or working on any problem, if ordered thereto by the Will. In fact, the Yogis, and their advanced students have mastered this art to such a surprising extent that they find it unnecessary to do the drudgery of thinking in the conscious field, and prefer to relegate such mental work to the sub-conscious, reserving their conscious work for the consideration of digested information and thought presented to them by the sub-conscious mind.

Their directions to their students cover a great deal of ground, and extend over a long period of time, and many of the directions are quite complicated and full of detail. But we think that we can give our students an abbreviated and condensed idea in a few pages of the lesson. And the remaining lessons of the course will also throw additional light on the subject of sub-conscious mental action, in connection with other subjects.

The Yogi takes the student when the latter is much bothered by a consideration of some knotty and perplexing philosophical subject. He bids the student relax every muscle,—take the tension from every nerve—throw aside all mental strain, and then wait a few moments. Then the student is instructed to grasp the subject which he has had before his mind firmly and fixedly before his mental vision, by means of concentration. Then he is instructed to pass it on to the sub-conscious mentality by an effort of the Will, which effort is aided by forming a mental picture of the subject as a material substance, *or bundle of thought,* which is being bodily lifted up and dropped down a mental hatch-way, or trap-door, in which it sinks from sight. The student is then instructed to say to the sub-conscious mentality: "I wish this subject thoroughly analyzed, arranged, classified (and whatever else is desired) and then the results handed back to me. Attend to this."

The student is taught to speak to the sub-conscious mentality just as if it were a separate entity of being, which had been employed to do the work. He is also taught that *confident expectation* is an important part of the process, and that the degree of success depends upon the degree of this confident expectation.

In obstinate cases, the student is taught to use the Imagination freely, until he is able to make a mental image or picture of the sub-conscious mind doing what is required of it. This process clears away a mental path for the feet of the sub-conscious mind, which it will choose thereafter, as it prefers to follow the line of least resistance.

Of course much depends upon practice—practice makes perfect, you know, in everything else, and sub-consciousing is no exception to the rule.

The student gradually acquires a proficiency in the art of sub-consciousing, and thereafter devotes his time to acquiring new facts for mental digestion, rather than bestowing it upon the mechanical act of thinking.

But a very important point to be remembered is that the Will-power back of the transferred thought-material, which Will-power is the cause of the subconscious action, depends very greatly upon the attention and interest given to the acquired material. This mass of thought-material which is to be digested, and threshed out by the sub-conscious mind, must be well saturated with interest and attention, in order to obtain the best results. In fact interest and attention are such important aids to the Will, that any consideration of the development and acquirement of Will-power is practically a development and acquirement of attention and interest. The student is referred to previous lessons in this course in which the importance of interest and attention is explained and described.

In acquiring the mass of thought-material which is to be passed on to the sub-conscious digestion, one must concentrate a great degree of interest and attention upon each item of thought-material gathered up. The gathering of this thought-material is a matter of the greatest importance, and must not be lightly passed by. One cannot hastily gather together all sorts of thought-material, and then expect the subconscious mind to do its work properly—it will not, in fact, and the student proceeding upon any such erroneous supposition is doomed to disappointment.

The proper way to proceed, is to take up each bit of thought-material in turn, and examine it with the greatest possible interest, and consequently the greatest attention, and then after having fairly saturated it with this interested attention, place it with the pile of material which, after a while, is to be passed on to the sub-conscious mentality. Then take up the next bit of material, and after giving it similar treatment, pass it along to the pile also. Then after a while when you have gathered up the main facts of the case, proceed to consider the mass as a whole, with interest and attention, giving it as it were a "general treatment." Then drop it down the trap-door into the sub-conscious mind, with a strong command, "Attend to this thought-material," coupled with a strong expectant belief that your order will be obeyed.

The idea underlying this treatment of the thought-material with interest and attention is that by so doing a strong "Mental Image" is created, which may be easily handled by the sub-conscious mind. Remember that you are passing on "thoughts" for the sub-consciousness to act upon, and that the more tangible and real these thoughts are, the better can they be handled. Therefore any plan that will build these thoughts up into "real" things is the plan to pursue. And attention and interest produce just this result.

If we may be pardoned for using a homely and commonplace illustration we would say that the idea may be grasped by the illustration of boiling an egg, whereby the fluid "white" and "yolk" becomes solid and real. Also the use of a shaving brush by a man, by which the thin lather is gradually worked up into a rich, thick, creamy mass, is an illustration. Again, the churning of butter is a favorite illustration of the Hindus, who thus call the attention of their students to the fact that thought-material if worked upon with attention and interest become "thought-forms" that may be handled by the mind just as the hands handle a material object. We ask you to think of these illustrations, for when you once grasp the idea that we wish to convey to you, you will have the secret of great thinking powers within your grasp.

And this power of sub-consciousing is not confined alone to the consideration of philosophical questions. On the contrary it is applicable to every field of human thought, and may be properly employed in any and all of them. It is useful in solving the problems of every-day life and work, as well as to the higher flights of the human mind. And we wish every one of our students to realize that in this simple lesson we are giving them the key to a great mental power.

To realize just what we are offering to you, we would remind you of the old fairy tales of all races, in which there is to be found one or more tales telling of some poor cobbler, or tailor, or carpenter, as the case may be, who had by his good deeds, gained favor with the "brownies" or good fairies, who would come each night when the man and his family were asleep, and proceed to complete the work that the artisan had laid out for the morrow. The pieces of leather would be made into shoes; the cloth would be sewed into garments; the wood would be joined, and nailed together into boxes, chairs, benches and what not. But in each case the rough materials were prepared by the artisan himself during the day.

Well, that is just what we are trying to introduce to you. A clan of mental brownies, loving and kindly disposed toward you, who are anxious and willing to help you in your work. All you have to do is to give them the proper materials, and tell then what you want done, and they will do the rest. But these mental brownies are a part of your own mentality, remember, and no alien and foreign entities, as some have imagined.

A number of people who have accidentally discovered this power of the sub-conscious mind to work out problems, and to render other valuable service to its owner, have been led to suppose that the aid really came from some other entity or intelligence. Some have thought that the messages came from friends in the spirit land, and others have believed that some high intelligence—God or his angels—was working in their behalf. Without discussing spirit communication, or Divine messages, in both of which we believe (with certain provisional reservations) we feel justified in saying that the majority of cases of this kind may be referred to the sub-conscious workings of one's own mentality.

Each of us has "a friend" in our own mind—a score of them in fact, who delight in performing services for us, if we will but allow them to do so. Not only have we a Higher Self to whom we may turn for comfort and aid in times of deep distress and necessity, but we have these invisible mental workers on the sub-conscious plane, who are very willing and glad to perform much of our mental work for us, if we will but give them the material in proper shape.

It is very difficult to impart specific directions for obtaining these results, as each case must depend to a great extent upon the peculiar circumstances surrounding it. But we may say that the main thing needed is to "lick into shape" the material, and then pass it on to the sub-conscious mind in the manner spoken of a few moments ago. Let us run over a few cases wherein this principle may be applied.

Let us suppose that you are confronted with a problem consisting of an uncertainty as to which of two or more courses to adopt in some affair of life. Each course seems to have advantages and disadvantages, and you seem unable to pass upon the matter clearly and intelligently. The more you try the more perplexed and worried do you become. Your mind seems to tire of the matter, and manifests a state which may be called "mental nausea." This state will be apparent to any one who has had much "thinking" to do. The average person, however, persists in going over the matter, notwithstanding the tired condition of the mind, and its evident distaste for a further consideration of the subject. They will keep on forcing it back to the mind for consideration, and even at night time will keep thrashing away at the subject. Now this course is absurd. The mind recognizes that the work should be done by another part of itself—its digestive region, in fact—and naturally rebels at the finishing-up machinery being employed in work unsuited for it.

According to the Sub-consciousing plan, the best thing for the man to do would be for him first to calm and quiet his mind. Then he should arrange the main features of the problem, together with the minor details in their proper places. Then he should pass them slowly before him in review, giving a strong interest and attention to each fact and detail, as it passes before him, *but without the slightest attempt to form a decision, or come to a conclusion*. Then, having given the matter an interested and attentive review, let him *Will* that it pass on to his sub-conscious mind, forming the mental image of dropping it through the trap-door, and at the same time giving the command of the Will, "Attend to this for me!"

Then dismiss the matter from your conscious mind, by an effort of command of the Will. If you find it difficult to do this, you may soon acquire the mastery by a frequent assertion, "I have dismissed this matter from my conscious mind, and my sub-conscious mind will attend to it for me." Then, endeavor to create a mental feeling of perfect trust and confidence in the matter, and avoid all worry or anxiety about it. This may be somewhat difficult at the first trial, but will become a natural feeling after you have gained the confidence arising from successful results in several cases. The matter is one of practice, and, like anything else that is new, must be acquired by perseverance and patience. It is well worth the time and trouble, and once acquired will be regarded as something in the nature of a treasure discovered in an unexpected place. The sense of tranquillity and content—of calm and confidence—that comes to one who has practiced this plan, will of itself be worth all the trouble, not to speak of the main result. To one who has acquired this method, the old worries, frettings, and general "stewed up" feeling, will seem like a relic of barbarism. The new way opens up a world of new feelings and content.

In some cases the matter will be worked out by the sub-conscious mind in a very short time, and in fact we have known cases in which the answer would be flashed back almost instantly, almost like an inspiration. But in the majority of cases more or less time is required. The sub-conscious mind works very rapidly, but it takes time to arrange the thought-material properly, and to shape it into the desired forms. In the majority of cases it is well to let the matter rest until the next day—a fact that gives us a clue to the old advice to "sleep over" an important proposition, before passing a final decision.

If the matter does not present itself the following day, bring it up again before the conscious mind for review. You will find that it has shaped itself up considerably, and is assuming definite form and clearness. But right here—and this is important—do not make the mistake of again dissecting it, and meddling with it, and trying to arrange it with your conscious mind. But, instead, give it attention and interest in its new form, and then pass it back again to the sub-conscious mind for further work. You will find an improvement each time you examine it. But, right here another word of caution. Do not make the mistake of yielding to the impatience of the beginner, and keep on repeatedly bringing up the matter to see what is being done. Give it time to have the work done on it. Do not be like the boy who planted seeds, and who each day would pull them up to see whether they had sprouted, and how much.

Sooner or later, the sub-conscious mind will, of its own choice, lift up the matter and present it to you in its finished shape for the consideration of the conscious mind. The sub-conscious mind does not insist that you shall adopt its views, or accept its work, but merely hands out to you the result of its sorting, classifying and arranging. The choice and will still remains yours, but you will often find that there is seen to be one plan or path that stands out clearly from the others, and you will very likely adopt that one. The secret is that the sub-conscious mind with its wonderful patience and care has analyzed the matter, and has separated things before apparently connected. It has also found resemblances and has combined things heretofore considered opposed to each other. In short it has done for you all that you could have done with the expenditure of great work and time, and done it well. And then it lays the matter before you for your consideration and verdict.

Its whole work seems to have been in the nature of assorting, dissecting, analyzing, and arranging the evidence, and then presenting it before you in a clear, systematic shape. It does not attempt to exercise the judicial prerogative or function, but seems to recognize that its work ceases with the presentation of the edited evidence, and that of the conscious mind begins at the same point.

Now, do not confuse this work with that of the Intuition, which is a very different mental phase or plane. This sub-conscious working, just mentioned, plays an entirely different part. It is a good servant, and does not try to be more. The Intuition, on the contrary, is more like a higher friend—a friend at court, as it were, who gives us warnings and advice.

In our directions we have told you how to make use of this part of the mind, consciously and knowingly, so as to obtain the best results, and to get rid of worry and anxiety attendant upon unsettled questions. But, in fact, every one of us makes more or less use of this part of the mind unconsciously, and not realizing the important part it plays in our mental life. We are perplexed about a matter and keep it "on our minds" until we are forced to lay it aside by reason of some other demand, or when we sink to sleep. Often to our surprise we will find that when we next think of it the matter has somehow cleared up and straightened itself out, and we seem to have learned something about it that we did not know before. We do not understand it, and are apt to dismiss it as "just one of those things." In these lessons we are attempting to explain some of "those things," and to enable you to use them consciously and understandingly, instead of by chance, instinctively, and clumsily. We are teaching you Mastery of the Mind.

Now to apply the rule to another case. Suppose you wish to gather together all the information that you possess relating to a certain subject. In the first place it is certain that you know a very great deal more about any subject than you think you do. Stored away in the various recesses of the mind, or memory if you prefer that term, are stray bits of information and knowledge concerning almost any subject. But these bits of information are not associated with each other. You have never attempted to think attentively upon the particular question before you, and the facts are not correlated in the mind. It is just as if you had so many hundred pounds of anything scattered throughout the space of a large warehouse, a tiny bit here, and a tiny bit there, mixed up with thousands of other things.

You may prove this by sitting down some time and letting your thoughts run along the line of some particular subject, and you will find emerging into the field of consciousness all sorts of information that you had apparently forgotten, and each fitting itself into its proper place. Every person has had experiences of this kind. But the work of gathering together the scattered scraps of knowledge is more or less tedious for the conscious mind, and the sub-conscious mind will do the work equally well with the wear and tear on the attention. In fact, it is the sub-conscious mind that *always* does the work, even when you think it is the conscious mind. All the conscious mind does is to hold the attention firmly upon the object before it, and then let the sub-consciousness pass the material before it. But this holding the attention is tiresome work, and it is not necessary for it to expend its energies upon the details of the task, for the work may be done in an easier and simpler way.

The best way is to follow a plan similar to the one mentioned a few pages back. That is, to fix the interested attention firmly upon the question before you, until you manage to get a clear, vivid impression of *just what you want answered.* Then pass the whole matter into the sub-conscious mind with the command "Attend to this," and then leave it. Throw the whole matter off of your mind, and let the sub-conscious work go on. If possible let the matter run along until the next morning and then take it up for consideration, when, if you have proceeded properly you will find the matter worked out, arranged in logical sequence, so that your conscious attention will be able to clearly review the string of facts, examples, illustrations, experiences, etc., relating to the matter in question.

Now, many of you will say that you would like this plan to work in cases in which you have not the time to sleep over it. In such cases we will say that it is possible to cultivate a rapid method of sub-consciousing, and in fact many business men and men of affairs have stumbled upon a similar plan, driven to the discovery by necessity. They will give a quick, comprehensive, strong flash of attention upon the subject, getting right to the heart of it, and then will let it rest in the sub-conscious mind for a moment or two, killing a minute or two of time n "preliminary conversation," until the first flash of answer comes to them. After the first flash, and taking hold of the first loose end of the subject that presents itself to them, they will unwind a string of information and "talk" about the subject that will surprise even themselves. Many lawyers have acquired this knowledge, and are what is known as "resourceful." Such men are often confronted with questions of conditions utterly unsuspected by them a moment before. Practice has taught them the folly of fear and loss of confidence at such moments, and has also impressed upon them the truth that something within them will come to the rescue. So, presenting a confident air, they will manage to say a few platitudes or commonplaces, while the sub-conscious mind is most rapidly gathering its materials for the answer. In a moment an opening thought "flashes upon" the man, and as he continues idea after idea passes before his conscious and eager attention, sometimes so rapidly that it is almost impossible to utter them and lo! the danger is over, and a brilliant success is often snatched from the jaws of an apparent failure and defeat. In such cases the mental demand upon the sub-conscious mind is not voiced in words, but is the result of a strong mental need. However, if one gives a quick verbal command "*Attend to this*," the result will be heightened.

We have known of cases of men prominent in the world's affairs who made a practice of smoking a cigar during important business interviews, not because they particularly cared for tobacco, but because they had learned to appreciate the value of a moment's time for the mind to "gather itself together," as one man expressed it. A question would be asked, or a proposition advanced suddenly, demanding an immediate answer. Under the watchful eyes of the other party the questioned party tried not to show by his expression any indication of searching for an answer, for obvious reasons. So, instead, he would take a long puff at the cigar, then a slow attentive look at the ashes on its tip, and then another moment consumed in flicking the ash into the receptacle, and then came the answer, slowly, "Well, as to that—" or some other words of that kind, prefacing the real answer which had been rapidly framed by the sub-conscious mind in time to be uttered in its proper place. The few moments of time gained had been sufficient for the sub-conscious mind to gather up its materials, and the matter to be shaped properly, without any appearance of hesitation on the part of the answerer. All of this required practice, of course, but the principle may be seen through it all and in every similar case. The point is that the man, in such cases, sets some hidden part of his mind to work for him, and when he begins to speak the matter is at least roughly "licked into shape for him."

Our students will understand, of course, that this is not advice to smoke cigars during interviews of importance, but is merely given to illustrate the principle. We have known other men to twirl a lead pencil in their fingers in a lazy sort of fashion, and then drop it at the important moment. But we must cease giving examples of this kind, lest we be accused of giving instructions in worldly wisdom, instead of teaching the use of the mind. The impressive pause of the teacher, before answering his pupil's question, is also an example of the workings of this law. One often says "stop, let me think a moment," and during his pause he does not really consciously think at all, but stares ahead in a dreamy fashion, while his sub-conscious mind does the work for him, although he little suspects the nature of the operation. One has but to look around him to realize the importance and frequent application of this truth.

And not only may the sub-conscious mind be used in the directions indicated on preceding pages, but in nearly every perplexity and problem of life may it be called upon for help. These little sub-conscious brownies are ever at our disposal, and seem to be happy to be of service to us.

And so far from being apt to get us in a position of false dependence, it is calculated to make us self-confident—for we are calling upon a part of *ourselves*, not upon some outside intelligence. If those people who never feel satisfied unless they are getting "advice" from others would only cultivate the acquaintance of this little "home adviser" within them, they would lose that dependent attitude and frame of mind, and would grow self-confident and fearless. Just imagine the confidence of one who feels that he has within him a source of knowledge equal to that of the majority of those with whom he is likely to come in contact, and he feels less afraid to face them, and look them fearlessly in the eyes. He feels that his "mind" is not confined to the little field of consciousness, but is an area infinitely greater, containing a mass of information undreamed of. Everything that the man has inherited, or brought with him from past lives—everything that he has read, heard or seen, or experienced in this life, is hidden away there in some quarter of that great sub-conscious mind, and, if he will but give the command, the "essence" of all that knowledge is his. The details may not be presented to his consciousness (often it is not, for very good occult reasons) by the result, or essence of the knowledge will pass before his attention, with sufficient examples and illustrations, or arguments to enable him to make out "a good case" for himself.

In the next lesson we will call your attention to other features and qualities of this great field of mind, showing you how you can put it to work, and Master it. Remember, always, the "I" is the Master. And its Mastery must always be remembered and asserted over all phases and planes of the mind. Do not be a slave to the sub-conscious, but be its MASTER.

MANTRAM (OR AFFIRMATION).

I have within me a great area of Mind that is under my command, and subject to my Mastery. This Mind is friendly to me, and is glad to do my bidding, and obey my orders. It will work for me when I ask it, and is constant, untiring, and faithful. Knowing this I am no longer afraid, ignorant or uninformed. The "I" is master of it all, and is asserting its authority. "I" am master over Body, Mind, Consciousness, and Sub-consciousness. I am "I"—a Centre of Power, Strength, and Knowledge. I am "I"—and "I" am Spirit, a fragment from the Divine Flame.

THE ELEVENTH LESSON.

SUBCONSCIOUS CHARACTER BUILDING.

In our last lesson (the Tenth Lesson) we called your attention to the wonderful work of the sub-conscious regions of mentation in the direction of the performance of Intellectual work. Great as are the possibilities of this field of mentation in the direction named, they are equaled by the possibilities of building up character by similar methods.

Every one realizes that one may change his character by a strenuous course of repression and training, and nearly all who read these lines have modified their characteristics somewhat by similar methods. But it is only of late years that the general public have become aware that Character might be modified, changed, and sometimes completely altered by means of an intelligent use of the sub-conscious faculties of the mind.

The word "Character" is derived from ancient terms meaning "to mark," "to engrave," etc., and some authorities inform us that the term originally arose from the word used by the Babylonian brickmakers to designate the trade mark impressed by them upon their bricks, each maker having his own mark. This is interesting, in view of the recent theories regarding the cultivation of characteristics which may be found in the current Western works on psychology. But these theories are not new to the Yogi teachers of the East, who have employed similar methods for centuries past in training their students and pupils. The Yogis have long taught that a man's character was, practically, the crude character-stuff possessed by him at his birth, modified and shaped by outside influences in the case of the ordinary man, and by deliberate self-training and shaping by the wise man. Their pupils are examined regarding their characteristics, and then directed to repress the undesirable traits, and to cultivate the desirable ones.

The Yogi practice of Character Building is based upon the knowledge of the wonderful powers of the sub-conscious plane of the mind. The pupil is not required to pursue strenuous methods of repression or cultivation, but, on the contrary, is taught that such methods are opposed to nature's plans, and that the best way is to imitate nature and to gradually unfold the desired characteristics by means of focusing the will-power and attention upon them. The weeding out of undesirable characteristics is accomplished by the pupil cultivating the characteristics directly opposed to the undesirable ones. For instance, if the pupil desires to overcome Fear, he is not instructed to concentrate on Fear with the idea of killing it out, but, instead, is taught to mentally deny that he has Fear, and then to concentrate his attention upon the ideal of Courage. When Courage is developed, Fear is found to have faded away. The positive always overpowers the negative.

In the word "ideal" is found the secret of the Yogi method of sub-conscious character building. The teachings are to the effect that "ideals" may be built up by the bestowal of attention upon them. The student is given the example of a rose bush. He is taught that the plant will grow and flourish in the measure that care and attention is bestowed upon it and *vice versa.* He is taught that the ideal of some desired characteristic is a mental rosebush, and that by careful attention it will grow and put forth leaves and flowers. He is then given some minor mental trait to develop, and is taught to dwell upon it in thought—to exercise his imagination and to mentally "see" himself attaining the desired quality. He is given mantrams or affirmation to repeat, for the purpose of giving him a mental center around which to build an ideal. There is a mighty power in words, used in this way, providing that the user always thinks of the meaning of the words, and makes a mental picture of the quality expressed by them, instead of merely repeating them parrot fashion.

The Yogi student is trained gradually, until he acquires the power of conscious direction of the sub-conscious mind in the building up process, which power comes to anyone—Oriental or Occidental—who will take the trouble to practice. In fact, nearly everyone possesses and actively uses this power, although he may not be aware of it. One's character is largely the result of the quality of thoughts held in the mind, and of the mental pictures or ideals entertained by the person. The man who constantly sees and thinks of himself as unsuccessful and down-trodden is very apt to grow ideals of thought forms of these things until his whole nature is dominated by them, and his every act works toward the objectification of the thoughts. On the contrary, the man who makes an ideal of success and accomplishment finds that his whole mental nature seems to work toward that result—the objectification of the ideal. And so it is with every other ideal. The person who builds up a mental ideal of Jealousy will be very apt to objectify the same, and to unconsciously create condition that will give his Jealousy food upon which to feed. But this particular phase of the subject, properly belongs to our next lesson. This Eleventh Lesson is designed to point out the way by which people may mould their characters in any way they desire—supplanting undesirable characteristics by desirable ones, and developing desirable ideals into active characteristics. The mind is plastic to him who knows the secret of its manipulation.

The average person recognizes his strong and weak points of character, but is very apt to regard them as fixed and unalterable, or practically so. He thinks that he "is just as the Lord made him," and that is the end of it. He fails to recognize that his character is being unconsciously modified every day by association with others, whose suggestions are being absorbed and acted upon. And he fails to see that he is moulding his own character by taking interest in certain things, and allowing his mind to dwell upon them. He does not realize that he himself is really the maker of himself, from the raw and crude material given him at his birth. He makes himself negatively or positively. Negatively, if he allows himself to be moulded by the thoughts and ideals of others, and positively, if he moulds himself. Everyone is doing one or the other—perhaps both. The weak man is the one who allows himself to be made by others, and the strong man is the one who takes the building process in his own hands.

The process of Character-building is so delightfully simple that its importance is apt to be overlooked by the majority of persons who are made acquainted with it. It is only by actual practice and the experiencing of results that its wonderful possibilities are borne home to one.

The Yogi student is early taught the lesson of the power and importance of character building by some strong practical example. For instance, the student is found to have certain tastes of appetite, such as a like for certain things, and a corresponding dislike for others. The Yogi teacher instructs the student in the direction of cultivating a desire and taste for the disliked thing, and a dislike for the liked thing. He teaches the student to fix his mind on the two things, but in the direction of imagining that he likes the one thing and dislikes the other. The student is taught to make a mental picture of the desired conditions, and to say, for instance, "I loathe candy—I dislike even the sight of it," and, on the other hand, "I crave tart things—I revel in the taste of them," etc., etc., at the same time trying to reproduce the taste of sweet things accompanied with a loathing, and a taste of tart things, accompanied with a feeling of delight. After a bit the student finds that his tastes are actually changing in accordance with his thoughts, and in the end they have completely changed places. The truth of the theory is then borne home to the student, and he never forgets the lesson.

In order to reassure readers who might object to having the student left in this condition of reversed tastes, we may add that the Yogi teachers then teach him to get rid of the idea of the disliked thing, and teach him to cultivate a liking for all wholesome things, their theory being that the dislike of certain wholesome eatables has been caused by some suggestion in childhood, or by some prenatal impression, as wholesome eatables are made attractive to the taste by Nature. The idea of all this training, however, is not the cultivation of taste, but practice in mental training, and the bringing home to the student the truth of the fact that his nature is plastic to his Ego, and that it may be moulded at will, by concentration and intelligent practice. The reader of this lesson may experiment upon himself along the lines of the elementary Yogi practice as above mentioned, if he so desires. He will find it possible to entirely change his dislike for certain food, etc., by the methods mentioned above. He may likewise acquire a liking for heretofore distasteful tasks and duties, which he finds it necessary to perform.

The principle underlying the whole Yogi theory of Character Building by the sub-conscious Intellect, is that the Ego is Master of the mind, and that the mind is plastic to the commands of the Ego. The Ego or "I" of the individual is the one real, permanent, changeless principle of the individual, and the mind, like the body, is constantly changing, moving, growing, and dying. Just as the body may be developed and moulded by intelligent exercises, so may the mind be developed and shaped by the Ego if intelligent methods are followed.

The majority of people consider that Character is a fixed something, belonging to a man, that cannot be altered or changed. And yet they show by their everyday actions that at heart they do not believe this to be a fact, for they endeavor to change and mould the characters of those around them, by word of advice, counsel, praising or condemnation, etc.

It is not necessary to go into the matter of the consideration of the causes of character in this lesson. We will content ourselves by saying that these causes may be summed up, roughly, as follows: (1) Result of experiences in past lives; (2) Heredity; (3) Environment; (4) Suggestion from others; and (5) Auto-suggestion. But no matter how one's character has been formed, it may be modified, moulded, changed, and improved by the methods set forth in this lesson, which methods are similar to what is called by Western writers, "Auto-suggestion."

The underlying idea of Auto-suggestion is the "willing" of the individual that the changes take place in his mind, the willing being aided by intelligent and tried methods of creating the new ideal or thought-form. The first requisite for the changed condition must be "desire" for the change. Unless one really desires that the change take place, he is unable to bring his Will to bear on the task. There is a very close connection between Desire and Will. Will is not usually brought to bear upon anything unless it is inspired by Desire. Some people connect the word Desire with the lower inclinations, but it is equally applicable to the higher. If one fights off a low inclination or Desire, it is because he is possessed of a higher inclination or Desire. Many Desires are really compromises between two or more conflicting Desires—a sort of average Desire, as it were.

Unless one desires to change his character he will not make any move toward it. And in proportion to the strength of the desire, so will be the amount of will-power that is put in the task. The first thing for one to do in character building is to "want to do it." And if he finds that the "want" is not sufficiently strong to enable him to manifest the perseverance and effort necessary to bring it to a successful conclusion, then he should deliberately proceed to "build up the desire."

Desire may be built up by allowing the mind to dwell upon the subject until a desire is created. This rule works both ways, as many people have found out to their sorrow and misery. Not only may one build up a commendable desire in this way, but he may also build up a reprehensible one. A little thought will show you the truth of this statement. A young man has no desire to indulge in the excesses of a "fast" life. But after a while he hears, or reads something about others leading that sort of life, and he begins to allow his mind to dwell upon the subject, turning it around and examining it mentally, and going over it in his imagination. After a time he begins to find a desire gradually sending forth roots and branches, and if he continues to water the thing in his imagination, before long he will find within himself a blossoming inclination, which will try to insist upon expression in action. There is a great truth behind the words of the poet:

"Vice is a monster of so frightful mien,
That to be hated needs but to be seen.
Yet seen too oft, familiar with her face,
We first endure, then pity, and then embrace."

And the follies and crimes of many a man have been due to the growing of desire within his mind, through this plan of planting the seed, and then carefully watering and tending to it—this cultivation of the growing desire. We have thought it well to give this word of warning because it will throw light upon many things that may have perplexed you, and because it may serve to call your attention to certain growing weeds of the mind that you have been nourishing.

But remember, always, that the force that leads downward may be transmuted and made to lead upward. It is just as easy to plant and grow wholesome desires as the other kind. If you are conscious of certain defects and deficiencies in your character (and who is not?) and yet find yourself not possessed of a strong enough desire to make the changes necessary, then you should commence by planting the desire seed and allowing it to grow by giving it constant care and attention. You should picture to yourself the advantages of acquiring the desirable traits of character of which you have thought. You should frequently go over and over them in your mind, imaging yourself in imagination as possessing them. You will then find that the growing desire will make headway and that you will gradually begin to "want to" possess that trait of character more and more. And when you begin to "want to" hard enough, you will find arising in your consciousness a feeling of the possession of sufficient Will-power to carry it through. Will follows the

Desire. Cultivate a Desire and you will find back of it the Will to carry it through. Under the pressure of a very strong Desire men have accomplished feats akin to miracles.

If you find yourself in possession of desires that you feel are hurtful to you, you may rid yourself of them by deliberately starving them to death, and at the same time growing opposite desires. By refusing to think of the objectionable desires you refuse them the mental food upon which alone they can thrive. Just as you starve a plant by refusing it nourishing soil and water, so may you starve out an objectionable desire by refusing to give it mental food. *Remember this, for it is most important.* Refuse to allow the mind to dwell upon such desires, and resolutely turn aside the attention, *and, particularly, the imagination*, from the subject. This may call for the manifestation of a little will-power in the beginning, but it will become easier as you progress, and each victory will give you renewed strength for the next fight. But do not temporize with the desire—do not compromise with it—refuse to entertain the idea. In a fight of this kind each victory gives one added strength, and each defeat weakens one.

And while you are refusing to entertain the objectionable guest you must be sure to grow a desire of an entirely opposite nature—a desire directly opposed to the one you are starving to death. Picture the opposite desire, and think of it often. Let your mind dwell upon it lovingly and let the imagination help to build it up into form. Think of the advantages that will arise to you when you fully possess it, and let the imagination picture you as in full possession of it, and acting out your new part in life strong and vigorous in your new found power.

All this will gradually lead you to the point where you will "want to" possess this power. Then you must be ready for the next step which is "Faith" or "Confident Expectation."

Now, faith or confident expectation is not made to order in most persons, and in such cases one must acquire it gradually. Many of you who read these lines will have an understanding of the subject that will give you this faith. But to those who lack it, we suggest that they practice on some trivial phases of the mental make-up, some petty trait of character, in which the victory will be easy and simple. From this stage they should work up to more difficult tasks, until at last they gain that faith or confident expectation that comes from persevering practice.

The greater the degree of faith or confident expectation that one carries with him in this task of character building, the greater will be his success. And this because of well established psychological laws. Faith or confident expectation clears away the mental path and renders the work easier, while doubt or lack of faith retards the work, and acts as obstacles and stumbling blocks. Strong Desire, and Faith, or confident expectation are the first two steps. The third is Will-power.

By Will-power we do not mean that strenuous, clenching-of-fist-and-frowning-brow thing that many think of when they say "Will." Will is not manifested in this way. The true Will is called into play by one realizing the "I" part of himself and speaking the word of command from that center of power and strength. It is the voice of the "I." And it is needed in this work of character building.

So now you are ready for work, being possessed of (1) Strong Desire; (2) Faith or Confident Expectation; and (3) Will-power. With such a triple-weapon nothing but Success is possible.

Then comes the actual work. The first thing to do is to lay the track for a new Character Habit. "Habit?" you may ask in surprise. Yes, Habit! For that word gives the secret of the whole thing. Our characters are made up of inherited or acquired habits. Think over this a little and you will see the truth of it. You do certain things without a thought, because you have gotten into the habit of doing them. You act in certain ways because you have established the habit. You are in the habit of being truthful, honest, virtuous, because you have established the habit of being so. Do you doubt this? Then look around you—or look within your own heart, and you will see that you have lost some of your old habits of action, and have acquired new ones. The building up of Character is the building up of Habits. And the changing of Character is the changing of Habits. It will be well for you to settle this fact in your own mind, for it will give you the secret of many things connected with the subject.

And, remember this, that Habit is almost entirely a matter of the sub-conscious mentality. It is true that Habits originate in the conscious mind, but as they are established they sink down into the depths of the sub-conscious mentality, and thereafter become "second nature," which, by the way, is often more powerful than the original nature of the person. The Duke of Wellington said that habit was as strong as ten natures, and he proceeded to drill habits into his army until they found it natural to act in accordance with the habits pounded into them during the drills. Darwin relates an interesting instance of the force of habit over the reason. He found that his habit of starting back at the sudden approach of danger was so firmly established that no will-power could enable him to keep his face pressed up against the cage of the cobra in the Zoological Gardens when the snake struck at him, although he knew the glass was so thick that there could be no danger, and although he exerted the full force of his will. But we venture to say that one could overcome even this strongly ingrained habit, by gradually training the sub-conscious mentality and establishing a new habit of thought and action.

It is not only during the actual process of "willing" the new habit that the work of making the new mental path goes on. In fact, the Yogis believe that the principal part of the work goes on sub-consciously between the intervals of commend, and that the real progress is made in that way, just as the real work of solving the problem is performed sub-consciously, as related in our last lesson. As an example, we may call your attention to some instances of the cultivation of physical habits. A physical task learned in the evening is much easier to perform the following-morning than it was the night before, and still easier the following Monday morning than it was on the Saturday afternoon previous. The Germans have a saying that "we learn to skate in summer, and to swim in winter," meaning that the impression passed on to the subconscious mentality deepens and broadens during the interval of rest. The best plan is to make frequent, sharp impressions, and then to allow reasonable periods of rest in order to give the sub-conscious mentality the opportunity to do its work. By "sharp" impressions we mean impressions given under *strong attention*, as we have mentioned in some of the earlier lessons of this series.

A writer has well said: "Sow an act, reap a habit; sow a habit, reap a character; sow a character, reap a destiny," thus recognizing habit as the source of character. We recognize this truth in our training of children, forming goods habits of character by constant repetition, by watchfulness, etc. Habit acts as a *motive* when established, so that while we think we are acting without motive we may be acting under the strong motive power of some well established habit. Herbert Spencer has well said: "The habitually honest man does what is right, not consciously because he 'ought' but with simple satisfaction; and is ill at ease till it is done." Some may object that this idea of Habit as a basis of Character may do away with the idea of a developed moral conscientiousness, as for instance, Josiah Royce who says: "The establishment of organized habit is never in itself enough to ensure the growth of an enlightened moral conscientiousness" but to such we would say that one must "want to" cultivate a high character before he will create the habits usual to the same, and the "want to" is the sign of the "moral conscientiousness," rather than the habit. And the same is true of the "ought to" side of the subject. The "ought to" arises in the conscious mind in the beginning, and inspires the cultivation of the habit, although the latter after a while becomes automatic, a matter of the sub-conscious mentality, without any "ought to" attachment. It then becomes a matter of "like to."

Thus we see that the moulding, modifying, changing, and building of Character is largely a matter of the establishing of Habits. And what is the best way to establish Habits? becomes our next question. The answer of the Yogi is: "Establish a Mental Image, and then build your Habit around it." And in that sentence he has condensed a whole system.

Everything we see having a form is built around a mental image—either the mental image of some man, some animal, or of the Absolute. This is the rule of the universe, and in the matter of character-building we but follow a well established rule. When we wish to build a house, we first think of "house" in a general way. Then we begin to think of "what kind" of a house. Then we go into details. Then we consult an architect, and he makes us a plan, which plan is his mental image, suggested by our mental image. Then, the plan once decided upon, we consult the builder, and at last the house stands completed—an objectified Mental Image. And so it is with every created thing—all manifestation of a Mental Image.

And so, when we wish to establish a trait of Character, we must form a clear, distinct Mental Image of what we wish to be. This is an important step. Make your picture clear and distinct, and fasten it in your mind. Then begin to build around it. Let your thoughts dwell upon the mental picture. Let your imagination see yourself as possessed of the desired trait, and *acting it out.* Act it out in your imagination, over and over again, as often as possible, persevering, and continuously, seeing yourself manifesting the trait under a variety of circumstances and conditions. As you continue to do this you will find that you will gradually begin to express the thought in action—to objectify the subjective mental image. It will become "natural" for you to act more and more in accordance with your mental image, until at last the new habit will become firmly fixed in your mind, and will become your natural mode of action and expression.

This is no vague, visionary theory. It is a well known and proven psychological fact, and thousands have worked marvelous changes in their character by its means.

Not only may one elevate his moral character in this way, but he may mould his "work-a-day" self to better conform to the needs of his environment and occupation. If one lacks Perseverance, he may attain it; if one is filled with Fear, he may supplant it with Fearlessness; if one lacks Self-confidence, he may gain it. In fact, there is no trait that may not be developed in this way. People have literally "made themselves over" by following this method of character-building. The great trouble with the race has been that persons have not realized that they *could* do these things. They have thought that they were doomed to remain just the creatures that they found themselves to be. They did not realize that the work of creation was not ended, and that they had within themselves a creative power adapted to the needs of their case. When man first realizes this truth, and proves it by practice, he becomes another being. He finds himself superior to environment, and training—he finds that he may ride over these things. He makes *his own environment*, and *he trains himself.*

In some of the larger schools in England and the United States, certain scholars who have developed and manifested the ability to control themselves and their actions are placed on the roll of a grade called the "Self-governed grade." Those in this grade act as if they had memorized the following words of Herbert Spencer: "In the supremacy of self-control consists one of the perfections of the ideal man. Not to be impulsive—not to be spurred hither and thither by each desire—but to be self-restrained, self-balanced, governed by the just decision of the feelings in council assembled * * * that it is which moral education strives to produce." And this is the desire of the writer of this lesson—to place each student in the "Self-governed class."

We cannot attempt, in the short space of a single lesson, to map out a course of instruction in Character Building adapted to the special needs of each individual. But we think that what we have said on the subject should be sufficient to point out the method for each student to map out a course for himself, following the general rules given above. As a help to the student, however, we will give a brief course of instruction for the cultivation of one desirable trait of character. The general plan of this course may be adapted to fit the requirements of *any other case*, if intelligence is used by the student. The case we have selected is that of a student who has been suffering from "a lack of Moral Courage—a lack of Self-Confidence—an inability to maintain my poise in the presence of other people—an inability to say 'No!'—a feeling of Inferiority to those with whom I come in contact." The brief outline of the course of practice given in this case is herewith given:

PRELIMINARY THOUGHT. You should fix firmly in your mind the fact that you are the Equal of any and every man. You come from the same source. You are an expression of the same One Life. In the eyes of the Absolute you are the equal of any man, even the highest in the land. Truth is "Things as God sees them"—and in Truth you and the man are equal, and, at the last, One. All feelings of Inferiority are illusions, errors, and lies, and have no existence in Truth. When in the company of others remember this fact and realize that the Life Principle in you is talking to the Life Principle in them. Let the Life Principle flow through you, and endeavor to forget your personal self. At the same time, endeavor to see that same Life Principle, behind and beyond the personality of the person in whose presence you are. He is by a personality hiding the Life Principle, just as you are. Nothing more—nothing less! You are both One in Truth. Let the conscious of the "I" beam forth and you will experience an uplift and sense of Courage, and the other will likewise feel it. You have within you the Source of Courage, Moral and Physical, and you have naught to Fear—Fearlessness is your Divine Heritage, avail yourself of it. You have Self-Conscience, for the Self is the "I" within you, not the petty personality, and you must have confidence in that "I." Retreat within yourself until you feel the presence of the "I," and then will you have a Self-Confidence that nothing can shake or disturb. Once having attained the permanent consciousness of the "I," you will have poise. Once having realized that you are a Center of Power, you will have no difficulty in saying "No!" when it is right to do so. Once having realized your true nature—your Real Self—you will lose all sense of Inferiority, and will know that you are a manifestation of the One Life and have behind you the strength, power, and grandeur of the Cosmos. Begin by realizing YOURSELF, and then proceed with the following methods of training the mind.

WORD IMAGES. It is difficult for the mind to build itself around an idea, unless that idea be expressed in words. A word is the center of an idea, just as the idea is the center of the mental image, and the mental image the center of the growing mental habit. Therefore, the Yogis always lay great stress upon the use of words in this way. In the particular case before us, we should suggest the holding before you of a few words crystallizing the main thought. We suggest the words "I Am"; Courage; Confidence; Poise; Firmness; Equality. Commit these words to memory, and then endeavor to fix in your mind a clear conception of the meaning of each word, so that each may stand for a Live Idea when you say it. Beware of parrot-like or phonographic repetition. Let each word's meaning stand out clearly before you, so that when you repeat it you may *feel* its meaning. Repeat the words over frequently, when opportunity presents itself, and you will soon begin to notice that they act as a strong mental tonic upon you, producing a bracing, energizing effect. And each time you repeat the words, understandingly, you have done something to clear away the mental path over which you wish to travel.

PRACTICE. When you are at leisure, and are able to indulge in "day dreams" without injury to your affairs of life, call your imagination into play and endeavor to picture yourself as being possessed of the qualities indicated by the words named. Picture yourself under the most trying circumstances, making use of the desired qualities, and manifesting them fully. Endeavor to picture yourself as acting out your part well, and exhibiting the desired qualities. Do not be ashamed to indulge in these day-dreams, for they are the prophecies of the things to follow, and you are but rehearsing your part before the day of the performance. Practice makes perfect, and if you accustom yourself to acting in a certain way in imagination, you will find it much easier to play your part when the real performance occurs. This may seem childish to many of you, but if you have an actor among your acquaintances, consult him about it, and you will find that he will heartily recommend it. He will tell you what practice does for one in this direction, and how repeated practice and rehearsals may fix a character so firmly in a man's mind that he may find it difficult to divest himself of it after a time. Choose well the part you wish to play—the character you wish to be yours—and then after fixing it well in your mind, practice, practice, practice. Keep your ideal constantly before you, and endeavor to grow into it. And you will succeed, if you exercise patience and perseverance.

But, more than this. Do not confine your practice to mere private rehearsal. You need some "dress rehearsals" as well—rehearsals in public. Therefore, after you get well started in your work, manage to exercise your growing character-habits in your everyday life. Pick out the little cases first and "try it on them."

You will find that you will be able to overcome conditions that formerly bothered you much. You will become conscious of a growing strength and power coming from within, and you will recognize that you are indeed a changed person. Let your thought express itself in action, whenever you get a good chance. But do not try to force chances just to try your strength. Do not, for instance, try to force people to ask for favors that you may say "No!" You will find plenty of genuine tests without forcing any. Accustom yourself to looking people in the eye, and feeling the power that is back of you, and within you. You will soon be able to see through their personality, and realize that it is just one portion of the One Life gazing at another portion, and that therefore there is nothing to be afraid of. A realization of your Real Self will enable you to maintain your poise under trying circumstances, if you will but throw aside your false idea about your personality. Forget yourself—your little personal self—for a while, and fix your mind on the Universal Self of which you are a part. All these things that have worried you are but incidents of the Personal Life, and are seen to be illusions when viewed from the standpoint of the Universal Life.

Carry the Universal Life with you as much as possible into your everyday life. It belongs there as much as anywhere, and will prove to be a tower of strength and refuge to you in the perplexing situations of your busy life.

Remember always that the Ego is master of the mental states and habits, and that the Will is the direct instrument of the Ego, and is always ready for its use. Let your soul be filled with the strong Desire to cultivate those mental habits that will make you Strong. Nature's plan is to produce Strong Individual expressions of herself, and she will be glad to give you her aid in becoming strong. The man who wishes to strengthen himself will always find great forces back of him to aid him in the work, for is he not carrying out one of Nature's pet plans, and one which she has been striving for throughout the ages. Anything that tends to make you realize and express your Mastery, tends to strengthen you, and places at your disposal Nature's aid. You may witness this in everyday life—Nature seems to like *strong* individuals, and delights in pushing them ahead. By Mastery, we mean mastery over your own lower nature, as well as over outside nature, of course. The "I" is Master—forget it not, O student, and assert it constantly. Peace be with you.

MANTRAM (OR AFFIRMATION).

I am the Master of my Mental Habits—I control my Character. I Will to be Strong, and summon the forces of my Nature to my aid.

THE TWELFTH LESSON.

SUB-CONSCIOUS INFLUENCES.

In this lesson we wish to touch upon a certain feature of sub-conscious mentation that has been much dwelt upon by certain schools of western writers and students during the past twenty years, but which has also been misunderstood, and, alas, too often misused, by some of those who have been attracted to the subject. We allude to what has been called the "Power of Thought." While this power is very real, and like any other of the forces of nature may be properly used and applied in our every day life, still many students of the power of the Mind have misused it and have stooped to practices worthy only of the followers of the schools of "Black Magic." We hear on all sides of the use of "treatments" for selfish and often base ends, those following these practices seeming to be in utter ignorance of the occult laws brought into operation, and the terrible reaction inevitably falling to the lot of those practicing this negative form of mental influence. We have been amazed at the prevailing ignorance concerning the nature and effects of this improper use of mental force, and at the same time, at the common custom of such selfish, improper uses. This, more particularly, when the true occultist knows that these things are not necessary, even to those who seek "Success" by mental forces. There is a true method of the use of mental forces, as well as an improper use, and we trust that in this lesson we may be able to bring the matter sharply and clearly before the minds of our students.

In our first course (The Fourteen Lessons) in the several lessons entitled, respectively, "Thought Dynamics," "Telepathy, etc.," and "Psychic Influence," we have given a general idea of the effect of one mind upon other minds, and many other writers have called the attention of the Western world to the same facts. There has been a general awakening of interest in this phase of the subject among the Western people of late years, and many and wonderful are the theories that have been advanced among the conflicting schools regarding the matter. But, notwithstanding the conflicting theories, there is a general agreement upon the fundamental facts. They all agree that the mental forces may be used to affect oneself and others, and many have started in to use these mental forces for their own selfish ends and purposes, believing that they were fully justified in so doing, and being unaware of the web of psychic causes and effects which they were weaving around them by their practices.

Now, at the beginning, let us impress upon the minds of our students the fact that while it is undoubtedly true that people who are unaware of the true sources of strength within them, may be, and often are affected by mental force exerted by others, it is equally true that no one can be adversely affected in this way providing he realizes the "I" within himself, which is the only Real part of him, and which is an impregnable tower of strength against the assaults of others. There is no cause for all of this fear that is being manifested by many Western students of thought-power, who are in constant dread of being "treated" adversely by other people. The man or woman who realizes the "I" within, may by the slightest exercise of the Will surround himself with a mental aura which will repel adverse thought-waves emanating from the minds of others. Nay, more than this—the habitual recognition of the "I," and a few moments' meditation upon it each day, will of itself erect such an aura, and will charge this aura with a vitality that will turn back adverse thought, and cause it to return to the source from which it came, where it will serve the good purpose of bringing to the mistaken mind originating it, the conviction that such practices are hurtful and to be avoided.

This realization of the "I," which we brought out in the first few lessons of the present series, is the best and only real method of self-protection. This may be easily understood, when we remind you that the whole phenomena of mental influencing belongs to the "illusion" side of existence—the negative side—and that the Real and Positive side must of necessity be stronger. Nothing can affect the Real in you—and the nearer you get to the Real, in realization and understanding, the stronger do you become. *This is the whole secret*. Think it over.

But, there are comparatively few people who are able to rest firmly in the "I" consciousness all the time and the others demand help while they are growing. To such, we would say "Creep as close the Realization of the I, as possible, and rest your spiritual feet firmly upon the rock of the Real Self." If you feel that people, circumstances, or things are influencing you unduly, stand up boldly, and deny the influence. Say something like this, "I DENY the power or influence of persons, circumstances, or things to adversely affect me. I ASSERT my Reality, Power and Dominion over these things." These words may seem very simple, but when uttered with the consciousness of the Truth underlying them, they become as a mighty force. You will understand, of course, that there is no magic or virtue in the words themselves—that is, in the grouping of the letters forming the words, or the sounds of the words—the virtue resting in the *idea* of which the words are the expression. You will be surprised at the effect of this STATEMENT upon depressing, or adverse influences surrounding you. If you—*you* who are reading these words now—feel yourself subject to any adverse or depressing influences, will then stand up erect, throwing your shoulders back, raising your head, and looking boldly and fearlessly ahead, and repeat these words firmly, and with faith, you will feel the adverse influences disappearing. You will almost see the clouds falling back from you. Try it now, before reading further, and you will become conscious of a new strength and power.

You are perfectly justified in thus denying adverse influence. You have a perfect right to drive back threatening or depressing thought-clouds. You have a perfect right to take your stand upon the Rock of Truth—your Real Self—and demand your Freedom. These negative thoughts of the world in general, and of some people in particular, belong to the dark side of life, and you have a right to demand freedom from them. You do not belong to the same idea of life, and it is your privilege—yes, your duty—to repel them and bid them disappear from your horizon. You are a Child of Light, and it is your right and duty to assert your freedom from the things of darkness. You are merely asserting the Truth when you affirm your superiority and dominion over these dark forces. And in the measure of your Recognition and Faith, will be the power at your disposal. Faith and Recognition renders man a god. If we could but fully recognize and realize just what we are, we could rise above this entire plane of negative, dark world of thought. But we have become so blinded and stupefied with the race-thought of fear and weakness, and so hypnotized with the suggestions of weakness that we hear on all sides of us, that even the best of us find it hard to avoid occasionally sinking back into the lower depths of despair and discouragement. But, let us remember this, brothers and sisters, that these periods of "back-sliding" become less frequent, and last a shorter time, as we proceed. Bye-and-bye we shall escape them altogether.

Some may think that we are laying too much stress upon the negative side of the question, but we feel that what we have said is timely, and much needed by many who read these lessons. There has been so much said regarding this negative, adverse power of thought, that it is well that all should be taught that it is in their power to rise above this thing— that the weapon for its defeat is already in their hand.

The most advanced student may occasionally forget that he is superior to the adverse influence of the race-thought, and other clouds of thought influence that happen to be in his neighborhood. When we think of how few there are who are sending forth the positive, hopeful, thought-waves, and how many are sending forth continually the thoughts of discouragement, fear, and despair, it is no wonder that at times there comes to us a feeling of discouragement, helplessness, and "what's the use." But we must be ever alert, to stand up and *deny these things out of existence* so far as our personal thought world is concerned. There is a wonderful occult truth in the last sentence. We are the makers, preservers, and destroyers of our personal thought-world. We may bring into it that which we desire to appear; we may keep there what we wish, cultivating, developing and unfolding the thought-forms that we desire; we may destroy that which we wish to keep out. The "I" is the master of its thought-world. Think over this great truth, O student! By Desire we call into existence—by affirmation we preserve and encourage—by Denial we destroy. The Hindus in their popular religious conceptions picture the One Being as a Trinity, composed of Brahma, the Creator; Vishnu, the Preserver, and Siva, the Destroyer—not three gods, as is commonly supposed, but a Trinity composed of three aspects of Deity or Being. This idea of the threefold Being is also applicable to the Individual—"as above so below." The "I" is the Being of the Individual, and the thought-world is its manifestation. It creates, preserves, and destroys—as it Will. Carry this idea with you, and realize that your individual thought-world is your own field of manifestation. In it you are constantly creating—constantly preserving—constantly destroying. And if you can destroy anything in your own thought-world you remove it from its field of activity, so far as you are concerned. And if you create anything in your own thought-world, you bring it into active being, so far as you are concerned. And if you preserve anything, you keep it by you in effect and full operation and influence in your life. This truth belongs to the higher phases of the subject, for its explanation is inextricably bound up in the explanation of the "Thing-in-Itself"—the Absolute and Its Manifestations. But even what we have said above, should give to the alert student sufficient notice to cause him to grasp the facts of the case, and to apply the principles in his own life.

If one lives on the plane of the race-thought, he is subject to its laws, for the law of cause and effect is in full operation on each plane of life. But when one raises himself above the race-thought, and on to the plane of the Recognition of the Real Self—The "I"—then does he extricate himself from the lower laws of cause and effect, and places himself on a higher plane of causation, in which he plays a much higher part. And so we are constantly reminding you that your tower of strength and refuge lies on the higher plane. But, nevertheless, we must deal with the things and laws of the lower plane, because very few who read these lessons are able to rest entirely upon the higher plane. The great majority of them have done no more than to lift themselves partially on to the higher plane, and they are consequently living on both planes, partly in each, the consequence being that there is a struggle between the conflicting laws of the two planes. The present stage is one of the hardest on the Path of Attainment, and resembles the birth-pains of the physical body. But you are being born into a higher plane, and the pain after becoming the most acute will begin to ease, and in the end will disappear, and then will come peace and calm. When the pain becomes the most acute, then be cheered with the certainty that you have reached the crisis of your new spiritual birth, and that you will soon gain peace. And then you will see that the peace and bliss will be worth all the pain and struggle. Be brave, fellow followers of The Path—Deliverance is nigh. Soon will come the Silence that follows the Storm. The pain that you are experiencing—ah, well do we know that you are experiencing the pain—is not punishment, but is a necessary part of your growth. All Life follows this plan—the pains of labor and birth ever precede the Deliverance. Such is Life—and Life is based upon Truth—and all is well with the world. We did not intend to speak of these things in this lesson, but as we write there comes to us a great cry for help and a word of encouragement and hope, from the Class which is taking this course of lessons, and we feel bound to respond as we have done. Peace be with you—one and all.

And, now we will begin our consideration of the laws governing what we have called "Sub-conscious Influence."

All students of the Occult are aware of the fact that men may be, and are, largely influenced by the thoughts of others. Not only is this the case in instances where thoughts are directed from the mind of one person to the mind of another, but also when there is no special direction or intention in the thought sent forth. The vibrations of thoughts linger in the astral atmosphere long after the effort that sent forth the thought has passed. The astral atmosphere is charged with the vibrations of thinkers of many years past, and still possesses sufficient vitality to affect those whose minds are ready to receive them at this time. And we all attract to us thought vibrations corresponding in nature with those which we are in the habit of entertaining. The Law of Attraction is in full operation, and one who makes a study of the subject may see instances of it on all sides.

We invite to ourselves these thought vibrations by maintaining and entertaining thoughts along certain lines. If we cultivate a habit of thinking along the lines of Cheerfulness, Brightness and Optimism, we attract to ourselves similar thought vibrations of others and we will find that before long we will find all sorts of cheerful thoughts pouring into our minds from all directions. And, likewise, if we harbor thoughts of Gloom, Despair, Pessimism, we lay ourselves open to the influx of similar thoughts which have emanated from the minds of others. Thoughts of Anger, Hate, or Jealousy attract similar thoughts which serve to feed the flame and keep alive the fire of these low emotions. Thoughts of Love tend to draw to ourselves the loving thoughts of others which tend to fill us with a glow of loving emotion.

And not only are we affected in this way by the thoughts of others, but what is known as "Suggestion" also plays an important part in this matter of sub-conscious influence. We find that the mind has a tendency to reproduce the emotions, moods, shades of thought, and feelings of other persons, as evidenced by their attitude, appearance, facial expression, or words. If we associate with persons of a gloomy temperament, we run the risk of "catching" their mental trouble by the law of suggestion, unless we understand this law and counteract it. In the same way we find that cheerfulness is contagious, and if we keep in the company of cheerful people we are very apt to take on their mental quality. The same rule applies to frequenting the company of unsuccessful or successful people, as the case may be. If we allow ourselves to take up the suggestions constantly emanating from them, we will find that our minds will begin to reproduce the tones, attitudes, characteristics, dispositions and traits of the other persons, and before long we will be living on the same mental plane. As we have repeatedly said, these things are true only when we allow ourselves to "take on" the impressions, but unless one has mastered the law of suggestion, and understands its principles and operations he is more or less apt to be affected by it. All of you readily recall the effect of certain persons upon others with whom they come in contact. One has a faculty of inspiring with vigor and energy those in whose company he happens to be. Another depresses those around him, and is avoided as a "human wet-blanket." Another will cause a feeling of uneasiness in those around him, by reason of his prevailing attitude of distrust, suspicion, and low cunning. Some carry an atmosphere of health around them, while others seem to be surrounded with a sickly aura of disease, even when their physical condition does not seem to indicate the lack of health. Mental states have a subtle way of impressing themselves upon us, and the student who will take the trouble to closely observe those with whom he comes in contact will receive a liberal education along these lines.

There is of course a great difference in the degree of suggestibility among different persons. There are those who are almost immune, while at the other end of the line are to be found others who are so constantly and strongly impressed by the suggestions of others, conscious or unconscious, that they may be said to scarcely have any independent thought or will of their own. But nearly all persons are suggestible to a greater or lesser degree.

It must not be supposed from what we have said that all suggestions are "bad," harmful, or undesirable. Many suggestions are very good for us, and coming at the right time have aided us much. But, nevertheless, it is well to always *let your own mind pass upon* these suggestions, before allowing them to manifest in your sub-conscious mind. Let the final decision be your own—and not the will of another—although you may have considered outside suggestions in connection with the matter.

Remember always that YOU are an Individual, having a mind and Will of your own. Rest firmly upon the base of your "I" consciousness, and you will find yourself able to manifest a wonderful strength against the adverse suggestions of others. Be your own Suggestor—train and influence your sub-conscious mind Yourself, and do not allow it to be tampered with by the suggestions of others. Grow the sense of Individuality.

There has been much written of recent years in the Western world regarding the effect of the Mental Attitude upon Success and attainment upon the material plane. While much of this is nothing but the wildest imagining, still there remains a very firm and solid substratum of truth underlying it all.

It is undoubtedly true that one's prevailing mental attitude is constantly manifesting and objectifying itself in his life. Things, circumstances, people, plans, all seem to fit into the general ideal of the strong mental attitude of a man. And this from the operation of mental law along a number of lines of action.

In the first place, the mind when directed toward a certain set of objects becomes very alert to discover things concerning those objects—to seize upon things, opportunities, persons, ideas, and facts tending to promote the objects thought of. The man who is looking for facts to prove certain theories, invariably finds them, and is also quite likely to overlook facts tending to disprove his theory. The Optimist and the Pessimist passing along the same streets, each sees thousands of examples tending to fit in with his idea. As Kay says: "When one is engaged in seeking for a thing, if he keep the image of it clearly before the mind, he will be very likely to find it, and that too, probably, where it would otherwise have escaped his notice. So when one is engaged in thinking on a subject, thoughts of things resembling it, or bearing upon it, and tending to illustrate it, come up on every side. Truly, we may well say of the mind, as has been said of the eye, that 'it perceives only what it brings within the power of perceiving.'" John Burroughs has well said regarding this that "No one ever found the walking fern who did not have the walking fern in his mind. A person whose eye is full of Indian relics picks them up in every field he walks through. They are quickly recognized because the eye has been commissioned to find them."

When the mind is kept firmly fixed upon some ideal or aim, its whole and varied powers are bent toward the realization and manifestation of that ideal. In thousands of ways the mind will operate to objectify the subjective mental attitude, a great proportion of the mental effort being accomplished along sub-conscious lines. It is of the greatest importance to one who wishes to succeed in any undertaking, to keep before his mind's eye a clear mental image of that which he desires. He should picture the thing desired, and himself as securing it, until it becomes almost real. In this way he calls to his aid his entire mental force and power, along the sub-conscious lines, and, as it were, makes a clear path over which he may walk to accomplishment. Bain says regarding this: "By aiming at a new construction, we must clearly conceive what is aimed at. Where we have a very distinct and intelligible model before us, we are in a fair way to succeed; in proportion as the ideal is dim and wavering, we stagger or miscarry." Maudsley says: "We cannot do an act voluntarily unless we know what we are going to do, and we cannot know exactly what we are going to do until we have taught ourselves to do it." Carpenter says: "The continued concentration of attention upon a certain idea gives it a dominant power, not only over the mind, but over the body." Muller says: "The idea of our own strength gives strength to our movements. A person who is confident of effecting anything by muscular efforts will do it more easily than one not so confident of his own power." Tanner says: "To believe firmly is almost tantamount in the end to accomplishment. Extraordinary instances are related showing the influence of the will over even the involuntary muscles."

Along the same lines, many Western writers have added their testimony to the Yogi principle of the manifestation of thought into action. Kay has written: "A clear and accurate idea of what we wish to do, and how it is to be effected, is of the utmost value and importance in all the affairs of life. A man's conduct naturally shapes itself according to the ideas in his mind, and nothing contributes more to success in life than having a high ideal and keeping it constantly in view. Where such is the case one can hardly fail in attaining it. Numerous unexpected circumstances will be found to conspire to bring it about, and even what seemed at first to be hostile may be converted into means for its furtherance; while by having it constantly before the mind he will be ever ready to take advantage of any favoring circumstances that may present themselves." Along the same lines, Foster has written these remarkable words: "It is wonderful how even the casualties of life seem to bow to a spirit that will not bow to them, and yield to subserve a design which they may, in their first apparent tendency, threaten to frustrate. When a firm, decisive spirit is recognized, it is curious to see how the space clears around a man and leaves him room and freedom." Simpson has said: "A passionate desire and an unwearied will can perform impossibilities, or what seem to be such to the cold and feeble." And Maudsley gives to aspiring youth a great truth, when he says: "Thus it is that aspirations are often prophecies, the harbingers of what a man shall be in a condition to perform." And we may conclude the paragraph by quoting Lytton: "Dream, O youth, dream manfully and nobly, and thy dreams shall be prophets."

This principle of the power of the Mental Image is strongly impressed upon the mind of the *chela*, or student, by the Yogi teachers. The student is taught that just as the house is erected in accordance with the plan of the architect, so is one's life built in accordance with the prevailing Mental Image. The mind sub-consciously moulds itself around the prevailing mental image or attitude, and then proceeds to draw upon the outer world for material with which to build in accordance with the plan. Not only is one's character built in this way, but the circumstances and incidents of his life follow the same rule. The Yogi student is instructed into the mysteries of the power of the mind in this direction, not that he may make use of it to build up material success, or to realize his personal desires—for he is taught to avoid these things—but he is fully instructed, nevertheless, that he may understand the workings of the law around him. And it is a fact well known to close students of the occult, that the few who have attained extraordinarily high degrees of development, make use of this power in order to help the race. Many a world movement has been directed by the mind, or minds, of some of these advanced souls who were able to see the ideal of evolution ahead of the race, and by visualizing the same, and concentrating upon it in meditation, actually hastened the progress of the evolutionary wave, and caused to actually manifest that which they saw, and upon which they had meditated.

It is true that some occultists have used similar plans to further their own selfish personal ends—often without fully realizing just what power they were employing—but this merely illustrates the old fact that the forces of Nature may be used rightly and wrongly. And it is all the more reason why those who are desirous of advancing the race—of assisting in the evolution of the world—should make use of this mighty power in their work. Success is not reprehensible, notwithstanding the fact that many have interpreted and applied the word in such a matter as to make it appear as if it had no other meaning or application other than the crude, material selfish one generally attributed to it, by reason of its misuse. The Western world is playing its part in the evolution of the race, and its keynote is "Accomplishment." Those who have advanced so high that they are able to view the world of men, as one sees a valley from a mountain peak, recognize what this strenuous Western life means. They see mighty forces in operation—mighty principles being worked out by those who little dream of the ultimate significance of that which they are doing. Mighty things are before the Western world to-day—wonderful changes are going on—great things are in the womb of time, and the hour of birth draws near. The men and women in the Western world feel within them the mighty urge to "accomplish" something—to take an active part in the great drama of life. And they are right in giving full expression to this urge, and are doing well in using every legitimate means in the line of expression. And this idea of the Mental Attitude, or the Mental Image, is one of the greatest factors in this striving for Success.

In this lesson we do not purpose giving "Success Talks" for our students. These lessons are intended to fill another field, and there are many other channels of information along the lines named. What we wish to do is to point out to our students the meaning of all this strenuous striving of the age, in the Western world, and the leading principle employed therein. The great achievements of the material world are being accomplished by means of the Power of the Mind. Men are beginning to understand that "Thought manifests itself in Action," and that Thought attracts to itself the things, persons and circumstances in harmony with itself. The Power of Mind is becoming manifest in hundreds of ways. The power of Desire, backed by Faith and Will, is beginning to be recognized as one of the greatest of known dynamic forces. The life of the race is entering into a new and strange stage of development and evolution, and in the years to come MIND will be seen, more clearly and still more clearly, to be the great principle underlying the world of material things and happenings. That "All is Mind" is more than a dreamy, metaphysical utterance, is being recognized by the leaders in the world's thought.

As we have said, great changes are before the world and the race, and every year brings us nearer to the beginning of them. In fact, the beginning is already upon us. Let any thinker stop and reflect over the wonderful changes of the past six years—since the dawning of the Twentieth Century, and he will be dull indeed if he sees not the trend of affairs. We are entering into a new Great Cycle of the race, and the old is being prepared for being dropped off like an old worn out husk. Old conventions, ideals, customs, laws, ethics, and things sociological, economical, theological, philosophical, and metaphysical have been outgrown, and are about to be "shed" by the race. The great cauldron of human thought is bubbling away fiercely, and many things are rising to its surface. Like all great changes, the good will come only with much pain—all birth is with pain. The race feels the pain and perpetual unrest, but knows not what is the disease nor the remedy. Many false cases of diagnosis and prescription are even now noticeable, and will become still more in evidence as the years roll by. Many self-styled saviours of the race—prescribers for the pain of the soul and mind—will arise and fall. But out of it all will come that for which the race now waits.

The changes that are before us are as great as the changes in thought and life described in the late novel by H. G. Wells, entitled "*In the Days of the Comet.*" In fact, Mr. Wells has indicated in that story some of the very changes that the advanced souls of the race have informed their students are before the race—the prophetic insight of the writer named seems marvelous, until one realizes that even that writer is being used as a part of the mental machinery of The Change itself. But the change will not come about by reason of the new gas caused by the brushing of the earth's surface by a passing comet. It will come from the unfolding of the race mind, the process being now under way. Are not the signs of mental unrest and discomfort becoming more and more apparent as the days go by? The pain is growing greater, and the race is beginning to fret and chafe, and moan. It knows not what it wants, but it knows that it feels pain and wants something to relieve that pain. The old things are beginning to totter and fall, and ideas rendered sacred by years of observance are being brushed aside with a startling display of irreverence. Under the surface of our civilization we may hear the straining and groaning of the ideas and principles that are striving to force their way out on to the plane of manifestation.

Men are running hither and thither crying for a leader and a savior. They are trying this thing, and that thing, but they find not that which they seek. They cry for Satisfaction, but it eludes them. And yet all this search and disappointment is part of the Great Change, and is preparing the race for That-which-must-Come. And yet the relief will not come from any Thing or Things. It will come from Within. Just as when, in Well's story, things righted themselves when the vapor of the comet had cleared men's minds, so will Things take their new places when the mind of the race becomes cleared by the new unfoldment that is even now under way. Men are beginning to feel each other's pains—they find themselves unsatisfied by the old rule of "every man for himself, and the devil take the hindmost"—it used to content the successful, but now it doesn't seem to be so satisfying. The man on top is becoming lonesome, and dissatisfied, and discontented—his success seems to appall him, in some mysterious manner. And the man underneath feels stirring within himself strange longings and desires, and dissatisfaction. And new frictions are arising, and new and startling ideas are being suddenly advanced, supported and opposed.

And the relations between people seem to be unsatisfactory. The old rules, laws, and bonds are proving irksome. New, strange, and wild thoughts are coming into the minds of people, which they dare not utter to their friends—and yet these same friends are finding similar ideas within themselves. And somehow, underneath it all is to be found a certain Honesty—yes, there is where the trouble seems to come, *the world is tiring of hypocrisy and dishonesty in all human relations*, and is crying aloud to be led back, someway, to Truth and Honesty in Thought and Action. But it does not see the way out! And it will not see the way out, until the race-mind unfolds still further. And the pain of the new unfoldment is stirring the race to its depths. From the deep recesses of the race-mind are rising to the surface old passions, relics from the cave-dweller days, and all sorts of ugly mental relics of the past. And they will continue to rise and show themselves until at last the bubbling pot will begin to quiet down, and then will come a new peace, and the best will come to the surface—the essence of all the experiences of the race.

To our students, we would say: During the struggle ahead of the race, play well your part, doing the best you can, living each day by itself, meeting each new phase of life with confidence and courage. Be not deluded by appearances, nor follow after strange prophets. Let the evolutionary processes work themselves out, and do you fall in with the wave without struggling, and without overmuch striving. The Law is working itself out well—of that be assured. Those who have entered into even a partial understanding and recognition of the One Life underlying, will find that they will be as the chosen people during the changes that are coming to the race. They have attained that which the race is reaching toward in pain and travail. And the force behind the Law will carry them along, for they will be the leaven that is to lighten the great mass of the race in the new dispensation. Not by deed, or by action, but by Thought, will these people leaven the mass. The Thought is even now at work, and all who read these words are playing a part in the work, although they may know it not. If the race could realize this truth of the One Life underlying, to-day, the Change would occur in a moment, but it will not come in that way. When this understanding gradually dawns upon the race—this new consciousness—then will Things take their proper places, and the Lion and the Lamb lie down together in peace.

We have thought it well to say these things in this the last lesson of this course. They are needed words—they will serve to point out the way to those who are able to read. "*Watch and wait for the Silence that will follow the Storm.*"

In this series of lessons we have endeavored to give you a plain, practical presentation of some of the more important features of "Raja Yoga." But this phase of the subject, as important and interesting as it is, is not the highest phase of the great Yoga teachings. It is merely the preparation of the soil of the mind for what comes afterward. The phase called "Gnani Yoga"—the Yoga of Wisdom—is the highest of all the various phases of Yoga, although each of the lower steps is important in itself. We find ourselves approaching the phase of our work for which we have long wished. Those who have advised and directed this work have counseled us to deal with the less advanced and simpler phases, in order to prepare the minds of those who might be interested, so that they would be ready for the higher teachings. At times we have felt an impatience for the coming of the day when we would be able to teach the highest that has come to us. And now the time seems to have come. Following this course, we will begin a series of lessons in "GNANI YOGA"—the Yoga of Wisdom—in which we will pass on to our students the highest teachings regarding the Reality and its Manifestations—the One and the Many. The teachings that "All is Mind" will be explained in such a manner as to be understood by all who have followed us so far. We will be able to impart to you the higher truths about Spiritual Evolution, sometimes called "Reincarnation," as well as Spiritual Cause and Effect, often called "Karma." The highest truths about these important subjects are often obscured by popular misconceptions occasioned by partial teaching. We trust that you—our students—will wish to follow us still higher—higher than we have ventured so far, and we assure you that there is a Truth to be seen and known that is as much higher than the other phases upon which we have touched, as those phases have been higher than the current beliefs of the masses of the race. We trust that the Powers of Knowledge may guide and direct us that we may be able to convey our message so that it may be accepted and understood. We thank our students who have traveled thus far with us, and we assure them that their loving sympathy has ever been a help and an inspiration to us.

Peace be with you.

The End.

A SERIES OF
Lessons in Gnani Yoga
(The Yoga of Wisdom.)

BY YOGI RAMACHARAKA.

THIS BOOK GIVES THE HIGHEST YOGI TEACHINGS REGARDING

THE ABSOLUTE AND ITS MANIFESTATIONS.

INDEX

LESSON PAGE

THE FIRST LESSON

THE ONE.

The Yogi Philosophy may be divided into several great branches, or fields. What is known as "Hatha Yoga" deals with the physical body and its control; its welfare; its health; its preservation; its laws, etc. What is known as "Raja Yoga" deals with the Mind; its control; its development; its unfoldment, etc. What is known as "Bhakti Yoga" deals with the Love of the Absolute—God. What is known as "Gnani Yoga" deals with the scientific and intellectual knowing of the great questions regarding Life and what lies back of Life—the Riddle of the Universe.

Each branch of Yoga is but a path leading toward the one end—unfoldment, development, and growth. He who wishes first to develop, control and strengthen his physical body so as to render it a fit instrument of the Higher Self, follows the path of "Hatha Yoga." He who would develop his will-power and mental faculties, unfolding the inner senses, and latent powers, follows the path of "Raja Yoga." He who wishes to develop by "knowing"—by studying the fundamental principles, and the wonderful truths underlying Life, follows the path of "Gnani Yoga." And he who wishes to grow into a union with the One Life by the influence of Love, he follows the path of "Bhakti Yoga."

But it must not be supposed that the student must ally himself to only a single one of these paths to power. In fact, very few do. The majority prefer to gain a rounded knowledge, and acquaint themselves with the principles of the several branches, learning something of each, giving preference of course to those branches that appeal to them more strongly, this attraction being the indication of *need*, or requirement, and, therefore, being the hand pointing out the path.

It is well for every one to know something of "Hatha Yoga," in order that the body may be purified, strengthened, and kept in health in order to become a more fitting instrument of the Higher Self. It is well that each one should know something of "Raja Yoga," that he may understand the training and control of the mind, and the use of the Will. It is well that every one should learn the wisdom of "Gnani Yoga," that he may realize the wonderful truths underlying life—the science of Being. And, most assuredly every one should know something of Bhakti Yogi, that he may understand the great teachings regarding the Love underlying all life.

We have written a work on "Hatha Yoga," and a course on "Raja Yoga" which is now in book form. We have told you something regarding "Gnani Yoga" in our Fourteen Lessons, and also in our Advanced Course. We have written something regarding "Bhakti

Yoga" in our Advanced Course, and, we hope, have taught it also all through our other lessons, for we fail to see how one can teach or study any of the branches of Yoga without being filled with a sense of Love and Union with the Source of all Life. To know the Giver of Life, is to love him, and the more we know of him, the more love will we manifest.

In this course of lessons, of which this is the first, we shall take up the subject of "Gnani Yoga"—the Yoga of Wisdom, and will endeavor to make plain some of its most important and highest teachings. And, we trust that in so doing, we shall be able to awaken in you a still higher realization of your relationship with the One, and a corresponding Love for that in which you live, and move and have your being. We ask for your loving sympathy and cooperation in our task.

Let us begin by a consideration of what has been called the "Questions of Questions"—the question: "What is Reality?" To understand the question we have but to take a look around us and view the visible world. We see great masses of something that science has called "matter." We see in operation a wonderful something called "force" or "energy" in its countless forms of manifestations. We see things that we call "forms of life," varying in manifestation from the tiny speck of slime that we call the Moneron, up to that form that we call Man.

But study this world of manifestations by means of science and research—and such study is of greatest value—still we must find ourselves brought to a point where we cannot progress further. Matter melts into mystery—Force resolves itself into something else—the secret of living-forms subtly elude us—and mind is seen as but the manifestation of something even finer. But in losing these things of appearance and manifestation, we find ourselves brought up face to face with a Something Else that we see must underlie all these varying forms, shapes and manifestations. And that Something Else, we call Reality, because it is Real, Permanent, Enduring. And although men may differ, dispute, wrangle, and quarrel about this Reality, still there is one point upon which they must agree, and that is that *Reality is One*—that underlying all forms and manifestations there must be a *One* Reality from which all things flow. And this inquiry into this One Reality is indeed the Question of Questions of the Universe.

The highest reason of Man—as well as his deepest intuition—has always recognized that this Reality or Underlying Being must be but ONE, of which all Nature is but varying degrees of manifestation, emanation, or expression. All have recognized that Life is a stream flowing from One great fount, the nature and name of which is unknown—some have said unknowable. Differ as men do about theories regarding the nature of this one, they all agree that it can be but One. It is only when men begin to name and analyze this One, that confusion results.

Let us see what men have thought and said about this One—it *may* help us to understand the nature of the problem.

The materialist claims that this one is a something called Matter—self-existent—eternal—infinite—containing within itself the potentiality of Matter, Energy and Mind. Another school, closely allied to the materialists, claim that this One is a something called Energy, of which Matter and Mind are but modes of motion. The Idealists claim that the One is a something called Mind, and that Matter and Force are but ideas in that One Mind. Theologians claim that this One is a something called a personal God, to whom they attribute certain qualities, characteristics, etc., the same varying with their creeds and dogmas. The Naturistic school claims that this One is a something called Nature, which is constantly manifesting itself in countless forms. The occultists, in their varying schools, Oriental and Occidental, have taught that the One was a Being whose Life constituted the life of all living forms.

All philosophies, all science, all religions, inform us that this world of shapes, forms and names is but a phenomenal or shadow world—a show-world—back of which rests Reality, called by some name of the teacher. But remember this, *all philosophy that counts* is based upon some form of monism—Oneness—whether the concept be a known or unknown god; an unknown or unknowable principle; a substance; an Energy, or Spirit. There is but One—there can be but One—such is the inevitable conclusion of the highest human reason, intuition or faith.

And, likewise, the same reason informs us that this One Life must permeate all apparent forms of life, and that all apparent material forms, forces, energies, and principles must be emanations from that One, and, consequently "of" it. It may be objected to, that the creeds teaching a personal god do not so hold, for they teach that their God is the creator of the Universe, which he has set aside from himself as a workman sets aside his workmanship. But this objection avails naught, for where could such a creator obtain the material for his universe, except from himself; and where the energy, except from the same source; and where the Life, unless from his One Life. So in the end, it is seen that there must be but One—not two, even if we prefer the terms God *and* his Universe, for even in this case the Universe must have proceeded from God, and can only live, and move and act, and think, by virtue of his Essence permeating it.

In passing by the conceptions of the various thinkers, we are struck by the fact that the various schools seem to manifest a one-sidedness in their theories, seeing only that which fits in with their theories, and ignoring the rest. The Materialist talks about Infinite and Eternal Matter, although the latest scientific investigations have shown us Matter fading into Nothingness—the Eternal Atom being split into countless particles called Corpuscles or Electrons, which at the last seem to be nothing but a unit of Electricity, tied up in a "knot in the Ether"—although just what the Ether is, Science does not dare to guess. And Energy, also seems to be unthinkable except as operating through matter, and always seems to be acting under the operation of Laws—and Laws without a Law giver, and a Law giver without mind or something higher than Mind, is unthinkable. And Mind, as we know it, seems to be bound up with matter and energy in a wonderful combination, and is seen to be subject to laws outside of itself, and to be varying, inconstant, and changeable, which attributes cannot be conceived of as belonging to the Absolute. Mind as we know it, as well as Matter and Energy, is held by the highest occult teachers to be but an appearance and a relativity of something far more fundamental and enduring, and we are compelled to fall back upon that old term which wise men have used in order to describe that Something Else that lies back of, and under, Matter, Energy and Mind—and that word is "Spirit."

We cannot tell just what is meant by the word "Spirit," for we have nothing with which to describe it. But we can think of it as meaning the "essence" of Life and Being—the Reality underlying Universal Life.

Of course no name can be given to this One, that will fitly describe it. But we have used the term "The Absolute" in our previous lessons, and consider it advisable to continue its use, although the student may substitute any other name that appeals to him more strongly. We do not use the word God (except occasionally in order to bring out a shade of meaning) not because we object to it, but because by doing so we would run the risk of identifying The Absolute with some idea of a personal god with certain theological attributes. Nor does the word "Principle" appeal to us, for it seems to imply a cold, unfeeling, abstract thing, while we conceive the Absolute Spirit or Being to be a warm, vital, living, acting, feeling Reality. We do not use the word Nature, which many prefer, because of its materialistic meaning to the minds of many, although the word is very dear to us when referring to the outward manifestation of the Absolute Life.

Of the real nature of The Absolute, of course, we can know practically nothing, because it transcends all human experience and Man has nothing with which he can measure the Infinite. Spinoza was right when he said that "to define God is to deny him," for any attempt to define, is, of course an attempt to limit or make finite the Infinite. To define a thing is to identify it with something else—and where is the something else with which to identify the Infinite? The Absolute cannot be described in terms of the Relative. It is not Something, although it contains within itself the reality underlying Everything. It cannot be said to have the qualities of any of its apparently separated parts, for it is the ALL. It is all that really IS.

It is beyond Matter, Force, or Mind as we know it, and yet these things emanate from it, and must be within its nature. For what is in the manifested must be in the manifestor—

no stream can rise higher than its source—the effect cannot be greater than the cause—you cannot get something out of nothing.

But it is hard for the human mind to take hold of That which is beyond its experience—many philosophers consider it impossible—and so we must think of the Absolute in the concepts and terms of its highest manifestation. We find Mind higher in the scale than Matter or Energy, and so we are justified in using the terms of Mind in speaking of the Absolute, rather than the terms of Matter or Energy—so let us try to think of an Infinite Mind, whose powers and capacities are raised to an infinite degree—a Mind of which Herbert Spencer said that it was "a mode of being as much transcending intelligence and will, as these transcend mere mechanical motion."

While it is true (as all occultists know) that the best information regarding the Absolute come from regions of the Self higher than Intellect, yet we are in duty bound to examine the reports of the Intellect concerning its information regarding the One. The Intellect has been developed in us for use—for the purpose of examining, considering, thinking—and it behooves us to employ it. By turning it to this purpose, we not only strengthen and unfold it, but we also get certain information that can reach us by no other channel. And moreover, by such use of the Intellect we are able to discover many fallacies and errors that have crept into our minds from the opinions and dogmas of others—as Kant said: "The chief, and perhaps the only, use of a philosophy of pure reason is a negative one. It is not an organon for extending, but a discipline for limiting! Instead of discovering truth, its modest function is to guard against error." Let us then listen to the report of the Intellect, as well as of the higher fields of mentation.

One of the first reports of the Intellect, concerning the Absolute, is that it must have existed forever, and must continue to exist forever. There is no escape from this conclusion, whether one view the matter from the viewpoint of the materialist, philosopher, occultist, or theologian. The Absolute could not have sprung from Nothing, and there was no other cause outside of itself from which it could have emanated. And there can be no cause outside of itself which can terminate its being. And we cannot conceive of Infinite Life, or Absolute Life, dying. So the Absolute must be Eternal—such is the report of the Intellect.

This idea of the Eternal is practically unthinkable to the human mind, although it is forced to believe that it must be a quality of the Absolute. The trouble arises from the fact that the Intellect is compelled to see everything through the veil of Time, and Cause and Effect. Now, Cause and Effect, and Time, are merely phenomena or appearances of the relative world, and have no place in the Absolute and Real. Let us see if we can understand this.

Reflection will show you that the only reason that you are unable to think of or picture a Causeless Cause, is because everything that you have experienced in this relative world of the senses has had a cause—something from which it sprung. You have seen Cause and Effect in full operation all about you, and quite naturally your Intellect has taken it for granted that there can be nothing uncaused—nothing without a preceding cause. And the Intellect is perfectly right, so far as Things are concerned, for all Things are relative and are therefore caused. But back of the caused things must lie THAT which is the Great Causer of Things, and which, not being a Thing itself, cannot have been caused—cannot be the effect of a cause. Your minds reel when you try to form a mental image of That which has had no cause, because you have had no experience in the sense world of such a thing, and there fail to form the image. It is out of your experience, and you cannot form the mental picture. But yet your mind is compelled to believe that there must have been an Original One, that can have had no cause. This is a hard task for the Intellect, but in time it comes to see just where the trouble lies, and ceases to interpose objections to the voice of the higher regions of the self.

And, the Intellect experiences a similar difficulty when it tries to think of an Eternal—a That which is above and outside of Time. We see Time in operation everywhere, and take it for granted that Time is a reality—an actual thing. But this is a mistake of the senses. There is no such thing as Time, in reality. Time exists solely in our minds. It is merely a form of perception by which we express our consciousness of the Change in Things.

We cannot think of Time except in connection with a succession of changes of things in our consciousness—either things of the outer world, or the passing of thought-things through our mind. A day is merely the consciousness of the passing of the sun—an hour or minute merely the subdivision of the day, or else the consciousness of the movement of the hands of the clock—merely the consciousness of the movement of Things—the symbols of changes in Things. In a world without changes in Things, there would be no such thing as Time. Time is but a mental invention. Such is the report of the Intellect.

And, besides the conclusions of pure abstract reasoning about Time, we may see many instances of the relativity of Time in our everyday experiences. We all know that when we are interested Time seems to pass rapidly, and when we are bored it drags along in a shameful manner. We know that when we are happy, Time develops the speed of a meteor, while when we are unhappy it crawls like a tortoise. When we are interested or happy our attention is largely diverted from the changes occurring in things—because we do not notice the Things so closely. And while we are miserable or bored, we notice the details in Things, and their changes, until the length of time seems interminable. A tiny insect mite may, and does, live a lifetime of birth, growth, marriage, reproduction, old age, and death, in a few minutes, and no doubt its life seems as full as does that of the elephant with his hundred years. Why? *Because so many things haze happened!* When we are conscious of many things happening, we get the impression and sensation of the length of time. The greater the consciousness of things, the greater the sensation of Time. When we are so interested in talking to a loved one that we forget all that is occurring about us, then the hours fly by unheeded, while the same hours seem like days to one in the same place who is not interested or occupied with some task.

Men have nodded, and in the second before awakening they have dreamed of events that seemed to have required the passage of years. Many of you have had experiences of this kind, and many such cases have been recorded by science. On the other hand, one may fall asleep and remain unconscious, but without dreams, for hours, and upon awakening will insist that he has merely nodded. Time belongs to the relative mind, and has no place in the Eternal or Absolute.

Next, the Intellect informs us that it must think of the Absolute as Infinite in Space—present everywhere—Omnipresent. It cannot be limited, for there is nothing outside of itself to limit it. There is no such place as Nowhere. Every place is in the Everywhere. And Everywhere is filled with the All—the Infinite Reality—the Absolute.

And, just as was the case with the idea of Time, we find it most difficult—if not indeed impossible—to form an idea of an Omnipresent—of That which occupies Infinite Space. This because everything that our minds have experienced has had dimensions and limits. The secret lies in the fact that Space, like Time, has no real existence outside of our perception of consciousness of the relative position of Things—material objects. We see this thing here, and that thing there. Between them is Nothingness. We take another object, say a yard-stick, and measure off this Nothingness between the two objects, and we call this measure of Nothingness by the term Distance. And yet we cannot have measured Nothingness—that is impossible. What have we really done? Simply this, determined how many lengths of yard-stick could be laid between the other two objects.

We call this process measuring Space, but Space is Nothing, and we have merely determined the relative position of objects. To "measure Space" we must have three Things or objects, *i.e.*, (l) The object from which we start the measure; (2) The object with which we measure; and (3) The object with which we end our measurement. We are unable to conceive of Infinite Space, because we lack the third object in the measuring process—the ending object. We may use ourselves as a starting point, and the mental yard-stick is always at hand, but where is the object at the other side of Infinity of Space by which the measurement may be ended? It is not there, and we cannot think of the end without it.

Let us start with ourselves, and try to imagine a million million miles, and then multiply them by another million million miles, a million million times. What have we done?

Simply extended our mental yard-stick a certain number of times to an imaginary point in the Nothingness that we call Space. So far so good, but the mind intuitively recognizes that beyond that imaginary point at the end of the last yard-stick, there is a capacity for an infinite extension of yard-sticks—an infinite capacity for such extension. Extension of what? Space? No! Yard-sticks! Objects! Things! Without material objects Space is unthinkable. It has no existence outside of our consciousness of Things. There is no such thing as Real Space. Space is merely an infinite capacity for extending objects. Space itself is merely a name for Nothingness. If you can form an idea of an object swept out of existence, and nothing to take its place, that Nothing would be called Space, the term implying the possibility of placing something there without displacing anything else.

Size, of course, is but another form of speaking of Distance. And in this connection let us not forget that just as one may think of Space being infinite in the direction of largeness, so may we think of it as being infinite in the sense of smallness. No matter how small may be an object thought of, we are still able to think of it as being capable of subdivision, and so on infinitely. There is no limit in this direction either. As Jakob has said: "The conception of the infinitely minute is as little capable of being grasped by us, as is that of the infinitely great. Despite this, the admission of the reality of the infinitude, both in the direction of greatness and of minuteness, is inevitable."

And, as Radenhausen has said: "The idea of Space is only an unavoidable illusion of our Consciousness, or of our finite nature, and does not exist outside of ourselves; the universe is infinitely small and infinitely great."

The telescope has opened to us ideas of magnificent vastness and greatness, and the perfected microscope has opened to us a world of magnificent smallness and minuteness. The latter has shown us that a drop of water is a world of minute living forms who live, eat, fight, reproduce, and die. The mind is capable of imagining a universe occupying no more space than one million-millionth of the tiniest speck visible under the strongest microscope—and then imagining such a universe containing millions of suns and worlds similar to our own, and inhabited by living forms akin to ours—living, thinking men and women, identical in every respect to ourselves. Indeed, as some philosophers have said, if our Universe were suddenly reduced to such a size—the relative proportions of everything being preserved, of course—then we would not be conscious of any change, and life would go on the same, and we would be of the same importance to ourselves and to the Absolute as we are this moment. And the same would be true were the Universe suddenly enlarged a million-million times. These changes would make no difference in reality. Compared with each other, the tiniest speck and the largest sun are practically the same size when viewed from the Absolute.

We have dwelt upon these things so that you would be able to better realize the relativity of Space and Time, and perceive that they are merely symbols of Things used by the mind in dealing with finite objects, and have no place in reality. When this is realized, then the idea of Infinity in Time and Space is more readily grasped.

As Radenhausen says: "Beyond the range of human reason there is neither Space nor Time; they are arbitrary conceptions of man, at which he has arrived by the comparison and arrangement of different impressions which he has received from the outside world. The conception of Space arises from the sequence of the various forms which fill Space, by which the external world appears to the individual man. The conception of Time arises from the sequence of the various forms which change in space (motion), by which the external world acts on the individual man, and so on. But externally to ourselves, the distinction between repletion of Space and mutation of Space does not exist, for each is in constant transmutation, whatever is is filling and changing at the same time—nothing is at a standstill," and to quote Ruckert: "The world has neither beginning nor end, in space nor in time. Everywhere is center and turning-point, and in a moment is eternity."

Next, the Intellect informs us that we must think of the Absolute as containing within Itself all the Power there is, because there can be no other source or reservoir of Power, and there can be no Power outside of the All-Power. There can be no Power outside of the Absolute to limit, confine, or conflict with It. Any laws of the Universe must have been imposed by It, for there is no other law-giver, and every manifestation of Energy, Force, or Power, perceived or evident in Nature must be a part of the Power of the Absolute working along lines laid down by it. In the Third Lesson, which will be entitled The Will-to-Live, we shall see this Power manifesting along the lines of Life as we know it.

Next, the Intellect informs us that it is compelled to think of the Absolute as containing within Itself all possible Knowledge or Wisdom, because there can be no Knowledge or Wisdom outside of It, and therefore all the Wisdom and Knowledge possible must be within It. We see Mind, Wisdom, and Knowledge manifested by relative forms of Life, and such must emanate from the Absolute in accordance with certain laws laid down by It, for otherwise there would be no such wisdom, etc., for there is nowhere outside of the All from whence it could come. The effect cannot be greater than the cause. If there is anything unknown to the Absolute, then it will never be known to finite minds. So, therefore, ALL KNOWLEDGE that Is, Has Been, or Can Be, must be NOW vested in the One—the Absolute.

This does not mean that the Absolute *thinks*, in any such sense as does Man. The Absolute must Know, without Thinking. It does not have to gather Knowledge by the process of Thinking, as does Man—such an Idea would be ridiculous, for from whence could the Knowledge come outside of itself. When man thinks he draws to himself Knowledge from the Universal source by the action of the Mind, but the Absolute has only itself to draw on. So we cannot imagine the Absolute compelled to Think as we do.

But, lest we be misunderstood regarding this phase of the subject, we may say here that the highest occult teachings inform us that the Absolute *does* manifest a quality somewhat akin to what we would call constructive thought, and that such "thoughts" manifest into objectivity and manifestation, and become Creation. Created Things, according to the Occult teachings are "Thoughts of God." Do not let this idea disturb you, and cause you to feel that you are nothing, because you have been called into being by a Thought of the Infinite One. Even a Thought of that One would be intensely real in the relative world—actually Real to all except the Absolute itself—and even the Absolute knows that the *Real* part of its Creations must be a part of itself manifested through its thought, for the Thought of the Infinite must be Real, and a part of Itself, for it cannot be anything else, and to call it Nothing is merely to juggle with words. The faintest Thought of the Infinite One would be far more real than anything man could create—as solid as the mountain—as hard as steel—as durable as the diamond—for, verily, even these are emanations of the Mind of the Infinite, and are things of but a day, while the higher Thoughts—the soul of Man—contains within itself a spark from the Divine Flame itself—the Spirit of the Infinite. But these things will appear in their own place, as we proceed with this series. We have merely given you a little food for thought at this point, in connection with the Mind of the Absolute.

So you see, good friends and students, that the Intellect in its highest efforts, informs us that it finds itself compelled to report that the One—the Absolute—That which it is compelled to admit really exists—must be a One possessed of a nature so far transcending human experience that the human mind finds itself without the proper concepts, symbols, and words with which to think of It. But none the less, the Intellect finds itself bound by its own laws to postulate the existence of such an One.

It is the veriest folly to try to think of the One as It is "in Itself"—for we have nothing but human attributes with which to measure it, and It so far transcends such measurements that the mental yard-sticks run out into infinity and are lost sight of. The highest minds of the race inform us that the most exalted efforts of their reason compels them to report that the One—in Itself—cannot be spoken of as possessing attributes or qualities capable of being expressed in human words employed to describe the Things of the relative world—and all of our words are such. All of our words originate from such ideas, and all of our ideas arise from our experience, directly or indirectly. So we are not equipped with words with which to think of or speak of that which transcends experience, although our Intellect informs us that Reality lies back of our experience.

Philosophy finds itself unable to do anything better than to bring us face to face with high paradoxes. Science in its pursuit of Truth finds it cunningly avoiding it, and ever escaping its net. And we believe that the Absolute purposely causes this to be, that in the end Man may be compelled to look for the Spirit within himself—the only place where he can come in touch with it. This, we think, is the answer to the Riddle of the Sphinx—"Look Within for that which Thou needest."

But while the Spirit may be discerned only by looking within ourselves, we find that once the mind realizes that the Absolute Is, it will be able to see countless evidences of its action and presence by observing manifested Life without. All Life is filled with the Life Power and Will of the Absolute.

To us Life is but One—the Universe is a living Unity, throbbing, thrilling and pulsating with the Will-to-Live of the Absolute. Back of all apparent shapes, forms, names, forces, elements, principles and substances, there is but One—One Life, present everywhere, and manifesting in an infinitude of shapes, forms, and forces All individual lives are but centers of consciousness in the One Life underlying, depending upon it for degree of unfoldment, expression and manifestation.

This may sound like Pantheism to some, but it is very different from the Pantheism of the schools and cults. Pantheism is defined as "the doctrine that God consists in the combined forces and laws manifested in the existing Universe," or that "the Universe taken or conceived as a whole is God." These definitions do not fit the conception of the Absolute, of the Yogi Philosophy—they seem to breathe but a refined materialism. The Absolute is not "the combined forces and laws manifested in the universe," nor "the universe conceived as a whole." Instead, the Universe, its forces and laws, even conceived as a whole, have no existence in themselves, but are mere manifestations of the Absolute. Surely this is different from Pantheism.

We teach that the Absolute is immanent in, and abiding in all forms of Life in the Universe, as well as in its forces and laws—all being but manifestations of the Will of the One. And we teach that this One is superior to all forms of manifestations, and that Its existence and being does not depend upon the manifestations, which are but effects of the Cause.

The Pantheistic Universe—God is but a thing of phenomenal appearance, but the Absolute is the very Spirit of Life—a Living, Existing Reality, and would be so even if every manifestation were withdrawn from appearance and expression—drawn back into the source from which it emanated. The Absolute is more than Mountain or Ocean—Electricity or Gravitation—Monad or Man—It is SPIRIT—LIFE—BEING—REALITY—the ONE THAT IS. Omnipotent, Omnipresent; Omniscient; Eternal;

Infinite; Absolute; these are Man's greatest words, and yet they but feebly portray a shadow thrown by the One Itself.

The Absolute is not a far-away Being directing our affairs at long range—not an absentee Deity—but an Immanent Life in and about us all—manifesting in us and creating us into individual centers of consciousness, in pursuance with some great law of being.

And, more than this, the Absolute instead of being an indifferent and unmoved spectator to its own creation, is a thriving, longing, active, suffering, rejoicing, feeling Spirit, partaking of the feelings of its manifestations, rather than callously witnessing them. It lives in us—with us—through us. Back of all the pain in the world may be found a great feeling and suffering love. The pain of the world is not punishment or evidence of divine wrath, but the incidents of the working out of some cosmic plan, in which the Absolute is the Actor, through the forms of Its manifestations.

The message of the Absolute to some of the Illumined has been, "All is being done in the best and only possible way—I am doing the best I can—all is well—and in the end will so appear."

The Absolute is no personal Deity—yet in itself it contains all that goes to make up all personality and all human relations. Father, Mother, Child, Friend, is in It. All forms of human love and craving for sympathy, understanding and companionship may find refuge in loving the Absolute.

The Absolute is constantly in evidence in our lives, and yet we have been seeking it here and there in the outer world, asking it to show itself and prove Its existence. Well may it say to us: "Hast thou been so long time with me, and hast thou not known me?" This is the great tragedy of Life, that the Spirit comes to us—Its own—and we know It not. We fail to hear Its words: "Oh, ye who mourn, I suffer with you and through you. Yea, it is I who grieve in you. Your pain is mine—to the last pang. I suffer all pain through you—and yet I rejoice beyond you, for I know that through you, and with you, I shall conquer."

And this is a faint idea of what we believe the Absolute to be. In the following lessons we shall see it in operation in all forms of life, and in ourselves. We shall get close to the workings of Its mighty Will—close to Its Heart of Love.

Carry with you the Central Thought of the Lesson: CENTRAL THOUGHT. There is but One Life in the Universe. And underlying that One Life—Its Real Self—Its Essence—Its Spirit—is The Absolute, living, feeling, suffering, rejoicing, longing, striving, in and through us. The Absolute is all that really Is, and all the visible Universe and forms of Life is Its expression, through Its Will. We lack words adequate to describe the nature of the Absolute, but we will use two words describing its inmost nature as best we see it. These two words are LIFE and LOVE, the one describing the outer, the other the inner nature. Let us manifest both Life and Love as a token of our origin and inner nature. Peace be with you.

THE SECOND LESSON

OMNIPRESENT LIFE.

In our First Lesson of this series, we brought out the idea that the human mind was compelled to report the fact that it could not think of The Absolute except as possessing the quality of Omnipresence—Present-Everywhere. And, likewise, the human mind is compelled to think that all there IS must be The Absolute, or *of* the Absolute. And if a thing is *of* the Absolute, then the Absolute must be *in* it, in some way—must be the *essence* of it. Granting this, we must then think that everything must be filled with the essence of Life, for Life must be one of the qualities of the Absolute, or rather what we call Life must be the outward expression of the essential Being of the Absolute. And if this be so, then it would follow that *everything in the Universe must be Alive.* The mind cannot escape this conclusion. And if the facts do not bear out this conclusion then we must be forced to admit that the entire basic theory of the Absolute and its emanations must fall, and be considered as an error. No chain is stronger than its weakest link, and if this link be too weak to bear the weight of the facts of the universe, then must the chain be discarded as imperfect and useless, and another substituted. This fact is not generally mentioned by those speaking and writing of All being One, or an emanation of the One, but it must be considered and met. If there is a single thing in the Universe that is "dead"—non-living—lifeless—then the theory must fall. If a thing is non-living, then the essence of the Absolute cannot be in it—it must be alien and foreign to the Absolute, and in that case the Absolute cannot be Absolute for there is something outside of itself. And so it becomes of the greatest importance to examine into the evidences of the presence of Life in all things, organic or inorganic. The evidence is at hand—let us examine it.

The ancient occultists of all peoples always taught that the Universe was Alive—that there was Life in everything—that there was nothing dead in Nature—that Death meant simply a change in form in the material of the dead bodies. They taught that Life, in varying degrees of manifestation and expression, was present in everything and object, even down to the hardest mineral form, and the atoms composing that form.

Modern Science is now rapidly advancing to the same position, and each months investigations and discoveries serve only to emphasize the teachings.

Burbank, that wonderful moulder of plant life, has well expressed this thought, when he says: "All my investigations have led me away from the idea of a dead material universe tossed about by various forces, to that of a universe which is absolutely all force, life, soul, thought, or whatever name we may choose to call it. Every atom, molecule, plant, animal or planet, is only an aggregation of organized unit forces, held in place by stronger forces, thus holding them for a time latent, though teeming with inconceivable power. All life on our planet is, so to speak, just on the outer fringe of this infinite ocean of force. The universe is not half dead, but all alive."

Science today is gazing upon a living universe. She has not yet realized the full significance of what she has discovered, and her hands are raised as if to shade her eyes from the unaccustomed glare that is bursting upon her. From the dark cavern of universal dead matter, she has stepped out into the glare of the noon-day sun of a Universe All-Alive even to its smallest and apparently most inert particle.

Beginning at Man, the highest form of Life known to us, we may pass rapidly down the scale of animal life, seeing life in full operation at each descending step. Passing from the animal to the vegetable kingdom, we still see Life in full operation, although in lessened degrees of expression. We shall not stop here to review the many manifestations of Life among the forms of plant-life, for we shall have occasion to mention them in our next lesson, but it must be apparent to all that Life is constantly manifesting in the sprouting of seeds; the putting forth of stalk, leaves, blossoms, fruit, etc., and in the enormous manifestation of force and energy in such growth and development. One may see the life force in the plant pressing forth for expression and manifestation, from the first sprouting of the seed, until the last vital action on the part of the mature plant or tree.

Besides the vital action observable in the growth and development of plants, we know, of course, that plants sicken and die, and manifest all other attributes of living forms. There is no room for argument about the presence of life in the plant kingdom.

But there are other forms of life far below the scale of the plants. There is the world of the bacteria, microbes, infusoria—the groups of cells with a common life—the single cell creatures, down to the Monera, the creatures lower than the single cells—the Things of the slime of the ocean bed.

These tiny Things—living Things—present to the sight merely a tiny speck of jelly, without organs of any kind. And yet they exercise all the functions of life—movement, nutrition, reproduction, sensation, and dissolution. Some of these elementary forms are all stomach, that is they are all one organ capable of performing all the functions necessary for the life of the animal. The creature has no mouth, but when it wishes to devour an object it simply envelopes it—wraps itself around it like a bit of glue around a gnat, and then absorbs the substance of its prey through its whole body.

Scientists have turned some of these tiny creatures inside out, and yet they have gone on with their life functions undisturbed and untroubled. They have cut them up into still tinier bits, and yet each bit lived on as a separate animal, performing all of its functions undisturbed. They are all the same all over, and all the way through. They reproduce themselves by growing to a certain size, and then separating into two, and so on. The rapidity of the increase is most remarkable.

Haekel says of the Monera: "The Monera are the simplest permanent cytods. Their entire body consists of merely soft, structureless plasm. However thoroughly we may examine them with the help of the most delicate reagents and the strongest optical instruments, we yet find that all the parts are completely homogeneous. These Monera are therefore, in the strictest sense of the word, 'organisms without organs,' or even in a strict philosophical sense they might not even be called organisms, since they possess no organs and since they are not composed of various particles. They can only be called organisms in so far as they are capable of exercising the organic phenomena of life, of nutrition, reproduction, sensation and movement."

Verworn records an interesting instance of life and mind among the *Rhizopods*, a very low form of living thing. He relates that the *Difflugia ampula*, a creature occupying a tiny shell formed of minute particles of sand, has a long projection of its substance, like a feeler or tendril, with which it searches on the bottom of the sea for sandy material with which to build the shell or outer covering for its offspring, which are born by division from the parent body. It grasps the particle of sand by the feeler, and passes it into its body by enclosing it. Verworn removed the sand from the bottom of the tank, replacing it by very minute particles of highly colored glass. Shortly afterward he noticed a collection of these particles of glass in the body of the creature, and a little later he saw a tiny speck of protoplasm emitted from the parent by separation. At the same time he noticed that the bits of glass collected by the mother creature were passed out and placed around the body of the new creature, and cemented together by a substance secreted by the body of the parent, thus forming a shell and covering for the offspring. This proceeding showed the presence of a mental something sufficient to cause the creature to prepare a shell for the offspring previous to its birth—or rather to gather the material for such shell, to be afterward used; to distinguish the proper material; to mould it into shape, and cement it. The scientist reported that a creature always gathered just exactly enough sand for its purpose—never too little, and never an excess. And this in a creature that is little more than a tiny drop of glue!

We may consider the life actions of the Moneron a little further, for it is the lowest form of so-called "living matter"—the point at which living forms pass off into non-living forms (so-called). This tiny speck of glue—an organism without organs—is endowed with the faculty called sensation. It draws away from that which is likely to injure it, and toward that which it desires—all in response to an elementary sensation. It has the instinct of self-preservation and self-protection. It seeks and finds its prey, and then eats, digests and assimilates it. It is able to move about by "false-feet," or bits of its body which it pushes forth at will from any part of its substance. It reproduces itself, as we have seen, by separation and self-division.

The life of the bacteria and germs—the yeasty forms of life—are familiar to many of us. And yet there are forms of life still below these. The line between living forms and non-living forms is being set back further and further by science. Living creatures are now known that resemble the non-living so closely that the line cannot be definitely drawn.

Living creatures are known that are capable of being dried and laid away for several years, and then may be revived by the application of moisture. They resemble dust, but are full of life and function. Certain forms of bacilli are known to Science that have been subjected to degrees of heat and cold that are but terms to any but the scientific mind.

Low forms of life called Diatoms or "living crystals" are known. They are tiny geometrical forms. They are composed of a tiny drop of plasm, resembling glue, covered by a thin shell of siliceous or sandy material. They are visible only through the microscope, and are so small that thousands of them might be gathered together on the head of a pin. They are so like chemical crystals that it requires a shrewd and careful observer to distinguish them. And yet they are alive, and perform all the functions of life.

Leaving these creatures, we enter the kingdom of the crystals, in our search for life. Yes, the crystals manifest life, as strange as this statement may appear to those who have not followed the march of Science. The crystals are born, grow, live, and may be killed by chemicals or electricity. Science has added a new department called "Plasmology," the purpose of which is the study of crystal life. Some investigators have progressed so far as to claim that they have discovered signs of rudimentary sex functioning among crystals. At any rate, crystals are born and grow like living things. As a recent scientific writer has said: "Crystallization, as we are to learn now, is not a mere mechanical grouping of dead atoms. It is a birth."

The crystal forms from the mother liquor, and its body is built up systematically, regularly, and according to a well defined plan or pattern, just as are the body and bones of the animal form, and the wood and bark of the tree. There is life at work in the growth of the crystal. And not only does the crystal grow, but it also reproduces itself by separation or splitting-off, just as is the case with the lower forms of life, just mentioned.

The principal point of difference between the growth and development of the crystals and that of the lower forms of life referred to is that the crystal takes its nourishment from the outside, and builds up from its outer surface, while the Monera absorbs its nourishment from within, and grows outwardly from within. If the crystal had a soft center, and took its nourishment in that way, it would be almost identical with the Diatom, or, if the Diatom grew from the outside, it would be but a crystal. A very fine dividing line.

Crystals, like living forms, may be sterilized and rendered incapable of reproduction by chemical process, or electrical discharges. They may also be "killed" and future growth prevented in this manner. Surely this looks like "Life," does it not?

To realize the importance of this idea of life among the crystals, we must remember that our hardest rocks and metals are composed of crystals, and that the dirt and earth upon which we grow and live are but crumbled rock and miniature crystals. Therefore the very dust under our feet is alive. *There is nothing dead.* There is no transformation of "dead matter" into live plant matter, and then into live animal matter. The chemicals are alive, and from chemical to man's body there is but a continuous change of shape and form of living matter. Any man's body, decomposing, is again resolved into chemicals, and the chain begins over again. Merely changes in living forms—that's all, so far as the bodies are concerned.

Nature furnishes us with many examples of this presence of life in the inorganic world. We have but to look around to see the truth of the statement that All is Alive. There is that which is known as the "fatigue of elasticity" in metals. Razors get tired, and require a rest. Tuning forks lose their powers of vibration, to a degree, and have to be given a vacation. 'Machinery in mills and manufactories needs an occasional day off. Metals are subject to disease and infection, and have been poisoned and restored by antidotes. Window glass, especially stained glass, is subject to a disease spreading from pane to pane.

Men accustomed to handling and using tools and machinery naturally drop into the habit of speaking of these things as if they were alive. They seem to recognize the presence of "feeling" in tools or machine, and to perceive in each a sort of "character" or personality, which must be respected, humored, or coaxed in order to get the best results.

Perhaps the most valuable testimony along these lines, and which goes very far toward proving the centuries-old theories of the Yogis regarding Omnipresent Life, comes from Prof. J. Chunder Bose, of the Calcutta University, a Hindu educated in the English

Universities, under the best teachers, and who is now a leading scientific authority in the western world, tie has given to the world some very valuable scientific information along these lines in his book entitled "*Response in the Living and Non-living*," which has caused the widest comment and created the greatest interest among the highest scientific authorities. His experiments along the lines of the gathering of evidence of life in the inorganic forms have revolutionized the theories of modern science, and have done much to further the idea that life is present everywhere, and that there is no such thing as dead matter.

He bases his work upon the theory that the best and only true test for the presence of life in matter is the response of matter to external stimulus. Proceeding from this fundamental theory he has proven by in-numerable experiments that so-called inorganic matter, minerals, metals, etc., give a response to such stimulus, which response is similar, if not identical, to the response of the matter composing the bodies of plants, animals, men.

He devised delicate apparatus for the measurement of the response to the outside stimulus, the degree, and other evidence being recorded in traces on a revolving cylinder. The tracings or curves obtained from tin and other metals, when compared with those obtained from living muscle, were found to be identical. He used a galvanometer, a very delicate and accurate scientific instrument, in his experiments. This instrument is so finely adjusted that the faintest current will cause a deflection of the registering needle, which is delicately swung on a tiny pivot. If the galvanometer be attached to a human nerve, and the end of the nerve be irritated, the needle will register.

Prof. Bose found that when he attached the galvanometer to bars of various metals they gave a similar response when struck or twisted. The greater the irritation applied to the metal, the greater the response registered by the instrument. The analogy between the response of the metal and that of the living muscle was startling. For instance, just as in the case of the living animal muscle or nerve matter, the response becomes fatigued, so in the case of the metal the curve registered by the needle became fainter and still fainter, as the bar became more and more fatigued by the continued irritation. And again, just after such fatigue the muscle would become rested, and would again respond actively, so would the metal when given a chance to recuperate.

Tetanus due to shocks constantly repeated, was caused and recovered. Metals recorded evidences of fatigue. Drugs caused identical effects on metals and animals—some exciting; some depressing; some killing. Some poisonous chemicals killed pieces of metal, rendering them immobile and therefore incapable of registering records on the apparatus. In some cases antidotes were promptly administered, and saved the life of the metal.

Prof. Bose also conducted experiments on plants in the same way. Pieces of vegetable matter were found to be capable of stimulation, fatigue, excitement, depression, poison. Mrs. Annie Besant, who witnessed some of these experiments in Calcutta, has written as follows regarding the experiments on plant life: "There is something rather pathetic in seeing the way in which the tiny spot of light which records the pulses in the plant, travels in ever weaker and weaker curves, when the plant is under the influence of poison, then falls into a final despairing straight line, and—stops. One feels as though a murder has been committed—as indeed it has."

In one of Prof. Bose's public experiments he clearly demonstrated that a bar of iron was fully as sensitive as the human body, and that it could be irritated and stimulated in the same way, and finally could be poisoned and killed. "Among such phenomena," he asks, "how can we draw the line of demarkation, and say, 'Here the physical ends, and there the physiological begins'? No such barrier exists." According to his theory, which agrees with the oldest occult theories, by the way, life is present in every object and form of Nature, and all forms respond to external stimulus, which response is a proof of the presence of life in the form.

Prof. Bose's great book is full of the most startling results of experiments. He proves that the metals manifest something like sleep; can be killed; exhibit torpor and sluggishness; get tired or lazy; wake up; can be roused into activity; may be stimulated, strengthened, weakened; suffer from extreme cold and heat; may be drugged or intoxicated, the different metals manifesting a different response to certain drugs, just as different men and animals manifest a varying degree of similar resistance. The response of a piece of steel subjected to the influence of a chemical poison shows a gradual fluttering and weakening until it finally dies away, just as animal matter does when similarly poisoned. When revived in time by an antidote, the recovery was similarly gradual in both metal and muscle. A remarkable fact is noted by the scientist when he tells us that the very poisons that kill the metals are themselves alive and may be killed, drugged, stimulated, etc., showing the same response as in the case of the metals, proving the existence in them of the same life that is in the metals and animal matter that they influence.

Of course when these metals are "killed" there is merely a killing of the metal as metal—the atoms and principles of which the metal is composed remaining fully alive and active, just as is the case with the atom of the human body after the soul passes out—the body is as much alive after death as during the life of the person, the activity of the parts being along the lines of dissolution instead of construction in that case.

We hear much of the claims of scientists who announce that they are on the eve of "*creating* life" from non-living matter. This is all nonsense—life can come only from life. Life from non-life is an absurdity. And all Life comes from the One Life underlying All.

But it is true that Science has done, is doing, and will do, something very much like "creating life," but of course this is merely changing the form of Life into other forms—the lesser form into the higher—just as one produces a plant from a seed, or a fruit from a plant. The Life is always there, and responds to the proper stimulus and conditions.

A number of scientists are working on the problem of generating living forms from inorganic matter. The old idea of "spontaneous generation," for many years relegated to the scrap-pile of Science, is again coming to the front. Although the theory of Evolution compels its adherents to accept the idea that at one time in the past living forms sprung from the non-living (so-called), yet it has been generally believed that the conditions which brought about this stage of evolution has forever passed. But the indications now all point to the other view that this stage of evolution is, and always has been, in operation, and that new forms of life are constantly evolving from the inorganic forms. "Creation," so-called (although the word is an absurdity from the Yogi point of view), is constantly being performed.

Dr. Charlton Bastian, of London, Eng., has long been a prominent advocate of this theory of continuous spontaneous generation. Laughed down and considered defeated by the leading scientific minds of a generation ago, he still pluckily kept at work, and his recent books were like bombshells in the orthodox scientific camp. He has taken more than five thousand photo-micrographs, all showing most startling facts in connection with the origin of living forms from the inorganic. He claims that the microscope reveals the development in a previously clear liquid of very minute black spots, which gradually enlarge and transform into bacteria—living forms of a very low order. Prof. Burke, of Cambridge, Eng., has demonstrated that he may produce in sterilized boullion, subjected to the action of sterilized radium chloride, minute living bodies which manifest growth and subdivision. Science is being gradually forced to the conclusion that living forms are still arising in the world by natural processes, which is not at all remarkable when one remembers that natural law is uniform and continuous. These recent discoveries go to swell the already large list of modern scientific ideas which correspond with the centuries-old Yogi teachings. When the Occult explanation that there is Life in everything, *inorganic as well as organic*, and that evolution is constant, is heard, then may we see that these experiments simply prove that the forms of life may be changed and developed—not that Life may be "created."

The chemical and mineral world furnish us with many instances of the growth and development of forms closely resembling the forms of the vegetable world. What is known as "metallic vegetation," as shown in the "lead tree," gives us an interesting example of this phenomenon. The experiment is performed by placing in a wide-necked bottle a clear acidulated solution of acetate of lead. The bottle is corked, a piece of copper wire being fastened to the cork, from which wire is suspended a piece of zinc, the latter hanging as nearly as possible in the center of the lead solution. When the bottle is corked the copper wire immediately begins to surround itself with a growth of metallic lead resembling fine moss. From this moss spring branches and limbs, which in turn manifest a growth similar to foliage, until at last a miniature bush or tree is formed. Similar "metallic vegetation" may be produced by other metallic solutions.

All of you have noticed how crystals of frost form on window panes in shapes of leaves, branches, foliage, flowers, blossoms, etc. Saltpeter when subjected to the effect of polarized light assumes forms closely resembling the forms of the orchid. Nature is full of these resemblances.

A German scientist recently performed a remarkable experiment with certain metallic salts. He subjected the salts to the action of a galvanic current, when to his surprise the particles of the salts grouped themselves around the negative pole of the battery, and then grew into a shape closely resembling a miniature mushroom, with tiny stem and umbrella top. These metallic mushrooms at first presented a transparent appearance, but gradually developed color, the top of the umbrella being a bright red, with a faint rose shade on the under surface. The stems showed a pale straw color. This was most interesting, but the important fact of the experiment consists in the discovery that these mushrooms have fine veins or tubes running along the stems, through which the nourishment, or additional material for growth, is transported, so that the growth is actually from the inside, just as is the case with fungus life. To all intents and purposes, these inorganic metallic growths were low forms of vegetable his.

But the search for Life does not end with the forms of the mineral world as we know them. Science has separated the material forms into smaller forms, and again still smaller. And if there is Life in the form composed of countless particles, then must there be Life in the particles themselves. For Life cannot come from non-Life, and if there be not Life in the particles, the theory of Omnipresent Life must fan. So we must look beyond the form and shape of the mineral—mist separate it into its constituent parts, and then examine the parts for indications of Life.

Science teaches us that all forms of matter are compiled of minute particles called molecules. A molecule is the smallest particle of matter that is possible, unless the chemical atoms composing the matter fly apart and the matter be resolved into its original elements. For instance, let us take the familiar instance of a drop of water. Let us divide and subdivide the drop, until at last we get to the smallest possible particle of water. That smallest possible particle would be a "molecule" of water. We cannot subdivide this molecule without causing its atoms of hydrogen and oxygen to fly apart—and then there would be no *water* at all. Well, these molecules manifest a something called Attraction for each other. They attract other molecules of the same kind, and are likewise attracted.

The operation of this law of attraction results in the formation of masses of matter, whether those masses be mountains of solid rock, or a drop of water, or a volume of gas. All masses of matter are composed of aggregations of molecules, held together by the law of attraction. This law of attraction is called Cohesion. This Cohesive Attraction is not a mere mechanical force, as many suppose, but is an exhibition of Life action, manifesting in the presence of the molecule of a "like" or "love" for the similar molecule. And when the Life energies begin to manifest on a certain plane, and proceed to mould the molecules into crystals, so that we may see the actual process under way, we begin to realize very clearly that there is "something at work" in this building up.

But wonderful as this may seem to those unfamiliar with the idea, the manifestation of Life among the atoms is still more so. The atom, you will remember, is the chemical unit which, uniting with other atoms, makes up the molecule. For instance, if we take two atoms of the gas called hydrogen and one atom of the gas called oxygen, and place them near each other, they will at once rush toward each other and form a partnership, which is called a molecule of water. And so it is with all atoms—they are continually forming partnerships, or dissolving them. Marriage and divorce is a part of the life of the atoms. These evidences of attraction and repulsion among the atoms are receiving much attention from careful thinkers, and some of the most advanced minds of the age see in this phenomena the corroboration of the old Yogi idea that there is Life and vital action in the smallest particles of matter.

The atoms manifest vital characteristics in their attractions and repulsions. They move along the lines of their attractions and form marriages, and thus combining they form the substances with which we are familiar. When they combine, remember, they do not lose their individuality and melt into a permanent substance, but merely unite and yet remain distinct. If the combination be destroyed by chemical action, electrical discharge, etc., the atoms fly apart, and again live their own separate lives, until they come in contact with other atoms with which they have affinities, and form a new union or partnership. In many chemical changes the atoms divorce themselves, each forsaking its mate or mates, and seeking some newer affinity in the shape of a more congenial atom. The atoms manifest a fickleness and will always desert a lesser attraction for a greater one. This is no mere bit of imagery, or scientific poetry. It is a scientific statement of the action of atoms along the lines of vital manifestation.

The great German scientist, Haekel, has said: "I cannot imagine the simplest chemical and physical processes without attributing the movement of the material particles to unconscious sensation. The idea of Chemical Affinity consists in the fact that the various chemical elements perceive differences in the qualities of other elements, and experience pleasure or revulsion at contact with them, and execute their respective movements on this ground." He also says: "We may ascribe the feeling of pleasure or pain (satisfaction or dissatisfaction) to all atoms, and thereby ascribe the elective affinities of chemistry to the attraction between living atoms and repulsion between hating atoms." He also says that "the sensations in animal and plant life are connected by a long series of evolutionary stages with the simpler forms of sensation that we find in the inorganic elements, and that reveal themselves in chemical affinity." Naegli says: "If the molecules possess something that is related, however distantly, to sensation, it must be comfortable for them to be able to follow their attractions and repulsions, and uncomfortable for them when they are forced to do otherwise."

We might fill page after page with quotations from eminent thinkers going to prove the correctness of the old Yogi teachings that Life is Omnipresent. Modern Science is rapidly advancing to this position, leaving behind her the old idea of "dead matter." Even the new theories of the electron—the little particles of electrical energy which are now believed to constitute the base of the atom—does not change this idea, for the electrons manifest attraction, and response thereto, and form themselves into groups composing the atom. And even if we pass beyond matter into the mystical Ether which Science assumes to be the material base of things, we must believe that there is life there too, and that as Prof. Dolbear says: "The Ether has besides the function of energy and motion, other inherent properties, out of which could emerge, under proper circumstances, other phenomena, such as life, mind, or whatever may be in the substratum," and, that as Prof. Cope has hinted, that the basis of Life lies back of the atoms and may be found in the Universal Ether.

Some scientists go even further, and assert that not only is Life present in everything, but that Mind is present where Life is. Verily, the dreams of the Yogi fathers are coming true, and from the ranks of the materialists are coming the material proofs of the spiritual teachings. Listen to these words from Dr. Saleeby, in his recent valuable scientific work, "*Evolution, the Master Key*." He says:

"Life is potential in matter; life-energy is not a thing unique and created at a particular time in the past. If evolution be true, living matter has been evolved by natural processes from matter which is, apparently, not alive. But if life is potential in matter, it is a thousand times more evident that Mind is potential in Life. The evolutionist is impelled to believe that Mind is potential in matter. (I adopt that form of words for the moment, but not without future criticism.) The microscopic cell, a minute speck of matter that is to become man, has in it the promise and the germ of mind. May we not then draw the inference that the elements of mind are present in those chemical elements—carbon, oxygen, hydrogen, nitrogen, sulphur, phosphorus, sodium, potassium, chlorine—that are found in the cell. Not only must we do so, but we must go further, since we know that each of these elements, and every other, is built up out of one invariable unit, the electron, and we must therefore assert that Mind is potential in the unit of Matter—the electron itself... It is to assert the sublime truth first perceived by Spinoza, that Mind and Matter are the warp and woof of what Goethe called 'the living garment of God.' Both are complementary expressions of the Unknowable Reality which underlies both."

There is no such thing as non-vital attraction or repulsion. All inclinations for or against another object, or thing, is an evidence of Life. Each thing has sufficient life energy to enable it to carry on its work. And as each form advances by evolution into a higher form, it is able to have more of the Life energy manifest through it. As its material machinery is built up, it becomes able to manifest a greater and higher degree of Life. It is not that one thing has a low life, or another a high life—this cannot be, for there is but One Life. It is like the current of electricity that is able to run the most delicate machinery or manifest a light in the incandescent lamp. Give it the organ or machinery of manifestation, and it manifests—give it a low form, and it will manifest a low degree—give it a high form, and it will manifest a high degree. The same steam power runs the clumsy engine, or the perfect apparatus which drives the most delicate mechanism. And so it is with the One Life—its manifestations may seem low and clumsy, or high and perfect—but it all depends upon the material or mental machinery through which it works. There is but One Life, manifesting in countless forms and shapes, and degrees. One Life underlying All—in All.

From the highest forms of Life down through the animal, vegetable and mineral kingdoms, we see Life everywhere present—Death an illusion. Back of all visible forms of material life there is still the beginnings of manifested life pressing forward for expression and manifestation. And underneath all is the Spirit of Life—longing, striving, feeling, acting.

In the mountain and the ocean—the flower and the tree—the sunset—the dawn—the suns—the stars—all is Life—manifestations of the One Life. Everything is Alive, quick with living force, power, action; thrilling with vitality; throbbing with feeling; filled with activity. All is from the One Life—and all that is from the One Life is Alive. There is no dead substance in the Universe—there can be none—for Life cannot Die. All is Alive. And Life is in All.

Carry with you this Central Thought of the Lesson:

CENTRAL THOUGHT: *There is but One Life, and its manifestations comprise all the forms and shapes of the Universe. From Life comes but Life—and Life can come only from Life. Therefore we have the right to expect that all manifestations of the One Life should be Alive. And we are not mocked in such belief. Not only do the highest Occult Teachings inform us that Everything is Alive, but Modern Science has proven to us that Life is present everywhere—even in that which was formerly considered dead matter. It now sees that even the atom, and what lies back of the atom, is charged with Life Energy and Action. Forms and shapes may change, and do change—but Life remains eternal and infinite. It cannot Die—for it is LIFE.*

Peace be with thee.

THE THIRD LESSON

THE CREATIVE WILL.

In our first lesson of this series, we stated that among the other qualities and attributes that we were compelled, by the laws of our reason, to think that the Absolute possessed, was that of Omnipotence or All-Power. In other words we are compelled to think of the One as being the source and fount of all the Power there is, ever has been, or ever can be in the Universe. Not only, as is generally supposed, that the Power of the One is greater than any other Power,—but more than this, that there can be no other power, and that, therefore, each and every, any and all manifestations or forms of Power, Force or Energy must be a part of the great one Energy which emanates from the One.

There is no escape from this conclusion, as startling as it may appear to the mind unaccustomed to it. If there is any power not from and of the One, from whence comes such power, for there is nothing else outside of the One? Who or what exists outside of the One that can manifest even the faintest degree of power of any kind? All power must come from the Absolute, and must in its nature be but one.

Modern Science has recognized this truth, and one of its fundamental principles is the Unity of Energy—the theory that all forms of Energy are, at the last, One. Science holds that all forms of Energy are interchangeable, and from this idea comes the theory of the Conservation of Energy or Correlation of Force.

Science teaches that every manifestation of energy, power, or force, from the operation of the law of gravitation, up to the highest form of mental force is but the operation of the One Energy of the Universe.

Just what this Energy is, in its inner nature, Science does not know. It has many theories, but does not advance any of them as a law. It speaks of the Infinite and Eternal Energy from which all things proceed, but pronounces its nature to be unknowable. But some of the latter-day scientists are veering around to the teachings of the occultists, and are now hinting that it is something more than a mere mechanical energy. They are speaking of it in terms of mind. Wundt, the German scientist, whose school of thought is called voluntarism, considers the motive-force of Energy to be something that may be called Will. Crusius, as far back as 1744 said: "Will is the dominating force of the world." And Schopenhauer based his fascinating but gloomy philosophy and metaphysics upon the underlying principle of an active form of energy which he called the Will-to-Live, which he considered to be the Thing-in-Itself, or the Absolute. Balzac, the novelist, considered a something akin to Will, to be the moving force of the Universe. Bulwer advanced a similar theory, and made mention of it in several of his novels

This idea of an active, creative Will, at work in the Universe, building up; tearing down; replacing; repairing; changing—always at work—ever active—has been entertained by numerous philosophers and thinkers, under different names and styles. Some, like Schopenhauer have thought of this Will as the final thing—that which took the place of God—the First Cause. But others have seen in this Will an active living principle emanating from the Absolute or God, and working in accordance with the laws impressed by Him upon it. In various forms, this latter idea is seen all through the history of philosophical thought. Cudsworth, the English philosopher, evolved the idea of a something called the "Plastic Nature," which so closely approaches the Yogi idea of the Creative Will, that we feel justified in quoting a passage from his book. He says:

"It seems not so agreeable to reason that Nature, as a distinct thing from the Deity, should be quite superseded or made to signify nothing, God Himself doing all things immediately and miraculously; from whence it would follow also that they are all done either forcibly and violently, or else artificially only, and none of them by any inward principle of their own.

"This opinion is further confuted by that slow and gradual process that in the generation of things, which would seem to be but a vain and idle pomp or a trifling formality if the moving power were omnipotent; as also by those errors and bungles which are committed where the matter is inept and contumacious; which argue that the moving power be not irresistible, and that Nature is such a thing as is not altogether incapable (as well as human art) of being sometimes frustrated and disappointed by the indisposition of matter. Whereas an omnipotent moving power, as it could dispatch its work in a moment, so would it always do it infallibly and irresistibly, no ineptitude and stubbornness of matter being ever able to hinder such a one, or make him bungle or fumble in anything.

"Wherefore, since neither all things are produced fortuitously, or by the unguided mechanism of matter, nor God himself may be reasonably thought to do all things immediately and miraculously, it may well be concluded that there is a Plastic Nature under him, which, as an inferior and subordinate instrument, doth drudgingly execute that part of his providence which consists in the regular and orderly motion of matter; yet so as there is also besides this a higher providence to be acknowledged, which, presiding over it, doth often supply the defects of it, and sometimes overrules it, forasmuch as the Plastic Nature cannot act electively nor with discretion."

The Yogi Philosophy teaches of the existence of a Universal Creative Will, emanating from the Absolute—infilled with the power of the Absolute and acting under established natural laws, which performs the active work of creation in the world, similar to that performed by "Cudsworth's Plastic Nature," just mentioned. This Creative Will is not Schopenhauer's Will-to-Live. It is not a Thing-in-itself, but a vehicle or instrument of the Absolute. It is an emanation of the mind of the Absolute—a manifestation in action of its Will—a mental product rather than a physical, and, of course, saturated with the life-energy of its projector.

This Creative Will is not a mere blind, mechanical energy or force—it is far more than this. We can explain it only by referring you to the manifestation of the Will in yourself. You wish to move your arm, and it moves. The immediate force may seem to be a mechanical force, but what is back of that force—what is the essence of the force? The Will! All manifestations of energy—all the causes of motion—all forces—are forms of the action of the Will of the One—the Creative Will—acting under natural laws established by the One, ever moving, acting, forcing, urging, driving, leading. We do not mean that every little act is a thought of the moment on the part of the Absolute, and a reaching out of the Will in obedience to that thought. On the contrary, we mean that the One set the Will into operation as a whole, conceiving of laws and limitations in its action, the Will constantly operating in obedience to that conception, the results manifesting in what we call natural law; natural forces, etc. Besides this, the Absolute is believed to manifest its Will specially upon occasions; and moreover permits its Will to be applied and used by the individual wills of individual Egos, under the general Law and laws, and plan of the One.

But you must not suppose that the Will is manifested only in the form of mechanical forces, cohesion, chemical attraction, electricity, gravitation, etc.

It does more than this. It is in full operation in all forms of life, and living things. It is present everywhere. Back of all forms of movement and action, we find a moving cause—usually a *Pressure*. This is true of that which we have been calling mechanical forces, and of all forms of that which we call Life Energy. Now, note this, this great Pressure that you will observe in all Life Action, is the Creative Will—the Will Principle of the One—bending toward the carrying out of the Great Plan of Life.

Look where we will, on living forms, and we may begin to recognize the presence of a certain creative energy at work—building up; moulding, directing; tearing down; replacing, etc.—always active in its efforts to create, preserve and conserve life. This visible creative energy is what the Yogi Philosophy calls "the Creative Will," and which forms the subject of this lesson. The Creative Will is that striving, longing, pressing forward, unfolding, progressing evolutionary effort, that all thoughtful people see in operation in all forms of life—throughout all Nature. From the lowest to the highest forms of life, the Effort, Energy, Pressure, may be recognized in action, creating, preserving, nourishing, and improving its forms. It is that Something that we recognize when we speak of "Nature's Forces" at work in plant growth and animal functioning. If you will but keep the word and idea—"NATURE"—before you, you will be able to more clearly form the mental concept of the Creative Will. The Creative Will is that which you have been calling "Nature at Work" in the growth of the plant; the sprouting of the seed; the curling and reaching of the tendril; the fertilization of the blossoms, etc. You have seen this Will at work, if you have watched growing things.

We call this energy "the Creative Will," because it is the objective manifestation of the Creative Energy of the Absolute—Its visible Will manifested in the direction of physical life. It is as much Will in action, as the Will that causes your arm to move in response to its power. It is no mere chance thing, or mechanical law—it is life action in operation.

This Creative Will not only causes movement in completed life, but all movement and action in life independent of the personal will of its individual forms. All the phenomena of the so-called Unconscious belong to it. It causes the body to grow; attends to the details of nourishment, assimilation, digestion, elimination, and all of the rest. It builds up bodies, organs, and parts, and keeps them in operation and function.

The Creative Will is directed to the outward expression of Life—to the objectification of Life. You may call this energy the "Universal Life Energy" if you wish, but, to those who know it, it is a Will—an active, living Will, in full operation and power, pressing forward toward the manifestation of objective life.

The Creative Will seems to be filled with a strong Desire to manifest. It longs to express itself, and to give birth to forms of activity. Desire lies under and in all forms of its manifestations. The ever present Desire of the Creative Will causes lower forms to be succeeded by higher forms—and is the moving cause of evolution—it is the Evolutionary Urge itself, which ever cries to its manifestations, "Move on; move upward."

In the Hindu classic, the "Mahabarata," Brahma created the most beautiful female being ever known, and called her Tillotama. He presented her in turn to all the gods, in order to witness their wonder and admiration. Siva's desire to behold her was so great that it developed in him four faces, in succession, as she made the tour of the assembly; and Indra's longing was so intense that his body became all eyes. In this myth may be seen exemplified the effect of Desire and Will in the forms of life, function and shape—all following Desire and Need, as in the case of the long neck of the giraffe which enables him to reach for the high branches of the trees in his native land; and in the long neck and high legs of the fisher birds, the crane, stork, ibis, etc.

The Creative Will finds within itself a desire to create suns, and they are formed. It desired planets to revolve around the suns, and they were thrown off in obedience to the law. It desired plant life, and plant life appeared, working from higher to lower form. Then came animal life, from nomad to man. Some of the animal forms yielded to the desire to fly, and wings appeared gradually, and we called it bird-life. Some felt a desire to burrow in the ground, and lo! came the moles, gophers, etc. It wanted a thinking creature, and Man with his wonderful brain was evolved. Evolution is more than a mere survival of the fittest; natural selection, etc. Although it uses these laws as tools and instruments, still back of them is that insistent urge—that ever-impelling desire—that ever-active Creative Will. Lamark was nearer right than Darwin when he claimed that Desire was back of it all, and preceded function and form. Desire wanted form and function, and produced them by the activity of the Creative Will.

This Creative Will acts like a living force—and so it is indeed—but it does not act as a reasoning, intellectual Something, in one sense—instead it manifests rather the "feeling," wanting, longing, instinctive phase of mind, akin to those "feelings" and resulting actions that we find within our natures. The Will acts on the Instinctive Plane.

Evolution shows us Life constantly pressing forward toward higher and still higher forms of expression. The urge is constantly upward and onward. It is true that some species sink out of sight their work in the world having been done, but they are succeeded by other species more in harmony with their environment and the needs of their times. Some races of men decay, but others build on their foundations, and reach still greater heights.

The Creative Will is something different from Reason or Intellect. But it underlies these. In the lower forms of life, in which mind is in but small evidence, the Will is in active operation, manifesting in Instinct and Automatic Life Action, so called. It does not depend upon brains for manifestation—for these lowly forms of life have no brains—but is in operation through every part of the body of the living thing.

Evidences of the existence of the Creative Will acting independently of the brains of animal and plant life may be had in overwhelming quantity if we will but examine the life action in the lower forms of life.

The testimony of the investigators along the lines of the Evolutionary school of thought, show us that the Life Principle was in active operation in lowly animal and plant life millions of years before brains capable of manifesting Thought were produced. Haekel informs us that during more than half of the enormous time that has elapsed since organic life first became evident, no animal sufficiently advanced to have a brain was in existence. Brains were evolved according to the law of desire or necessity, in accordance with the Great Plan, but they were not needed for carrying on the wonderful work of the creation and preservation of the living forms. And they are not today. The tiny infant, and the senseless idiot are not able to think intelligently, but still their life functions go on regularly and according to law, in spite of the absence of thinking brains. And the life work of the plants, and of the lowly forms of animal life, is carried on likewise. This wonderful thing that we call Instinct is but another name for the manifestation of the Creative Will which flows from the One Life, or the Absolute.

Even as far down the scale of life as the Monera, we may see the Creative Will in action. The Monera are but tiny bits of slimy, jelly-like substances—mere specks of glue without organs of any kind, and yet they exercise the organic phenomena of life, such as nutrition, reproduction, sensation and movement, all of which are usually associated with an organized structure. These creatures are incapable of thought in themselves, and the phenomenon is due to the action of the Will through them. This Instinctive impulse and action is seen everywhere, manifesting upon Higher and still higher lines, as higher forms of organisms are built up.

Scientists have used the term, "Appetency," defining it as, "the instinctive tendency of living organisms to perform certain actions; the tendency of an unorganized body to seek that which satisfies the wants of its organism." Now what is this tendency? It cannot be an effort of reason, for the low form of life has nothing with which to reason. And it is impossible to think of "purposive tendency" without assuming the existence of mental power of some kind. And where can such a power be located if not in the form itself? When we consider that the Will is acting in and through all forms of Life, from highest to lowest—from Moneron to Man—we can at once recognize the source of the power and activity. It is the Great Life Principle—the Creative Will, manifesting itself.

We can perhaps better form an idea of the Creative Will, by reference to its outward and visible forms of activity. We cannot see the Will itself—the Pressure and the Urge—but we can see its action through living forms. Just as we cannot see a man behind a curtain, and yet may practically see him by watching the movements of his form as he presses up against the curtain, so may we see the Will by watching it as it presses up against the living curtain of the forms of life. There was a play presented on the American stage a few years ago, in which one of the scenes pictured the place of departed spirits according to the Japanese belief. The audience could not see the actors representing the spirits, but they could see their movements as they pressed up close to a thin silky curtain stretched across the stage, and their motions as they moved to and fro behind the curtain were plainly recognized. The deception was perfect, and the effect was startling. One almost believed that he saw the forms of formless creatures. And this is what we may do in viewing the operation of the Creative Will—we may take a look at the moving form of the Will behind the curtain of the forms of the manifestation of life. We may see it pressing and urging here, and bending there—building up here, and changing there—always acting, always moving, striving, doing, in response to that insatiable urge and craving, and longing of its inner desire. Let us take a few peeps at the Will moving behind the curtain!

Commencing with the cases of the forming of the crystals, as spoken of in our last lesson, we may pass on to plant life. But before doing so, it may be well for us to take a parting look at the Will manifesting crystal forms. One of the latest scientific works makes mention of the experiments of a scientist who has been devoting much attention to the formation of crystals, and reports that he has noticed that certain crystals of organic compounds, instead of being built up symmetrically, as is usual with crystals, were "enation-morphic," that is, opposed to each other, in rights and lefts, like hands or gloves, or shoes, etc. These crystals are never found alone, but always form in pairs. Can you not see the Will behind the curtain here?

Let us look for the Will in plant-life. Passing rapidly over the wonderful evidences in the cases of the fertilization of plants by insects, the plant shaping its blossom so as to admit the entrance of the particular insect that acts as the carrier of its pollen, think for a moment how the distribution of the seed is provided for. Fruit trees and plants surround the seed with a sweet covering, that it may be eaten by insect and animal, and the seed distributed. Others have a hard covering to protect the seed or nut from the winter frosts, but which covering rots with the spring rains and allows the germ to sprout. Others surround the seed with a fleecy substance, so that the wind may carry it here and there and give it a chance to find a home where it is not so crowded. Another tree has a little pop-gun arrangement, by means of which it pops its seed to a distance of several feet.

Other plants have seeds that are covered with a burr or "sticky" bristles, which enables them to attach themselves to the wool of sheep and other animals, and thus be carried about and finally dropped in some spot far away from the parent plant, and thus the scattering of the species be accomplished. Some plants show the most wonderful plans and arrangements for this scattering of the seed in new homes where there is a better opportunity for growth and development, the arrangements for this purpose displaying something very much akin to what we would call "ingenuity" if it were the work of a reasoning mind. There are plants called cockle-burs whose seed-pods are provided with stickers in every direction, so that anything brushing against them is sure to pick them up. At the end of each sticker is a very tiny hook, and these hooks fasten themselves tightly into anything that brushes against it, animal wool, hair, or clothing, etc. Some of these seeds have been known to have been carried to other quarters of the globe in wool, etc., there to find new homes and a wider field.

Other plants, like the thistle, provide their seed with downy wings, by which the wind carries them afar to other fields. Other seeds have a faculty of tumbling and rolling along the ground to great distances, owing to their peculiar shape and formation. The maple provides its seed with a peculiar arrangement something like a propeller screw, which when the wind strikes the trees and looses the seed, whirls the latter through the air to a distance of a hundred yards or more. Other seeds are provided with floating apparatus, which enables them to travel many miles by stream or river, or rain washes. Some of these not only float, but actually swim, having spider-like filaments, which wriggle like legs, and actually propel the tiny seed along to its new home. A recent writer says of these seeds that "so curiously lifelike are their movements that it is almost impossible to believe that these tiny objects, making good progress through the water, are really seeds, and not insects."

The leaves of the Venus' Fly-trap fold upon each other and enclose the insect which is attracted by the sweet juice on the leaf, three extremely sensitive bristles or hairs giving the plant notice that the insect is touching them. A recent writer gives the following description of a peculiar plant. He says: "On the shores of Lake Nicaragua is to be found an uncanny product of the vegetable kingdom known among the natives by the expressive name of 'the Devil's Noose.' Dunstan, the naturalist, discovered it long ago while wandering on the shores of the lake. Attracted by the cries of pain and terror from his dog, he found the animal held by black sticky bands which had chafed the skin to bleeding point. These bands were branches of a newly-discovered carnivorous plant which had been aptly named the 'land octopus.' The branches are flexible, black, polished and without leaves, and secrete a viscid fluid."

You have seen flowers that closed when you touched them. You remember the Golden Poppy that closes when the sun goes down. Another plant, a variety of orchid, has a long, slender, flat stem, or tube, about one-eighth of an inch thick, with an opening at the extreme end, and a series of fine tubes where it joins the plant. Ordinarily this tube remains coiled up into a spiral, but when the plant needs water (it usually grows upon the trunks of trees overhanging swampy places) it slowly uncoils the little tube and bends it over until it dips into the water, when it proceeds to suck up the water until it is filled, when it slowly coils around and discharges the water directly upon the plant, or its roots. Then it repeats the process until the plant is satisfied. When the water is absent from under the plant the tube moves this way and that way until it finds what it wants—just like the trunk of an elephant. If one touches the tube or trunk of the plant while it is extended for water, it shows a great sensitiveness and rapidly coils itself up. Now what causes this life action? The plant has no brains, and cannot have reasoned out this process, nor even have acted upon them by reasoning processes. It has nothing to think with to such a high degree. It is the Will behind the curtain, moving this way and that way, and doing things.

There was once a French scientist named Duhamel. He planted some beans in a cylinder—something like a long tomato can lying on its side. He waited until the beans began to sprout, and send forth roots downward, and shoots upward, according to nature's invariable rule. Then he moved the cylinder a little—rolled it over an inch or two. The next day he rolled it over a little more. And so on each day, rolling it over a little each time. Well, after a time Duhamel shook the dirt and growing beans out of the cylinder, and what did he find? This, that the beans in their endeavor to grow their roots downward had kept on bending each day downward; and in their endeavor to send shoots upward, had kept on bending upward a little each day, until at last there had been formed two complete spirals—the one spiral being the roots ever turning downward, and the other the shoots ever bending upward. How did the plant know direction? What was the moving power. The Creative Will behind the curtain again, you see!

Potatoes in dark cellars have sent out roots or sprouts twenty and thirty feet to reach light. Plants will send out roots many feet to reach water. They know where the water and light are, and where to reach them. The tendrils of a plant know where the stake or cord is, and they reach out for it and twine themselves around it. Unwind them, and the next day they are found again twined around it. Move the stake or cord, and the tendril moves after it. The insect-eating plants are able to distinguish between nitrogenous and non-nitrogenous food, accepting the one and rejecting the other. They recognize that cheese has the same nourishing properties as the insect, and they accept it, although it is far different in feeling, taste, appearance and every other characteristic from their accustomed food.

Case after case might be mentioned and cited to show the operation of the Will in plant-life. But wonderful as are many of these cases, the mere action of the Will as shown in the *growing* of the plant is just as wonderful. Just imagine a tiny seed, and see it sprout and draw to itself the nourishment from water, air, light and soil, then upward until it becomes a great tree with bark, limbs, branches, leaves, blossoms, fruit and all. Think of this miracle, and consider what must be the power and nature of that Will that causes it.

The growing plant manifests sufficient strength to crack great stones, and lift great slabs of pavement, as may be noticed by examining the sidewalks of suburban towns and parks. An English paper prints a report of four enormous mushrooms having lifted a huge slab of paving stone in a crowded street overnight. Think of this exhibition of Energy and Power. This wonderful faculty of exerting force and motion and energy is fundamental in the Will, for indeed every physical change and growth is the result of motion, and motion arises only from force and pressure. Whose force, energy, power and motion? The Will's!

On all sides of us we may see this constant and steady urge and pressure behind living forces, and inorganic forms as well—always a manifestation of Energy and Power. And all this Power is in the Will—and the Will is but the manifestation of the All-Power—the Absolute. Remember this.

And this power manifests itself not only in the matter of growth and ordinary movements, but also in some other ways that seem quite mysterious to even modern Science. How is it that certain birds are able to fly directly against a strong wind, without visible movement of their wings? How do the buzzards float in the air, and make speed without a motion of the wing? What is the explanation of the movements of certain microscopic creatures who lack organs of movement? Listen to this instance related by the scientist Benet. He states that the Polycystids have a most peculiar manner of moving—a sort of sliding motion, to the right or left, upward, backward, sideways, stopping and starting, fast or slow, as it wills. It has no locomotive organs, and no movement can be seen to take place in the body from within or without. It simply slides. How?

Passing on to the higher animal life—how do eggs grow into chickens? What is the power in the germ of the egg? Can the germ think, and plan, and move, and grow into a chicken? Or is the Will at work there? And what is true in this case, is true of the birth and growth of all animal life—all animal life develops from a single germ cell. How, and Why?

There is a mental energy resident in the germ cell—of this there can be no doubt. And that mental energy is the Creative Will ever manifesting. Listen to these words from Huxley, the eminent scientist. He says:

"The student of Nature wonders the more and is astonished the less, the more conversant he becomes with her operations; but of all the perennial miracles she offers to his inspection, perhaps the most worthy of his admiration is the development of a plant or of an animal from its embryo. Examine the recently laid egg of some common animal, such as a salamander or a newt. It is a minute spheroid in which the best microscope will reveal nothing but a structureless sac, enclosing a glairy fluid, holding granules in suspension. But strange possibilities lie dormant in that semi-fluid globule. Let a moderate supply of warmth reach its watery cradle, and the plastic matter undergoes changes so rapid, and so purposelike in their succession, that one can only compare them to those operated by a skilled modeller upon a formless lump of clay. As with an invisible trowel, the mass is divided and subdivided into smaller and smaller portions, until it is reduced to an aggregation of granules not too large to build withal the finest fabrics of the nascent organism. And, then, it is as if a delicate finger traced out the line to be occupied by the spinal column, and moulded the contour of the body; pinching up the head at one end, the tail at the other, and fashioning flank and limb into due salamanderine proportions, in so artistic a way that, after watching the process hour by hour, one is almost involuntarily possessed by the notion that some more subtle aid to vision than the achromatic lens would show the hidden artist, with his plan before him, striving with skilful manipulation to perfect his work.

"As life advances and the young amphibian ranges the waters, the terror of his insect contemporaries, not only are the nutritious particles supplied by its prey (by the addition of which to its frame growth takes place) laid down, each in its proper spot, and in due proportion to the rest, as to reproduce the form, the color, and the size, characteristic of the parental stock; but even the wonderful powers of reproducing lost parts possessed by these animals are controlled by the same governing tendency. Cut off the legs, the tail, the jaws, separately or all together, and as Spallanzani showed long ago, these parts not only grow again, but the new limb is formed on the same type as those which were lost. The new jaw, or leg, is a newt's, and never by any accident more like that of a frog's."

In this passage from Huxley one may see the actual working of the Creative Will of the Universe,—moving behind the curtain—and a very thin curtain at that. And this wonderful work is going on all around us, all the time. Miracles are being accomplished every second—they are so common that we fail to regard them.

And in our bodies is the Will at work? Most certainly. What built you up from single cell to maturity? Did you do it with your intellect? Has not every bit of it been done without your conscious knowledge? It is only when things go wrong, owing to the violation of some law, that you become aware of your internal organs. And, yet, stomach and liver, and heart and the rest have been performing their work steadily—working away day and night, building up, repairing, nourishing, growing you into a man or woman, and keeping you sound and strong. Are you doing this with your reason or with your personal will? No, it is the great Creative Will of the Universe, Universe,—the expression of the purpose and power of the One, working in and through you. It is the One Life manifesting in you through its Creative Will.

And not only is this all. The Creative Will is all around us in every force, energy and principle. The force that we call mental power is the principle of the Will directed by our individual minds. In this statement we have a hint of the great mystery of Mental Force and Power, and the so-called Psychic Phenomena. It also gives us a key to Mental Healing. This is not the place to go into detail regarding these phases—but think over it a bit. This Will Power of the Universe, in all of its forms and phases, from Electricity to Thought-power, is always at the disposal of Man, within limits, and subject always to the laws of the Creative Will of the Universe. Those who acquire an understanding of the laws of any force may use it. And any force may be used or misused.

And the nearer in understanding and consciousness that we get to the One Life and Power, the greater will be our possible power, for we are thus getting closer and closer to the source of All Power. In these lessons we hope to be able to tell you how you may come into closer touch with this One Life of which you and all living things are but forms, shapes and channels of expression, under the operation of the Creative Will.

We trust that this lesson may have brought to your minds the realization of the Oneness of All—the fact that we are all parts of the one encircling unity, the heart-throbs and pulsations of which are to be felt even to the outer edge of the circle of life—in Man, in Monad, in Crystal, in Atom. Try to feel that inner essence of Creative Will that is within yourselves, and endeavor to realize your complete inner unity in it, with all other forms of life. Try to realize, as some recent writer has expressed it, "that all the living world is but mankind in the making, and that we are but part of the All." And also remember that splendid vistas of future unfoldment spread themselves out before the gaze of the awakened soul, until the mind fails to grasp the wondrous sight.

We will now close this lesson by calling your attention to its

CENTRAL THOUGHT.

There is but One Power in the Universe—One Energy—One Force. And that Power, Energy and Force is a manifestation of the One Life. There can be no other Power, for there is none other than the One from whom Power may come. And there can be no manifestation of Power that is not the Power of the One, for no other Power can be in existence. The Power of the One is visible in its manifestations to us in the natural laws and forces of Nature—which we call the Creative Will. This Creative Will is the inner moving power, urge and pressure behind all forms and shapes of Life. In atom, and molecule; in monad, in cell, in plant, in fish, in animal, in man,—the Life Principle or Creative Will is constantly in action, creating, preserving, and carrying on life in its functions. We may call this Instinct or Nature, but it is the Creative Will in action. This Will is back of all Power, Energy, or Force—be it physical, mechanical or mental force. And all Force that we use, consciously or unconsciously, comes from the One Great Source of Power. If we could but see clearly, we would know that back of us is the Power of the Universe, awaiting our intelligent uses, under the control of the Will of the All. There is nothing to be afraid of, for we are manifestations of the One Life, from which all Power proceeds, and the Real Self is above the effect, for it is part of the Cause. But over and above—under and behind—all forms of Being, Matter, Energy, Force and Power, is the ABSOLUTE—ever Calm; ever Peaceful; ever Content. In knowing this it becomes us to manifest that spirit of absolute Trust, Faith and Confidence in the Goodness and Ultimate Justice of That which is the only Reality there is.

Peace be with you.

THE FOURTH LESSON

THE UNITY OF LIFE.

In our First Lesson of this series we spoke of the One Reality underlying all Life. This One Reality was stated to be higher than mind or matter, the nearest term that can be applied to it being "Spirit." We told you that it was impossible to explain just what "Spirit" is, for we have nothing else with which to compare or describe it, and it can be expressed only in its own terms, and not in the terms applicable to its emanations or manifestations. But, as we said in our First Lesson, we may think of "Spirit" as meaning the "essence" of Life and Being—the Reality underlying Universal Life, and from which the latter emanates.

In the Second Lesson we stated that this "Spirit," which we called "The Absolute," expressed itself in the Universal Life, which Universal Life manifested itself in countless forms of life and activity. In the same lesson we showed you that the Universe is alive—that there is not a single dead thing in it—that there can be no such thing as a dead object in the Universe, else the theory and truth of the One underlying Life must fall and be rejected. In that lesson we also showed you that even in the world of inorganic things there was ever manifest life—in every atom and particle of inorganic matter there is the universal life energy manifesting itself, and in constant activity.

In the Third Lesson, we went still further into this phase of the general subject, and showed you that the Creative Will—that active principle of the Universal Life—was ever at work, building up new forms, shapes and combinations, and then tearing them down for the purpose of rebuilding the material into new forms, shapes, and combinations. The Creative Will is ever at work in its threefold function of creating, preserving and destroying forms—the change, however, being merely in the shape and form or combination, the real substance remaining unchanged in its inner aspect, notwithstanding the countless apparent changes in its objective forms. Like the great ocean the depths of which remain calm and undisturbed, and the real nature of which is unchanged in spite of the waves, and billows of surface manifestation, so does the great ocean of the Universal Life remain unchanged and unaltered in spite of the constant play of the Creative Will upon the surface. In the same lesson we gave you many examples of the Will in action—of its wondrous workings in the various forms of life and activity—all of which went to show you that the One Power was at work everywhere and at all times.

In our next lesson—the Fifth Lesson—we shall endeavor to make plain to you the highest teachings of the Yogi Philosophy regarding the One Reality and the Many Manifestations—the One and the Many—how the One apparently becomes Many—that great question and problem which lies at the bottom of the well of truth. In that lesson we shall present for your consideration some fundamental and startling truths, but before we reach that point in our teachings, we must fasten upon your mind the basic truth that all the various manifestations of Life that we see on all hands in the Universe are but forms of manifestation of One Universal Life which is itself an emanation of the Absolute.

Speaking generally, we would say to you that the emanation of the Absolute is in the form of a grand manifestation of One Universal Life, in which the various apparent separate forms of Life are but centers of Energy or Consciousness, the separation being more apparent than real, there being a bond of unity and connection underlying all the apparently separated forms. Unless the student gets this idea firmly fixed in his mind and consciousness, he will find it difficult to grasp the higher truths of the Yogi Philosophy. That all Life is One, at the last,—that all forms of manifestation of Life are in harmonious Unity, underlying—is one of the great basic truths of the Yogi Teaching, and all the students of that philosophy must make this basic truth their own before they may progress further. This grasping of the truth is more than a mere matter of intellectual conception, for the intellect reports that all forms of Life are separate and distinct from each other, and that there can be no unity amidst such diversity. But from the higher parts of the mind comes the message of an underlying Unity, in spite of all apparent diversity, and if one will meditate upon this idea he will soon begin to realize the truth, and will *feel* that he, himself, is but a center of consciousness in a great ocean of Life—that he and all other centers are connected by countless spiritual and mental filaments—and that all emerge from the One. He will find that the illusion of separateness is but "a working fiction of the Universe," as one writer has so aptly described it—and that All is One, at the last, and underlying all is One.

Some of our students may feel that we are taking too long a path to lead up to the great basic truths of our philosophy, but we who have traveled The Path, and know its rocky places and its sharp turns, feel justified in insisting that the student be led to the truth gradually and surely, instead of attempting to make short cuts across dangerous ravines and canyons. We must insist upon presenting our teachings in our own way—for this way has been tested and found good. We know that every student will come to realize that our plan is a wise one, and that he will thank us for giving him this gradual and easy approach to the wondrous and awful truth which is before us. By this gradual process, the mind becomes accustomed to the line of thought and the underlying principles, and also gradually discards wornout mental sheaths which have served their purposes, and which must be discarded because they begin to weigh heavily upon the mind as it reaches the higher altitudes of The Path of Attainment. Therefore, we must ask you to consider with us, in this lesson, some further teachings regarding the Unity of Life.

All the schools of the higher Oriental thought, as well as many of the great philosophical minds of the Western world, have agreed upon the conception of the Unity of Life—the Oneness of All Life. The Western thinkers, and many of the Eastern philosophers arrived at this conclusion by means of their Intellectual powers, greatly heightened and stimulated by concentration and meditation, which latter process liberated the faculties of the Spiritual Mind so that it passed down knowledge to the Intellect, which then seized upon the higher knowledge which it found within itself, and amplified and theorized upon the same. But among the Eastern Masters there are other sources of information open, and from these sources come the same report—the Oneness and Unity of Universal Life. These higher sources of information to which we have alluded, consist of the knowledge coming from those Beings who have passed on to higher planes of Life than ours, and whose awakened spiritual faculties and senses enable them to see things quite plainly which are quite dark to us. And from these sources, also, comes the message of the Oneness of Life—of the existence of a wonderful Universal Life including all forms of life as we know it, and many forms and phases unknown to us—many centers in the great Ocean of Life. No matter how high the source of inquiry, the answer is the same—"All Life is One." And this One Life includes Beings as much higher than ourselves, as we are higher than the creatures in the slime of the ocean-bed. Included in it are beings who would seem as archangels or gods to us, and they inform that beyond them are still higher and more radiant creatures, and so on to infinity of infinities. And yet all are but centers of Being in the One Life—all but a part of the great Universal Life, which itself is but an emanation of The Absolute.

The mind of man shrinks back appalled from the contemplation of such wonders, and yet there are men who dare to attempt to speak authoritatively of the attributes and qualities of "God," as if He, the Absolute, were but a magnified man. Verily, indeed, "fools rush in where angels fear to tread," as the poet hath said.

Those who will read our next lesson and thus gain an idea of the sublime conception of the Absolute held by the Yogi teachers may shudder at the presumption of those mortals who dare to think of the Absolute as possessing "attributes" and "qualities" like unto the meanest of things in this his emanated Universe. But even these spiritual infants are doing well—that is, they are beginning to *think*, and when man begins to *think* and *question*, he begins to progress. It is not the fact of these people's immature ideas that has caused these remarks on our part, but rather their tendency to set up their puny conceptions as the absolute truth, and then insisting upon forcing these views upon the outer world of men, whom they consider "poor ignorant heathen." Permit each man to think according to his light—and help him by offering to share with him the best that you possess—but do not attempt to force upon him your own views as absolute truth to be swallowed by him under threat of damnation or eternal punishment. Who are you that dares to speak of punishment and damnation, when the smell of the smoke of the hell of materialism is still upon your robes. When you realize just what spiritual infants you still are—the best of you—you will blush at these things. Hold fast to the best that you know—be generous to others who seem to wish to share your knowledge—but give without blame or feeling of superiority—for those whom you teach today may be your teachers tomorrow—there are many surprises of this kind along The Path. Be brave and confident, but when you begin to feel puffed up by your acquirement of some new bit of knowledge, let your prayer—*our* prayer, for we too are infants—be, "Lord, be merciful unto me, a fool!"

The above words are for us, the students of the Yogi Philosophy—the teachers of the same—for human nature is the same in spite of names, and we must avoid the "vanity of vanities"—Spiritual Pride and Arrogance—that fault which has sent many a soul tumbling headlong from a high position on The Path, and compelled it to again begin the journey, chastened and bruised. The fall of Lucifer has many correspondences upon the occult plane, and is, indeed, in itself an allegorical illustration of just this law. Remember, always, that you are but a Centre in the Ocean of Life, and that all others are Centres in the same ocean, and that underlying both and all of you is the same calm bed of Life and Knowledge, the property of all. The highest and the lowest are part of the same One Life—each of you has the same life blood flowing through your veins—you are connected with every other form of life, high or low, with invisible bonds, and none is separate from another. We are speaking, of course, to the personalities of the various students who are reading these words. The Real Self of each is above the need of such advice and caution, and those who are able to reach the Real Self in consciousness have no need for these words, for they have outlived this stage of error. To many, the consciousness of the One Life—the Universal Life—in which all are centres of consciousness and being—has come gradually as a final step of a long series of thought and reasoning, aided by flashes of truth from the higher regions of the mind. To others it has come as a great illumination, or flash of Truth, in which all things are seen in their proper relations and positions to each other, and all as phases of being in the One. The term "Cosmic Consciousness," which has been used in the previous series of these lessons, and by other writers, means this sudden flash of "knowing" in which all the illusionary dividing lines between persons and things are broken down and the Universal Life is seen to be actually existent as One Life. To those who have reached this consciousness by either route just mentioned—or by other routes—there is no sense of loss of individuality or power or strength. On the contrary there is always a new sense of increased power and strength and knowing—instead of losing Individuality, there is a sense of having found it. One feels that he has the whole Universe at his back, or within him, rather than that he has lost his identity in the great Ocean of Life.

While we are speaking of this phase of the subject, we should like to ask you if you have ever investigated and inquired into the real meaning of the much-used word "Individuality?" Have you ever looked up its origin and real meaning, as given by the standard authorities? We are sure that many of you have no real idea of the actual meaning of the term, as strange as this statement may appear to you at first glance. Stop now, and define the word to yourself, as you have been accustomed to think of it. Ninety-five people of a hundred will tell you that it means something like "a strong personality." Let us see about this.

Webster defines the word "Individual" as follows: "Not divided, or not to be divided; existing as one distinct being or object; single; one." The same authority informs us that the word arises from the Latin word *individuus*, meaning "indivisible; not divisible." Does not this help you to gain a clearer idea of the Individuality that knows itself to be a Centre of Consciousness in the One Life, rather than a separate, puny, insignificant thing apart from all other centres or forms of Life, or the source of Life? We think it will help to clear your mind of some of the fog that has not as yet lifted itself.

And while we are on the subject of definitions, let us take a little look at the word "Personality," that is generally believed to be a synonym of "Individuality," and is often so used. Webster tells us that the word "Person" originated from the Latin word *persona*, meaning "a mask used by actors," which word in turn arose from two other words, *per*, meaning "through," and *sonare*, meaning "to sound," the two combined words meaning "to sound through." The same authority informs us that the archaic meaning of the word was "a character or part, as in a play; an assumed character." If you will think of Personality as "a mask used by an actor," or as "a part in a play," or as something used to "sound through" or to speak through, by the real Individual behind the mask of Personality, then perhaps you will see a little further into the Mystery of Personality and Individuality.

Oh, dear students, be not deceived by the mask of Personality which you may happen to be wearing at this moment, or by the masks which are worn by those around you. Realize that back of your mask is the great Individual—the Indivisible—the Universal Life, in which you are a centre of consciousness and activity. This does not wipe out your identity—instead it gives you a greater and grander identity. Instead of your sinking into a Nirvana of extinction of consciousness, your consciousness so enlarges as you unfold, that you will in the end feel your identity to be the identity of the Universe. Instead of your gaining Nothingness, you gain Allness. All spiritual growth and unfoldment gives you a constantly increasing sense of relationship with, and agreement with, the All. You grow into Allness as you unfold. Be not deceived by this chatter about Nothingness, and loss of Individuality, in the Oriental thought, although some of the presentations of its teachings may so seem to mean at first reading. Remember always that Personality is the mask, and Individuality the Real One.

You have often heard persons, claiming to be acquainted with the teachings of Theosophy and other expositions of the Oriental Wisdom Religion (including our own presentation), asserting that the Oriental mind was ever bent upon attaining a final stage of Nothingness or Extinction in Nirvana. In addition to what we have said, and to what we shall say on this subject, let us quote from the inspired writer of the "*Secret Doctrine*" (a standard Theosophical work) when she says, in that work on page 286, Vol. I: "Is this annihilation, as some think? … To see in Nirvana annihilation, amounts to saying of a man plunged in a sound, dreamless sleep—one that leaves no impression on the physical memory and brain, because the sleeper's Higher Self is in its original state of absolute consciousness during these hours—that he too is annihilated. The latter simile answers only to one side of the question—the most material; since reabsorption is by no means such a dreamless sleep, but, on the contrary, absolute existence, an unconditional unity, or a state, to describe which human language is absolutely and hopelessly inadequate… Nor is the individuality—nor even the essence of the personality, if any be left behind—lost because re-absorbed." As J. Wm. Lloyd says, in connection with the above quotation, "This seems conclusive proof that Theosophy does not regard Nirvana as annihilation, but as an infinite enlargement of consciousness." And we would add that this is true not only as regards the Nirvana of the Theosophist, but also of the consciousness of the Unity of Life—the Universal Life. This too is not annihilation of individual consciousness, but an "infinite enlargement of consciousness" as this Western writer Lloyd has so well expressed it.

The very consciousness of Life that every man feels within him, comes not from something belonging exclusively to himself as a separate or personal thing. On the contrary, it belongs to his Individuality, not to his Personality, and is a phase of his consciousness or "awareness" of his relation to the One Universal Life which underlies his existence, and in which he is a center of consciousness. Do you grasp this idea? If not, meditate and concentrate upon it, for it is important. You must learn to *feel* the Life within you, and to know that it is the Life of the great Ocean of Universal Life upon the bosom of which you are borne as a centre of consciousness and energy. In this thought there is Power, Strength, Calm, Peace, and Wisdom. Acquire it, if you are wise. It is indeed a Gift from the Gods.

In this lesson we are not attempting to build up your idea of the Unity of Life by a series of arguments taken from a world of phenomena in which separateness and non-Unity is apparent. No such arguments would suffice, for it would be like trying to prove the existence and laws of color to a man born blind, by arguments taken from his world of darkness. On the contrary we are appealing to that region of the mind in which is stored the capacity for intuitively apprehending truth. We are endeavoring to speak in tones which will awaken a similar vibration in that part of your mentality, and if these vibrations be started into being, then will you be able to *feel* and *know* the truth, and then will your Intellect eagerly seize upon the new idea that it finds within itself, and will proceed to apply the same to the various problems that have been bothering you in the past.

This consciousness of Unity must come from the higher regions of the mind, for the Intellect alone knows it not,—it is out of its field. Just as one may not know that the earth is round by means of his senses which report quite the contrary, but may and does know this truth by abstract reasoning and higher intellectual effort; so may one know the truth that All Life is indeed One, at the last, and underlying, by the higher faculties of the mind, although his senses and ordinary intellectual processes fail to so inform him. The senses cannot inform man that the earth is round, *because they cannot see it as a whole, but only in part*—while the higher reasoning faculties are able to visualize the earth as a whole, and know it must be round. And the Intellect, in its ordinary field can see only separateness, and cannot report Oneness, but the Higher Mind sees Life as a Whole, and knows it to be One. And it is the Higher Mind that we are trying to bring into the field of consciousness in the appeal to you in this lesson. We trust that we may be successful—in fact we *know* that we shall be so, in many cases, for we know that the field is ready for the sowing of the seed—and that the call has been heard, and the message passed on to us to answer the call—else these words would not have been written.

The consciousness of the Unity of Life is something that must be experienced before the truth may be realized. It is not necessary for one to wait until he acquire full Cosmic Consciousness before he may realize, at least partially, the Oneness of All Life, for he may unfold gradually into the Cosmic Knowing, experiencing at each stage a fuller conception of the underlying Unity of Life, in which he is a centre of consciousness and manifestation. But there must be at least a partial unfoldment before one is able to *feel* the sense of Unity. To those who have not unfolded sufficiently to gain at least a glimmering of the truth, everything appears separate from every other thing, and there is no Unity of All. It is as if every leaf on a mighty tree were to consider itself a being separate and distinct from everything else in the world, failing to perceive its connection with the branch or limb, and tree, and its unity in being with every other leaf on the tree. After a bit the unfolding consciousness of the leaf enables it to perceive the stem that connects it with the twig. Then it begins to realize certain relationships, and feels its vital connection with the twig and the few other leaves attached to the same twig. Later on, it unfolds sufficiently to perceive that certain other leaf-bearing twigs are connected with the same branch, and it learns to feel its relationship with all twigs and leaves springing from that branch. Then again, a little later on, it begins to realize that other branches spring from the same limb as its branch, and the sense of relationship and dawning Unity begins to widen still further. And so it goes on, until at last, the tiny leaflet realizes that the life of the tree is the life of all of its parts—limbs, branches, twigs, leaves, blossoms, fruit, seed, etc., and that it, itself, is but a centre of expression in the One Life of the tree. Does the leaf feel less important and real from this discovery? We should say assuredly not, for it must feel that behind its tiny form and limited strength is the strength and vitality of the entire organism of the tree. It must know that the tree is ever at work extracting nourishment from the earth, air, and water, and transmitting that nourishment to its every part, including our little friend the leaflet. It knows that the sap will rise in the Spring to renew the manifestations of life, and it knows that although its leafy form may wither and die, still the essence of its life—its real Life—does not die but remains ever active and strong awaiting its chance for future expression and re-embodiment. Of course this figure of the leaf and the tree fails us if we attempt to carry it very far, but it will give us at least a partial idea of the relationship between the life of the person, and the One Life.

Some of the Oriental teachers have illustrated this idea to their students by various familiar examples and figures of speech. Some bid the student hold up his hand, and then point out to him that each finger is apparently separate and distinct if one does not look down to where it joins the hand. Each finger, if it had consciousness, might well argue that it was a separate individual, having no relationship with any other finger. It might prove this to its own satisfaction, and to that of its listeners, by showing that it could move itself without stirring the other fingers. And so long as its consciousness was confined to its upper two joints it would remain under the illusion of separateness. But when its consciousness at last permeated the depths of its being, it would find that it emerged from the same hand from which also sprung the other fingers, and that its real life and power was vested in the hand rather than in itself, and that although apparently separate and independent, it was really but a part of the hand. And when its consciousness, through the consciousness of the hand, broadened and widened, it would perceive its relationship with, and interdependence with, the whole body, and would also recognize the power of the brain, and its mighty Will.

Another favorite illustration of the Eastern teachers is the stream of water flowing over a rocky bed. They point to the stream before it comes to a rocky place, and show the *chela* (student) that it is One. Then they will move a little way down the stream and show him how the rocks and stones divide the stream into countless little streams, each of which might imagine itself a separate and distinct stream, until later on it again joins the main united stream, and finds that it was but a form of expression of the One.

Another illustration that is frequently used by the teachers, is that which bids the student consider himself as a minute cell, or "little-life" as the Hindus call it, in a body. It may be a cell in the blood performing the office of a carrier or messenger, or it may be a working cell in one of the organs of the body; or it may be a thinking cell in the brain. At any rate, the cell manifests capacity for thought, action and memory—and a number of secondary attributes quite wonderful in the way. (See "*Hatha Yoga*," Chapter XVIII.) Each cell might well consider itself as a separate individual—in a certain sense it *does*. It has a certain degree of something akin to consciousness, enabling it to perform its work correctly and properly, and is called upon at times to manifest something like judgment. It may well be excused for thinking of itself as a "person" having a separate life. The analogy between its illusions and that of the man when seen by a Master, is very close. But we know that the life of the cell is merely a centre of expression of the life of the body—that its consciousness is merely a part of the consciousness of the mind animating the body. The cell will die and apparently perish, but the *essence* of it will remain in the life of the person whose body it occupied, and nothing really dies or perishes. Would the cell feel any less real if it knew that behind its Personality as a cell, there was the Individuality of the Man—that its Real Self was the Man, not the cell? Of course, even this figure of speech can be carried only so far, and then must stop, for the personality of the man, when it is dissolved, leaves behind it an essence which is called Character, which becomes the property of the Ego and which accompanies it into after life according to the Law of Karma, of which we shall speak in future lessons. But back even of these attributes of Personality, is the Ego which exists in spite of Personality, and lives on and on throughout many Personalities, and yet learning the lessons of each, until at last it rises above Personality and enters into higher sphere of Knowing and Being.

Still another favorite illustration of the Hindu teachers is that of the sun beating down upon the ocean and causing a portion of the water to rise in the form of vapor. This vapor forms clouds which spread all over the earth, and which eventually condense in the form of rain drops, dew, etc. This rain and dew form streams, rivers, etc., and sooner or later every drop finds its way back to Mother Ocean which is its Real Self. Separate though the dewdrop be, yet it is a part of the Ocean, no matter how far distant it may be, and the attraction of the Ocean will surely, and without fail, draw it back to its bosom. And the dewdrop, if it could know the truth, would be so much happier and stronger, and braver if it could know that it was superior to accident, time and space, and that it could not escape its own good, and that nothing could prevent its final triumph and victory when at last "the dewdrop glides into the shining sea." How cheerfully it could have met its many changes of form. and the incidents of its journey, if it could have gotten rid of the illusion of separateness, and knew that instead of being a tiny insignificant dewdrop it was a part of the Mighty Ocean—in fact that its Real Self was that Ocean itself—and that the Ocean was continually drawing it toward it, and that the many changes, up and down, were in response to that mighty power of attraction which was slowly but irresistibly drawing it back Home to Rest, Peace, and Power.

As valuable as are all these illustrations, examples, and figures of speech, still all must of necessity fall short of the truth in the case of the Soul of Man—that wondrous something which has been built up by the Absolute after aeons and aeons of time, and which is destined to play an important part in the great Cosmic Drama which it has pleased the Absolute to think into existence. Drawing its Life from the Universal Life, it has the roots of its being still further back in the Absolute itself, as we shall see in the next lesson. Great and wonderful is it all, and our minds are but illy fitted to receive the truth, and must be gradually accustomed to the glare of the Sun. But it will come to all—none can escape his glorious destiny.

The Oriental writings are full of allusions to the underlying Oneness, in fact the entire Oriental philosophies rest upon it. You may find it everywhere if you will but look for it. The experience of Cosmic Consciousness, which is naught but a sudden or gradual "awareness" of the underlying Unity of Life, is evidenced everywhere in the *Upanishads*, that wonderful series of teachings in the Hindu classics. Every writer in the collection gives his evidence regarding this awareness of Unity and Oneness, and the experiences and mental characteristics arising from the same. The following quotations will give an idea of the prevalence of this thought:

"He that beholds all beings in the Self, and the Self in all things, he never turns away from it."

"When to a man who understands, the Self has become all things, what sorrow, what trouble, can there be to him who once beheld that unity."

The Hindu father explains to his son that the One Life is in all forms and shapes, points out object after object, saying to the boy: "*Tat tuam asi*, Thou art that; That thou art."

And the Mystics have added their testimony to that of others who have experienced this consciousness. Plotinus said: "Knowledge has three degrees: opinion, science, and illumination. The last is absolute knowledge founded upon the identity of the knowing mind with the known object."

And Eckhardt, the German mystic, has told his pupils that: "God is the soul of all things. He is the light that shines in us when the veil is rent."

And Tennyson, in his wonderful verse describing the temporary lifting of the veil for him, has described a phase of Cosmic Consciousness in the following words:

> "For knowledge is the swallow on the lake
> That sees and stirs the surface-shadow there,
> But never yet hath dippt into the abysm,
> The Abysm of all Abysms, beneath, within

The blue of sky and sea, the green of earth,
And in the million-millionth of a grain
Which cleft and cleft again for evermore
And ever vanishing, never vanishes. . .

And more, my son, for more than once when I
Sat all alone, revolving in myself
That word which is the symbol of myself,
The mortal symbol of the Self was loosed,
And past into the Nameless, as a cloud
Melts into Heaven. I touched my limbs, the limbs
Were strange, not mine—and yet no shadow of doubt,
But utter clearness, and through loss of Self
The gain of such large life as matched with ours
Were Sun to spark, unshadowable in words,
Themselves but shadows of a shadow-world."

And not only among the mystics and poets is this universal truth experienced and expressed, but among the great philosophers of all ages may we find this teaching of the Unity of Life originally voiced in the *Upanishads*. The Grecian thinkers have expressed the thought; the Chinese philosophers have added their testimony; the modern philosophers, Spinoza, Berkeley, Kant, Hegel, Schopenhauer, Hartman, Ferrier, Royce, although differing widely in their theories, all have expressed as a fundamental truth the Unity of Life—a One Life underlying. The basic teachings of the Vedas are receiving confirmation at the hands of Modern Science, which while calling itself Rationalistic and inclining to a Materialistic conception of the Universe, still finds itself compelled to say, "At the last, All is One."

And in nearly every human soul there is a secret chamber in which the text of this knowledge lies hidden, and in the rare moments in which the chamber door is opened in response to poetry, music, art, deep religious feeling, or those unaccountable waves of uplift that come to all, the truth is recognized for the moment and the soul feels at peace and is content in the feeling that it is at harmony with the All. The sense of Beauty, however expressed, when keenly experienced, has a tendency to lift us out of our consciousness of separateness into another plane of mind in which the keynote is Unity. The higher the human feeling, the nearer is the conscious realization of the underlying Unity.

This realization of the Unity of Life—the Oneness of Life—the Great Life—even when but faintly experienced, renders Life quite a different thing to the person. He feels no longer that he is a mere "part" of something that may be destroyed—or that he is a tiny personal something, separate from and opposed to all the rest of the Universe—but that he is, instead, a Unit of Expression—a Centre of Consciousness—in the Great One Life. He realizes that he has the Power, and Strength, and Life, and Wisdom of the Whole back of him, upon which he may learn to draw as he unfolds. He realizes that he is at Home, and that he cannot be thrust out, for there is no outside of the All. He feels within himself the certainty of infinite Life and being, for his Life is the all Life, and that cannot die. The petty cares, and worries, and griefs, and pains of everyday personal life are seen for what they are, and they cease to threaten and dominate him as of old. He sees the things of personality as merely the costume and trappings of the part in the play of life that he is acting out, and he knows that when he discards them he will still be "I."

When one really feels the consciousness of the One Life underlying, he acquires a confident trust and faith, and a new sense of freedom and strength comes to him, for is he not indeed delivered from the bondage of fear that has haunted him in his world of separateness. He feels within him the spiritual pulse of the Universal Life, and at once he thrills with a sense of new-found power and being. He becomes reconciled with Life in all its phases, for he knows these things as but temporary phases in the working out of some great Universal plan, instead of things permanent and fixed and beyond remedy. He begins to feel the assurance of Ultimate Justice and God, and the old ideas of Injustice and Evil begin to fade from him. He who enters into the consciousness of the Universal Life, indeed enters into a present realization of the Life Everlasting. All fear of being "lost" or "eternally damned" fades away, and one instinctively realizes that he is "saved" because he is of the One Life and cannot be lost. All the fear of being lost arises from the sense of illusion of separateness or apartness from the One Life. Once the consciousness of Unity is gained, fear drops from the soul like a wornout garment.

When the idea and consciousness of the Unity takes possession of one, he feels a new sense of cheerfulness and optimism entirely different from any other feeling that he has ever experienced. He loses that distrust and hardness which seems to cling to so many in this age who have arrived at the Intellectual stage of development, and have been unable to progress further. A new sense of peace and harmony comes to one, and illuminates his entire character and life. The bitterness engendered by the illusion of separateness is neutralized by the sweetness of the sense of Unity. When one enters into this consciousness he finds that he has the key to many a riddle of life that has heretofore perplexed him. Many dark corners are illuminated—many hard sayings are made clear. Paradoxes become understandable truths, and the pairs of opposites that dwell in all advanced intellectual conceptions, seem to bend around their ends and form themselves into a circle.

To the one who understands the Unity, all Nature seems akin and friendly. There is no sense of antagonism or opposition—everything is seen to fit into its place, and work out its appointed task in the Universal plan. All Nature is seen to be friendly, when properly understood, and Man regains that sense of harmonious environment and at-home-ness that he lost when he entered the stage of self-consciousness. The lower animal and the children feel this Unity, in their poor imperfect way, but Man lost this Paradise when he discovered Good and Evil. But Paradise Lost becomes Paradise Regained when Man enters into this new stage of consciousness. But unlike the animal or child, which instinctively feels the Unity, the awakened soul of man possesses the Unity consciousness, coupled with intelligent comprehension, and unfolding spiritual power. He has found that which he lost, together with the accumulated interest of the ages. This new kingdom of Consciousness is before the race. All must enter into it in time—all will enter into it—many are entering into it now, by gradual stages. This dawning sense of Unity is that which is causing the spiritual unrest which is now agitating the world, and Which in time will bring the race to a realization of the Fatherhood of God and the Brotherhood of Man, and his kinship to Every Living Thing. We are entering into this new cycle of human unfoldment, and the greatest changes are before the race. Ye who read these words are in the foremost ranks of the new dispensation, else you would not be interested in this subject. You are the leaven which is designed to lighten the heavy mass of the world-mind. Play well your parts. You are not alone. Mighty forces and great Intelligences are behind you in the work. Be worthy of them. Peace be with you.

Carry with you the Central Thought of this lesson:

CENTRAL THOUGHT. *There is but One Life—a Universal Life—in the world. This One Life is an emanation from the Absolute. It infills all forms, shapes and manifestations of Life, and is the Real Life that each imagines to be his personal property. There is but One—and you are centres of consciousness and expression in that One. There is a Unity and Harmony which becomes apparent to those who enter into the consciousness of the One Life. There is Peace and Calm in the thought. There is Strength and Power in the knowledge. Enter ye into your Kingdom of Power—possess yourselves of your Birthright of Knowledge. In the very center of your being you will find a holy of holies in which dwells the Consciousness of the One Life, underlying. Enter into the Silence of the Shrine within.*

THE FIFTH LESSON

THE ONE AND THE MANY.

As we have stated in previous Lessons, all philosophies which thinkers have considered worthy of respect, find their final expression of Truth in the fundamental thought that there is but *One Reality*, underlying all the manifold manifestations of shape and form. It is true that the philosophers have differed widely in their conception of that One, but, nevertheless, they have all agreed upon the logical necessity of the fundamental conception that there is, at least, but One Reality, underlying All.

Even the Materialists have conceded this conclusion, and they speak and think of a something called "Matter," as the One—holding that, inherent in Matter, is the potentiality of all Life. The school of Energists, holding that Matter in itself is non-existent, and that it is merely a mode of manifestation of a something called "Energy," asserts that this something called Energy is One, fundamental, real, and self-sufficient.

The various forms of Western religious thought, which hold to the various conceptions of a Personal Deity, also hold to a Oneness, inasmuch as they teach that in the beginning there was God, only, and that all the Universe has been *created* by Him. They do not go into details regarding this creation, and, unlike the Oriental teachers, they fail to distinguish between the conception of the *creation of shape and form*, on the one hand; and the *creation of the substance of these shapes and forms*, on the other hand. But, even accepting the premises of these people who hold to the Personal Deity conception, it will be seen that the Reason requires the acceptance of one or two ideas, *viz.*, (1) That the Deity created the substance of these shapes and forms from *Nothing*; or else (2) that he created them out of *his own substance*—out of Himself, in fact. Let us consider, briefly, these two conceptions.

In the first conception, *i.e.*, Creation from Nothing, we are brought face to face with an impregnable obstacle, inasmuch as the human reason positively refuses to think of Anything coming from Nothing. While it is perfectly true that the finite human mind cannot undertake to limit the powers of the Infinite; or to insist that the possibilities of the Divine Power must be measured and limited by the finite power of Man—still it must hearken to the report of its own highest faculties, and say "I cannot Think it," or else blindly accept the teachings of other finite minds which are equally unable to "Think it," and which have no superior sources of information. The Infinite Power has endowed us with reasoning faculties, and evidently expects us to use them to their full capacity—else the gift were a mockery. And in the absence of information from higher sources than the Reason, we must use the Reason in thinking of this matter, or else refuse to think of it at all.

In view of the above thought, let us then consider the report of the Reason, regarding this matter, And then, after having done so, let us apply the test of this report of the Reason, to the highest teaching of the Yogi Philosophy, and see how the latter stands the test. And, after having done this, we will apply the test of the Higher Consciousness to the same teachings. Remember this always, that while there is knowledge that transcends Reason—that is knowledge that comes from the Higher Regions of the Mind—still even such information of the Spiritual Mind *does not run contrary to Reason*, although it goes beyond it. There is harmony between the Spiritual Mind and the Highest Reason.

Returning to the consideration of the matter of Creation of Substance from Nothing, we again assert that *the Reason is unable to think of the creation of Something from Nothing*. It finds the statement unthinkable, and contrary to all the laws of thought. It is true that the Reason is compelled to accept as a final truth, many things that it cannot *understand* by reason of its finitude—but this is not one of them. There is no logical necessity for the Reason to accept any such conception as this—there is no warrant in the Reason for any such theory, idea or conclusion. Let us stop here, for a moment, and examine into this difference—it may help us to think clearer, hereafter.

We find it impossible to *understand* the fact of the Infinite Being having always existed—and Being without Cause. We find it impossible to conceive of the nature of an Eternal, Causeless, and Infinite Being—to conceive the *nature of*, such a Being, remember.

But, while this is so, still our Reason, by its own laws, compels us to think that there *must be* such a Being, so long as we think at all. For, if we think at all, we *must* think of there being a Fundamental Reality—and we *must* think of that Reality as being without Cause (because there can be no Cause for the First Cause); and we *must* think of that Reality as being Eternal (because It could not have sprung into Being from Nothing, and therefore must have always been); and we *must* think of that Reality as Infinite (because there is nothing outside of Itself to limit It). Think over this statement for a moment—until you grasp it fully.

But there is no such necessity, or compulsion, in the case of the question of Creation from Nothingness. On the contrary, the necessity and compulsion is all the other way. Not only is the Reason unable to *think of* Creation from Nothing—not only does all its laws forbid it to hold such a conception—but, more than this, it finds within itself a conception, full-grown and potent, which contradicts this idea. It finds within itself the strong certainty that *Whatever Really Is has Always Been*, and that all transient and finite shapes, forms, and manifestations, *must* proceed from that which is Real, Infinite, Causeless, and Infinite—and moreover *must be composed of the substance of that Reality*, for there is nothing else Real from which they could have been composed; and their composition from Nothing is unthinkable, for Nothing is Nothing, and always will be Nothing. "Nothing" is merely a name of denial of existence—an absolute denial of substantiality of any degree, kind or form—an absolute denial of Reality. And from such could come only Nothing—from Nothing, Nothing comes.

Therefore, finding within itself the positive report that All, and Anything There Is, must be composed of the Substance of the Reality, the Reason is compelled to think that the Universe is composed of the Substance of the One Reality—whether we call that One Reality, by the name of The Absolute; or whether we call it God. *We must believe that from this Absolute-God all things in the Universe have flown out, or been emanated, rather than created—begotten, rather than "made."*

This does not mean the Pantheistic idea that the Universe *is* God—but rather that God, while existing separate and apart from His Universe, in his Essence, and Being, is nevertheless *in* His Universe, and His Universe *in* Him. And this, no matter what conception of God or Deity is had—or whether one thinks of The Absolute as Principle. The Truth is the same—Truth no matter by what names it is called, or by what misconception it is surrounded. The Truth is that *One is in All, and All is in One*—such is the report of the highest Reason of Man—such is the report of the Illumined—such is the Highest Teachings that have come down to the race from the great souls that have trodden The Path of Attainment.

And now let us submit the Yogi Philosophy to these conceptions, and reports of the Reason. And let us discover just what more the Yogi Philosophy has to say concerning the *nature of* the Substance of the Divine, which infills all Life—and how it solves the Riddle of the Sphinx, concerning the One in All; and All in One. We hope to show you that the Riddle is capable of solution, and that the old Yogi teachers have long ago grasped that for which the human mind has ever sought. This phase of the Teachings is the highest, and it is usually hinted at, rather than expressed, in the writings on the subject—owing to danger of confusion and misconception. But in these Lessons we shall speak the Truth plainly, and without fear—for such is the Message which has been given us to deliver to our students—and we will perform the Right action, leaving the Result, or Fruits of the Action, where it belongs, according to the higher teachings found in the "*Bhagavad Gita*," and in the Higher Teachings of the Yogi Philosophy.

The fundamental Truth embedded in the Wisdom-Philosophies of the East—the Higher Yogi Teachings—is the impregnable doctrine of the One Self in the many selves—the many selves in the One Self. This fundamental Truth underlies all the Oriental Philosophies which are esoteric in their nature.

Notwithstanding the crude and often repulsive conceptions and practices of the masses of the people who represent the exoteric, or popular, phase of the teachings (and these two phases are to be found in *all* regions) still there is always this Inner Doctrine of the One Self, to be found to those who look for it.

Not only is this true among the Hindus; but even among the Mahommedans, of all countries, there is an Inner Circle of Mystics, known as the *Sufis*, holding to this Truth. And the inner teachings of the philosophies of all ages and races, have held likewise. And the highest thought of the philosophers of the Western races, has found refuge in this idea of the Over-soul, or Universal Self. But, it is only among the Yogis that we find an attempt made to explain the real nature of the manifestation of the One in Many—the holding of the Many forms in the One Self.

Before proceeding to the consideration of *how* the One becomes as Many, as expounded by the Higher Yogi Teachings, it becomes necessary to speak of a matter upon which there has been much confusion and misunderstanding, not only on the part of the students of various Oriental Philosophies, but also upon the part of some of the teachers themselves. We allude to the connection between THE ONE—THE ABSOLUTE—in Its ESSENCE—and that which has been called the One Life; the Universal Life, etc.

Many writers have spoken of the Universal Life, and The One, as being identical—but such is a grievous error, finding no warrant in the Highest Yogi Teachings. It is true that all living forms dwell in, and are infilled with the Universal Life—that All Life is One. We have taught this truth, and it is indeed Truth, without qualification. But there is still a Higher Truth—the Highest Truth, in fact—and that is, that even this Universal Life is not the One, but, instead, is in itself a manifestation of, and emanation from, THE ONE. There is a great difference here—-see that you perceive and understand it, before proceeding further.

THE ONE—THE ABSOLUTE—according to the Highest Teachings, is Pure Spirit, and not Life, Mind, or Being as we understand them in our finite and mortal expressions. But, still all Life, Mind, and Being, as we understand them, spring from, flow from, and emanate from, the One—and more than this, may be spoken of as *reflections* of the Life, Mind, and Being of The One, if we may be permitted to apply the names of finite manifestations to the Infinite Reality.

So, the Highest Teaching is that the Universal Life infilling all living things, is not, in itself, the Being and Life of THE ONE—but is rather a great fundamental emanation of The One, the manner and nature of which will be spoken of as we proceed. Remember this, please.

Leading up to the Supreme Idea of the One in All—All in One—let us examine into the report of the Reason upon the *nature of* the Substance—the Divine Substance—from which all living forms are shaped; and from which all that we know as Finite Mind is likewise composed. *How can these imperfect and finite forms be composed of a Divine and Perfect Substance?* This is the question that must occur to the minds of those who are capable of deep thought on the subject—and it is a question that must be answered. And it can be answered—and *is* answered in the Higher Yogi Philosophy. Let us examine the reports of the Reason, a little further—then shall we be ready for the Teachings.

Of what can the Substance of the Infinite be composed? Can it be Matter? Yes, if you are satisfied with the reasoning of the Materialists, and cannot see further into the Truth! These teach that Matter is God, and that God is Matter. But if you be among those who reject the Materialistic teachings, you will not be satisfied with this answer. Even if you incline toward a Non-mental Infinite, still if you are familiar with the results of modern scientific investigation, and know that Science has seen Matter resolve itself into something like Electric Energy, you will know that the Truth must lie behind and beyond Matter.

Then is it Pure Energy? you may ask. Pure Energy? what's that? Can you think of Energy apart from material manifestation? Have you ever known of such a thing? Do you not know that even the Electron Theory, which is attracting the attention of advanced Modern Science, and which holds that all things are composed of minute particles of Electric Energy, called Electrons, from which the Atoms are built—do you not know that even this theory recognizes the necessity of a "something like Matter, only infinitely finer," which they call the Ether, to enfold the Electric Energy as a unit—to give it a *body*, as it were? And can you escape from the fact that the most advanced scientific minds find confronting them—*the fact that in all Energy, and governing its actions, there 'is manifested "something like Mind*"?

And does not all this teach thinkers that just as Energy creates from itself, that which is called Matter, and then uses it as a vehicle of expression and action—so does this "Something like Mind" create from itself that which we call Energy, and proceeds to use it, with its accompanying phase of Matter, for its expression? Does not all advanced research show us that in all Matter and Energy there are evidences of the operation of this "Something like Mind"? And if this be so, are we not justified as regarding Matter and Energy as mere Effects—and to look to this "Something like Mind" as the more fundamental Substance? We think so—and Science is beginning to think so, too. And soon will Science be regarding with the most profound respect, the Metaphysical axiom that "All is Mind."

You will see by reference to our "*Advanced Course in Yogi Philosophy, etc.*," the general Yogi teachings regarding the Emanation of the One, known respectively as Mind, Energy, and Matter. You will see that the Yogis teach that Mind, Energy, and Matter comprise a threefold emanation of the Absolute. You will also see that it is taught that Mind was the Parent-Emanation—the Universal Mind; and that the Universal Energy was the Second-Emanation (proceeding from Mind); and that the Universal Matter was the

Third Emanation (proceeding from Energy) In the same book you will find that the Teaching is that above Matter, Energy, and Mind, is the Essence of the Absolute, which is called Spirit—the nature of which is non-understandable to the mind of Man, the highest conception of which is the highest manifestation of itself—Mind. But as we cannot comprehend spirit otherwise, we are justified in thinking of it as Something like Infinite Mind—Something as much higher than Finite Mind as that is higher than mere energy.

Now, then—we have seen the folly of thinking of the Divine Substance as Matter or Energy. And we have come to know it as Spirit, something like Mind, only infinitely higher, but which still may be thought of in terms of Infinite Mind, for we can have no higher terms in our thinking operations. So we may then assume that this Divine Nature or substance is SPIRIT, which we will think of as Infinite Mind, for want of a better form of conception.

We have seen the folly of thinking of the Divine Essential Substance as the Body of God. We have likewise seen the folly of thinking of it as the Vital Energy of God. And we have found that we could not escape thinking of it as the Spirit, or infinite Mind of God. Beyond this we cannot think intelligently.

But do you not see that all this exercise of the Reason has brought us to the point where we must think that this Divine Substance, which the Absolute-God uses in the manifestation of Universal Life; the Universe; and all the forms, and shapes, and manifestations of life and things in the Universe—this Divine Substance which must be *in* All Things—and *in which* All Things must rest, even as the bubble rests on the Ocean—that this can be nothing less than Spirit, and that this Spirit can be thought of only as Infinite Mind?

And, if this be so, then indeed must *All be Mind, and Mind be All*—meaning, of course, the Infinite Mind, not the finite manifestation that we *call* Mind.

Then, if this reasoning has been correct, then must we think that All Life—all the Universe—Everything except the Absolute itself—*must be held in the Infinite Mind of the Absolute*!

And, so, by the exercise of our Reason—by listening to, and examining its reports, we have been brought face to face—eye to eye—heart to heart—with the Teaching of the Illumined Ones, which has come down to us as the Highest Teaching of the Yogi Philosophy! For this, indeed, is the highest conception of Truth in the Yogi Teachings—this, that ALL MANIFESTATIONS AND EMANATIONS OF THE ABSOLUTE ARE MENTAL CREATIONS OF THE ABSOLUTE—THOUGHT-FORMS HELD IN THE

INFINITE MIND—THE INFINITE SPIRIT IN THEM—AND THEY IN THE INFINITE SPIRIT. _And that the only Real Thing about Man is THE SPIRIT involved in the Thought-Form, the rest is mere Personality, which changes and ceases to be. The Spirit in the Soul of Man, is the SOUL OF THE SOUL, which is never born; never changeth; never dieth—this is The Real Self of *Man, in which, indeed, he is "One with the Father."*

This is the point where the Reasoning Mind of Man has come to a sense of Agreement with the Highest Yogi Teachings. Let us now pass on to the Teachings themselves—let us listen to The Message of Truth.

In this consideration of the Highest Yogi Philosophy, and its teaching, we would again say to our students, that which we said to them in *"The Advanced Course"*—that we do not attempt to teach the "why" of the Manifestation of The Absolute, but rest content with delivering the Message of the Yogi Sages, which deals with the "how." As we stated in the lessons referred to, we incline to that school of the Higher Teachings, which holds that the "Why" of the Infinite Manifestation must, of necessity, rest with the Infinite alone, and that the finite mind cannot hope to answer the question. We hold that in all the Universal Mind, or in any of its Mind Manifestations, there is to be found no answer to this question! Wrapped in the Essence of the Absolute Spirit, alone, is this Final Answer!

The Sages, and Masters, from their high spiritual points of observation, possess many truths regarding the "how" side of the question that would appear almost like Infinite Wisdom itself, compared with our puny knowledge. But even these great souls report that they do not possess the answer to the Final Question—the "Why" of the Infinite Manifestation. And so we may be excused from attempting to answer it—and without shame or sense of shortcoming do we still say, to this question, "We do not know!"

In order that the Final Question may be fully understood let us consider it for a moment. We find the Question arising from the following condition:

The human Reason is compelled to admit that there is an Infinite, Eternal, Causeless REALITY underlying all forms of manifestation in the phenomenal world. It is likewise compelled to admit that this REALITY must comprise All that Really Is—and that there can be nothing Real outside of Itself. Arising from this is the Truth, that all forms of phenomenal manifestation, must emanate *from* the One Reality, for there is nothing else Real from which they could emanate. And the twin-Truth that these forms of manifestation, must also be *in* the Being of the One Reality, for there is nowhere outside of the All wherein they might find a place. So this One Reality is seen to be "That from which All Things flow"; and "That in which All Things live, and move and have their being."

Therefore All Things *emanate from*, and are *contained in* the One Reality. We shall consider "just how" later on, but the question which confronts us, and which has been called the "Final Question"—and that which we pronounce unanswerable—is this: "Why has the Infinite manifested and emanated Finite forms of being?" You will see the nature of the question when you stop to consider: (1) The Infinite cannot have Desire, for that is a Finite quality; (2) It cannot lack anything, for that would take away from its Infinity; (3) and even if it did lack anything, from whence could it expect to acquire it; for there is nothing outside of itself—if It lacks anything, it must continue to always lack it, for there is no outside source from which It could obtain anything which it does not already possess. And Desire would be, of course, a *wanting* for something which it lacked—so It could not Desire unless it Lacked—and it would know that Desire would be hopeless, even if indeed it did Lack.

So you see that if we regard the Infinite Reality as Perfect, we must drop all ideas of It Desiring or Lacking—and of it Growing or Improving—or of it obtaining more Power, or Knowledge. These ideas are ridiculous, for an Absolute, Infinite Reality, must possess All-Knowledge; All-Power; All-Presence, else it is not Absolute and Infinite. And, if It does not possess these attributes of Being, then It can never hope to acquire them, for there is Nowhere from whence they could be acquired—there is no Source outside of the All-Source. A Finite Thing, may lack, and desire, and improve and develop, for there is the Universal Source from which it may draw. But the Infinite has no Universal Source, for it is Its own Source. Do you see the nature of the Final Question? If not we will again state it—it is this:

"Why should the Infinite Reality, which possesses all that may be possessed, and which in itself is the only Source of Things—WHY should It Desire to manifest a Universe from and within Itself?"

A little consideration will show you that there is no intelligent answer to the "Why," either in your own minds, or in the writings and teachings of the greatest minds. The matter is important, to those who are confronted every day with some of the many attempts to answer this Final Question—it is well that our students inform them regarding the futility of such questioning. And with this end in view, we shall herein give a few of the wise "guesses" at the answer, and our reasons for considering them inadequate. We ask the student to consider carefully these remarks, for by so doing he will post himself, and will be saved much tedious and perplexing wandering along the dangerous places in the Swamp of Metaphysics, following the will-o'-the-wisp of Finite Mind masquerading as the Infinite Wisdom! Beware of the False Lights! They lead to the quagmire and quicksands of thought!

Let us now consider some of these "guesses" at the answer to the Final Question. Some thinkers have held that the Absolute was bound by a Divine Necessity to manifest itself as Many. The answer to this is that the Absolute could not be *bound* by anything, inner or outer, else it would not be Absolute and Infinite, but would be Relative and Finite. Another set of thinkers have held that the Absolute found within itself a Desire to Manifest as Many. From whence could come such an action-causing Desire? The Absolute could lack nothing, and there would be nothing for it to desire to gain, other than that which It already possessed. One does not desire things one already has, but only what he lacks.

Another school would tell us that the Infinite wished to *Express* itself in the phenomenal world. Why? Such a phenomenal world could only be reflection of Its power, witnessed only by Itself, and could contain nothing that was not already contained in the All. To what end would such a wish tend? What would be accomplished or gained? The Infinite All could not become anything more than It already was—so why the wish for expression? Some say that the whole phenomenal world is but *Maya*, or Illusion, and does not exist at all. Then who else than the Infinite caused the Illusion, and why the necessity? This answer only removes the question back one point, and does not really answer it. Some would say that the Universe is the "dream of the Infinite." Can we conceive the Infinite Being as exercising the finite faculty of "dreaming"—is not this childish?

Others would have us believe that the Absolute is indulging in a "game" or "play," when he makes Universes, and those inhabiting them. Can anyone really believe this of The Absolute—playing like a child, with men and women, worlds and suns, as Its blocks and tin-soldiers? Why should the Infinite "play"?—does It need amusement and "fun" like a child? Poor Man, with his attempts to read the Riddle of the Infinite!

We know of teachers who gravely instruct their pupils in the idea that the Absolute and Infinite One manifests Universes and Universal Life, and all that flows from them, because It wishes to "gain experience" through objective existence. This idea, in many forms has been so frequently advanced that it is worth while to consider its absurdity. In the first place, what "experience" could be gained by the Absolute and Infinite One? What could It expect to gain and learn, that it did not already know and possess? One can gain experience only from others, and outside things—not from oneself entirely separated from the outside world of things. And there would be no "outside" for the Infinite. These people would have us believe that The Absolute emanated a Universe from Itself—which could contain nothing except that which was obtained from Itself—and then proceeded to gain experience from it. Having no "outside" from which it could obtain experiences and sentences and sensations, it proceeded to make (from Itself) an imitation one—that is what this answer amounts to. Can you accept it?

The whole trouble in all of these answers, or attempted answers, is that the answerer first conceives of the Absolute-Infinite Being, as a Relative-Finite Man, and then proceeds to explain what this Big Man would do. This is but an exaggerated form of anthropomorphism—the conception of God as a Man raised to great proportions. It is but an extension of the idea which gave birth to the savage conceptions of Deity as a cruel chief or mighty warrior, with human passions, hates, and revenge; love, passions, and desires.

Arising from the same cause, and akin to the theories advanced above are similar ones, which hold that the Absolute cannot dwell alone, but must forever bring forth souls from Itself—this was the idea of *Plotinus*, the Greek philosopher. Others have thought that the Infinite was possessed of such a consuming love, that It manifested objects upon which it could bestow Its affections. Others have thought that It was lonesome, and desired companionship. Some have spoken of the Absolute as "sacrificing" itself, in becoming Many, instead of remaining One. Others have taught that the Infinite somehow has become entangled in Its Manifestations, and had lost the knowledge of Its Oneness—hence their teachings of "I Am God." Others, holding to a similar idea, tell us that the Infinite is deliberately "masquerading" as the Many, in order to fool and mystify Itself—a show of Itself; by Itself, and for Itself! Is not this Speculative Metaphysics run wild? Can one in calm thought so regard the Infinite and Absolute Being—All-Wise—Causeless—All-Powerful—All-Present—All-Possessing— Lacking Nothing—Perfect One—as acting and performing thus, and from these motives? Is not this as childish as the childishness of the savage, and barbarians, in their Mumbo-Jumbo conceptions? Let us leave this phase of the subject.

The Higher Yogi Teachings hold to no such ideas or theories. It holds that the Answer to the Secret is vested in the Infinite alone, and that finite "guesses" regarding the "Why" are futile and pitiful. It holds that while one should use the Reason to the full, still there are phases of Being that can be considered only in Love, Faith, and Confidence in THAT from which All Things flow, and in which we live and move and have our being. It recognizes that the things of the Spirit, are known by the Mind. It explores the regions of the Universal Mind to its utmost limits, fearlessly—but it pauses before the Closed Door of The Spirit, reverently and lovingly.

But, remember this—that while the Higher Yogi Teachings contain no "guess," or speculative theory, regarding the "Why" of the Divine Manifestation, still they do not deny the existence of a "Why". In fact, they expressly hold that the Absolute Manifestation of the Many is in pursuance of some wondrous Divine Plan, and that the Unfoldment of the Plan proceeds along well-established and orderly lines, and according to Law. They trust in the Wisdom and Love of the Absolute Being, and manifest a perfect Confidence, Trust and Peaceful Patience in the Ultimate Justice, and Final Victory of the

Divine Plan. No doubt disturbs this idea—it pays no attention to the apparent contradictions in the finite phenomenal world, but sees that all things are proceeding toward some far-away goal, and that "All is Well with the Universe".

But they do not think for a moment, or teach in the slightest degree, that all this Unfoldment, and Plan of the Universe, has for its object any advantage, benefit or gain to the Absolute—such a thought would be *folly*, for the Absolute is already Perfect, and Its Perfection cannot be added to, or taken away from. But they do positively teach that there is a great beneficial purpose in all the Plan, accruing in the end to the developed souls that have evolved through the workings of the plan. These souls do not possess the qualities of the Infinite—they are Finite, and thus are capable of receiving benefits; of growing, developing, unfolding, attaining. And, therefore, the Yogis teach that this building up of Great Souls seems to be the idea of the Infinite, so far as may be gained from an observation of the Workings of the Plan. The Absolute cannot *need these* Great Souls for Its own pleasure, and therefore their building-up must be for their own advantage, happiness and benefit.

The Yogis teach, on this subject, that there can be only ONE Real Perfect Being—Perfect without experience—Perfect from the Beginning—but only ONE! In other words, they teach that there can be no such thing as Absolute Perfection, outside of the Absolute Itself—and that not even the Absolute Being can create another Absolute Being, for in that case there would be no Absolute Being at all, but only *two Relative Beings*.

Think over this for a moment, and you will see its truth. The ABSOLUTE must always be "the One without a Second", as the Yogis express it—there cannot be *two* Perfect ones. And so, all Finite Beings, being Finite, must work their way up toward the plane of Perfection by The Path of Life, with all of its lessons, tasks, cares, pains, and strivings. This is the only way open to them—and even the Absolute cannot have it otherwise, and still be the Absolute. There is a fine point here—the Absolute is All-Powerful, but even that All-Power is not sufficient to enable It to destroy Its Absolute Being. And so, you who have wondered, perhaps you may now understand our words in the First Lesson of this series, in which we said that the message of the Absolute to some of the Illumined has been: "All is being done in the best and only possible way—I am doing the best I can—all is well—and in the end will so appear."

And, as we also said in that First Lesson: "The Absolute, instead of being an indifferent and unmoved spectator to its own creation, is a striving, longing, active, suffering, rejoicing, feeling Spirit, partaking of the feelings of Its manifestations, rather than callously witnessing them. It lives in us—with us—through us. Back of all the pain in the world, may be found a great feeling and suffering love." And in this thought there is comfort to the doubting soul—peace to the troubled mind.

In the Sixth Lesson, we shall proceed to deliver to you the further Message of Truth, concerning "how" the One Absolute manifests Its Mental Images as Universe; Universal Life; and Forms and Shapes; and Individualities, and Personalities. We had hoped to include the whole Message in this Fifth Lesson, but now find that we have merely laid the steps by which the student may reach the Essential Truth.

But, lest the student may be left in an uncertain state of mind, awaiting the conclusion of the consideration of the subject—and lest he may think that we intend teaching him that the Universe, and all in it, including himself are "Dreams," because we have said that All Things are Thought-Forms in the Mind of the Absolute—lest this misunderstanding may arise, we wish to add a few parting words to what we have said.

We wish to impress upon the mind of the student that though all Things are but Thought-Forms in the Mind of the Absolute Being, and that while it is true that the entire Universe of Universes is simply a Thought-Form held in the Mind of the Absolute—still this fact does not mean that all Things are "illusions" or "dreams." Remember this, now and forever, O Student—that that which is held in the Absolute Mind as a Thought-Form IS, and is all there IS, outside of the Absolute Itself. When the Absolute forms a Thought-Form, It forms it out of Its own mental substance—when the Absolute "holds anything in Its Mind," It holds it in Itself—for the Absolute is ALL-MIND.

The Absolute is not a material Being, from which Material Beings are created. It is a Spiritual Being—a Being whose Substance is akin to that which we call "Mind," only raised to Infinity and Absolute Perfection and Power. And this is the only way it can "create"—by creating a Thought-Form in Its Mental, or Spiritual Substance. The faintest "Thought" of the Absolute is more real and durable than anything that man can create—in fact, man can "create" nothing, for all the hard and real material he uses in his "creations," such as steel, diamonds, granite, are but some of the minor Forms, "thought" into being by the Absolute.

And also remember this, that the Absolute cannot "think" of anything, without putting Itself in that thing, as its Essence. Just as a man's Mental Images are not only *in* his mind, *but his mind is in them, also.*

Why, you doubting and timorous ones, does not even the finite "thinking" of Man manifest itself in physical and material changes of form and shape?—does not a man's every thought actually "create" physical forms and shapes, in his brain-cells and physical tissue? You who are reading these words—yea, *while* you are reading these words—are "creating" changes of form and shape in your brain-cells, and physical organism. Your mind is constantly at work, also, in building up your physical body, along the lines of the

Instinctive Mind (see previous series of lessons)—you are mentally creating in a miniature universe, every moment of your life. And yet, the idea of the Absolute "creating" a Universe by pure Thought, in Its own Mind, and thereafter causing the work of the Universe to proceed according to Law, by simply "Willing" it so, causes you to wonder, and perhaps to doubt.

O, ye of little faith, you would deny to the Absolute even the power you possess yourself. You plan things in your mind every day, and then proceed to cause them to appear in material manifestation, and yet you doubt the ability of the Absolute to do likewise. Why even the poets, or writers of fiction, create characters in their minds—and these seem so real, that even you imagine them to be actual entities, and you weep over their pains, and smile at their joys—and yet all this is on the finite plane. Why, even the "imaginations" of your petty finite, undeveloped minds, have sufficient power to make your physical bodies sick, or well, or even to cause you to "die," from some imagined ailment. And yet you doubt the power of the Absolute, to "think" things into being! You tiny students in the great Kindergarten of Life—you must learn better lessons from your little blocks and games. And you *will*—this is the Law.

And you who are filled with the sense of your smallness, and "unreality"—know you that so long as you are "held in the Mind of God," then so long are you "remembered" by Him. And so long as you are remembered by Him, no real harm can befall you, and your Reality is second only to His own. Even though you pass out of your mortal frame—doth he remember you in His Mind, and keeping you there, he holds you safe and unharmed. The greatest satisfaction that can come to one, is to be able to fully realize that he, or she, is held firmly IN THE MIND OF THE INFINITE BEING. To such comes the knowledge that in THAT LIFE there can be NO DEATH.

Peace be with you in this Realization. May you make it your own!

THE SIXTH LESSON

WITHIN THE MIND OF THE ONE.

In our last lesson we gave you the Inner Teachings of the Yogi Philosophy, relating to the real nature of the Universe, and all that is therein contained. We trust that you have pondered well and carefully the statements contained in that lesson, for in them is to be found the essence of the highest Yogi teachings. While we have endeavored to present these high truths to you in the simplest possible form, yet unless your minds have been trained to grasp the thought, you may have trouble in fully assimilating the essence of the teachings. But, be not discouraged, for your mind will gradually unfold like the flower, and the Sun of Truth will reach into its inmost recesses. Do not be troubled if your comprehension seems dull, or your progress slow, for all things will come to you in time. You cannot escape the Truth, nor can the Truth escape you. And it will not come to you one moment sooner than you are ready to receive it, nor will it be delayed one moment in its coming, when you are ready for it. Such is the Law, and none can escape it, nor alter it, nor modify it. All is Well, and All is Under the Law—nothing ever "happens."

To many, the thought that the Universe and all that is therein contained, are simply "Thought Forms" in the Infinite Mind—Mental Creations of the Absolute, may seem startling, and a sense of unreality may pervade one. This is inevitable, but the reaction will come. To some who have grasped this mighty truth there has come a feeling that "All is Nothing," which idea is embodied in their teachings and writings. But this is merely the Negative Phase of the Truth—there is a Positive Phase which comes as one advances.

The Negative Phase shows us that all that we have considered as real and permanent—the foundations of the Universe itself—is but a mental image in the mind of the Absolute, and therefore lacks the fundamental reality that we had previously associated with it. And realizing this, we are at first apt to feel that, indeed "all is nothing," and to fall into a state of apathy, and lack of desire to play our part in the world. But, then, happily the reaction sets in, sooner or later, and we begin to see the Positive Phase of the Truth. This Positive Phase shows us that while all the forms, shapes, and phenomena of the Universe are but parts of a great show-world, still the *essence of* all must be Reality, itself, else there would not be even the "appearance" of a Universe. Before a thing can be a Mental Image, there must be a Mind to hold that Mental Image, and a BEING to possess that Mind. And, the very essence of that BEING must pervade and be immanent in every Image in that Mind. Just as *You* are really in your Mental Images, as well as they in You, so must the Absolute be *in* Its Mental Images, or Creations, or Thought Forms, as truly as they are in the Mind of the Absolute. Do you see this plainly? Think well over it—ponder it well—for in it lies the Truth.

And so, this Positive Phase of the Truth, is far from depressing—it is the most stimulating conception one can hold, if he but grasps it in its entirety and fulness. Even if it be true that all these shapes, and forms, and appearances, and phenomena, and personalities, be but illusion as compared to the inner Reality—what of it? Are you not then assured that the Spirit within Yourself is the Spirit of the Absolute—that the Reality within You is the Reality of the Absolute—that you ARE, because the Absolute IS, and cannot be otherwise? Does not the Peace, and Calm, and Security, and Bliss that comes to you with this Realization, far more than counterbalance the petty nothings that you have discarded? We think that there can be but one answer to this, when you have fully Realized the Truth.

What gives you the greatest Satisfaction and Content in Life? Let us see. Well, there is the Satisfaction of Immortality. The human mind instinctively craves this. Well, what that even the highest finite conceptions of Future Life have given you, can compare with the assurance of Actual Being, in and of the Absolute? What are your petty conceptions of "heavens," "paradises," "happy-hunting-grounds," "divine regions of the blessed," and the other ideas of the various religious sects, when compared with the conceptions of your Infinite and Eternal Existence in Spirit—your relation with The One—that conception of Infinite Wisdom, Being, and Bliss? When you grasp this truth, you will see that you are "in Eternity right Now," and are Immortal even this moment, as you have always been.

Now, what we have said above is not intended to deny the "heaven-worlds," or planes. On the contrary, you will find much in the teachings regarding these, which the Yogis enter into with much detail. But, we mean that back of all the "heavens" and "celestial planes," there is a still higher state of being being—the "Absolute Being." Even the "heavens," and "heaven-worlds," and regions of the *Devas*, or Archangels, are but relative states—there is a state higher than even these exalted relative states, and that is the State of the Conscious Unity and Identity with the One. When one enters into that State, he becomes more than Man—more than gods—he is then "in the bosom of the Father."

And now, before proceeding to a consideration of the phenomenal manifestation of the Absolute—the evolving of the Universe in the Infinite Mind—we will again call your attention to the fact that underlies all the Universe of forms, shapes and appearances, and that is, as we stated in our last lesson:

All Manifestations and Emanations of the Absolute are Mental Creations of the Absolute—Thought-Forms held in the Infinite Mind—the Infinite Spirit in them—and they in the Infinite Spirit. And, the only Real Thing about Man is the Spirit involved in the Thought-Form—the rest is mere Personality, which changes and ceases to be. The Spirit in the Soul of Man, is the Soul of the Soul, which is never born; never changeth; never dieth—this is The Real Self of Man, in which, indeed, he is "One with the Father."

And, now let us consider the Yogi Teachings regarding the creation of the Universe, and the evolution of the living forms thereon. We shall endeavor to give you the story as plainly as may be, holding fast to the main thought, and avoiding the side-paths of details, etc., so far as is possible.

In the first place, we must imagine ourselves back to the beginning of a "Day of Brahm,"—the first dawn of that Day, which is breaking from the darkness of a "Night of Brahm." Before we proceed further, we must tell you something about these "Days and Nights of Brahm," of which you have seen much mention in the Oriental writings.

The Yogi Teachings contain much regarding the "Days and Nights of Brahm;" the "In-breathing and Out-breathing of the Creative Principle;" the periods of "*Manvantara*," and the periods of "*Pralaya*." This thought runs through all the Oriental thought, although in different forms, and with various interpretations. The thought refers to the occult truth that there is in Cosmic Nature alternate periods of Activity and Inactivity—Days and Nights—In-breathings and Out-breathings—Wakefulness and Sleep. This fundamental law manifests in all Nature, from Universes to Atoms. Let us see it now in its application to Universes.

At this point we would call the attention of the student that in many of the presentations of the Hindu Teachings the writers speak as if the Absolute, *Itself*, were subject to this law of Rhythm, and had Its Periods of Rest and Work, like Its manifestations. This is incorrect. The highest teachings do not so hold, although at first glance it would so appear. The teaching really is that while the Creative Principle manifests this rhythm, still even this principle, great though it be, is a manifestation of the Absolute, and not the Absolute itself. The highest Hindu teachings are firm and unmistakable about this point.

And, another point, in which there is much mistaken teaching. In the periods of Creative Inactivity in a Universe it must not be supposed that there is no Activity anywhere. On the contrary, there is never a cessation of Activity on the part of the Absolute. While it is Creative Night in one Universe, or System of Universes, there is intense activity of Mid-Day in others. When we say "The Universe" we mean the Universe of Solar Systems—millions of such systems—that compose the particular universe of which we have any knowledge. The highest teachings tell us that this Universe is but one of a System of Universes, millions in number—and that this System is but one, in a higher System, and so on and on, to infinity. As one Hindu Sage hath said: "Well do we know that the Absolute is constantly creating Universes in Its Infinite Mind—and constantly destroying them—and, though millions upon millions of aeons intervene between creation and destruction, yet doth it seem less than the twinkle of an eye to The Absolute One."

And so the "Day and Night of Brahm" means only the statement of the alternating periods of Activity and Inactivity in some one particular Universe, amidst the Infinite Universality. You will find a mention of these periods of Activity and Inactivity in the "*Bhagavad Gita*," the great Hindu epic. The following quotations, and page references, relate to the edition published by the Yogi Publication Society, which was compiled and adapted by the writer of these lessons. In that edition of the "*Bhagavad Gita*," on page 77, you will find these words attributed to *Krishna*, the Absolute One in human incarnation:

"The worlds and universes—yea, even the world of Brahm, a single day of which is like unto a thousand *Yugas* (four billion years of the earth), and his night as much—these worlds must come and go… The Days of Brahm are succeeded by the Nights of Brahm.

In these Brahmic Days all things emerge from invisibility, and become visible. And, on the coming of the Brahmic Night, all visible things again melt into invisibility. The Universe having once existed, melteth away; and lo! is again re-created."

And, in the same edition, on page 80, we find these words, attributed to the same speaker:

"At the end of a *Kalpa*—a Day of Brahm—a period of Creative Activity—I withdraw into my nature, all things and beings. And, at the beginning of another *Kalpa*, I emanate all things and beings, and re-perform my creative act."

We may say here, in passing, that Modern Science now holds to the theory of periods of Rhythmic Change; of Rise and Fall; of Evolution and Dissolution.

It holds that, beginning at some time in the past aeons of time, there was the beginning of an upward or evolutionary movement, which is now under way; and that, according to the law of Nature, there must come a time when the highest point will be reached, and then will come the beginning of the downward path, which in time must come to an end, being succeeded by a long period of inactivity, which will then be followed by the beginning of a new period of Creative Activity and Evolution—"a Day of Brahm."

This thought of this law of Rhythm, in its Universal form, has been entertained by the thinkers of all times and races. Herbert Spencer expressly held to it in his "First Principles," expressing it in many ways akin to this: "Evolution must come to a close in complete equilibrium or rest;" and again, "It is not inferable from the general progress towards equilibrium, that a state of universal quiescence or death will be reached; but that if a process of reasoning ends in that conclusion, a further process of reasoning points to renewals of activity and life;" and again, "Rhythm in the totality of changes—alternate eras of evolution and dissolution." The Ancient Western Philosophers also indulged in this idea. Heraclitus taught that the universe manifested itself in cycles, and the Stoics taught that "the world moves in an endless cycle, through the same stages." The followers of Pythagoras went even further, and claimed that "the succeeding worlds resemble each other, down to the minutest detail," this latter idea, however—the idea of the "Eternal Recurrence"—while held by a number of thinkers, is not held by the Yogi teachers, who teach infinite progression—an Evolution of Evolution, as it were. The Yogi teachings, in this last mentioned particular, are resembled more by the line of Lotze's thinking, as expressed in this sentence from his *Micro-cosmos:* "The series of Cosmic Periods, ... each link of which is bound together with every other; ... the successive order of these sections shall compose the unity of an onward-advancing melody." And, so through the pages of Heraclitus, the Stoics, the Pythagoreans, Empedocles, Virgil, down to the present time, in Nietzsche, and his followers, we find this thought of Universal Rhythm—that fundamental conception of the ancient Yogi Philosophy.

And, now, returning to the main path of our thought—let us stand here at the beginning of the dawn of a Day of Brahm. It is verily a beginning, for there is nothing to be seen—there is nothing but Space. No trace of Matter, Force or Mind, as we know these terms. In that portion of Infinite Space—that is, of course, in that "portion" of the Infinite Mind of the Absolute One, for even Space is a "conception" of that Mind, there is "Nothing." This is "the darkest moment, just before the dawn."

Then comes the breaking of the dawn of the Brahmic Day. The Absolute begins the "creation" of a Universe. And, how does It create? There can be no creation of something out of nothing. And except the Absolute Itself there is but Nothing.

Therefore The Absolute must create the Universe out of Its own "substance," if we can use the word "substance" in this connection. "Substance" means, literally, "that which stands under," being derived from the two Latin words, *sub*, meaning "under," and *stare*, meaning "to stand." The English word "understand" means, literally, "to stand under"—the two words really meaning the same. This is more than a coincidence.

So the Absolute must create the Universe from its own substance, we have seen. Well, what is this "substance" of the Absolute? Is it Matter? No! for Matter we know to be, in itself, merely a manifestation of Force, or Energy. Then, is it Force or Energy? No! because Force and Energy, in itself, cannot possess Mind, and we must think of the Absolute as possessing Mind, for it manifests Mind, and what is manifested must be in the Manifestor, or Manifesting Agent. Then this "substance" must be Mind? Well, yes, in a way—and yet not Mind as we know it, finite and imperfect. But something like Mind, only Infinite in degree and nature—something sufficiently greater than Mind as we know it, to admit of it being the Cause of Mind. But, we are compelled to think of it as "Infinite Mind," for our finite Minds can hold no higher conception. So we are content to say that this "substance" from which the Absolute must create the Universe is a something that we will call Infinite Mind. Fix this in your mind, please, as the first step in our conception.

But, how can the Infinite Mind be used to create finite minds, shapes, forms, and things, without it being lessened in quantity—how can you take something from something, and still have the original something left? An impossibility! And, we cannot think of the Absolute as "dividing Itself up" into two or more portions—for if such were the case, there would be two or more Absolutes, or else None. There cannot be two Absolutes, for if the Absolute were to divide itself so there would be no Absolute, but only two Relatives—two Finites instead of One Infinite. Do you see the absurdity?

Then how can this work of Creation be accomplished, in view of these difficulties which are apparent even to our finite minds? You may thresh this question over and over again in your minds—men have done so in all times—and you will not find the answer except in the fundamental Idea of the Yogi Teachings. And this Fundamental Idea is that the creation is purely a Mental Creation, and the Universe is the Mental Image, or Thought-Form, in the Mind of the Absolute—in the Infinite Mind, itself. No other "creation" is possible. And so this, say the Yogi Masters, this is the Secret of Universal Creation. The Universe is *of*, and *in*, the Infinite Mind, and this is the only way it could be so. So, fix in your mind this second step in our conception.

But then, you ask us, from whence comes Force, Matter, and Finite Mind?
Well asked, good student—your answer shall be forthcoming. Here it is.

Finite Mind; Force or Energy; and Matter; in themselves have no existence. They are merely Mental Images, or Thought-Forms in the Infinite Mind of the Absolute. Their whole existence and appearance depends upon their Mental Conception and Retention in the Infinite Mind. In It they have their birth, rise, growth, decline and death.

Then what is Real about ME, you may ask—surely I have a vivid consciousness of Reality—is this merely an illusion, or shadow? No, not so! that sense of Reality which you possess and which every creature or thing possesses—that sense of "I Am"—is the perception by the Mental Image of the Reality of its Essence—and that Essence is the Spirit. And that Spirit is the SUBSTANCE OF THE ABSOLUTE embodied in Its conception, the Mental Image. It is the perception by the Finite, of its Infinite Essence. Or, the perception by the Relative of its Absolute Essence. Or, the perception by You, or I, or any other man or woman, of the Real Self, which underlies all the sham self or Personality. It is the reflection of the Sun, in the dew-drop, and thousands of dew-drops—seemingly thousands of Suns, and yet but One. And yet, that reflection of the Sun in the dewdrop is more than a "reflection," for it is the substance of the Sun itself—and yet the Sun shines on high, one and undivided, yet manifesting in millions of dew-drops. It is only by figures of speech that we can speak of the Unspeakable Reality.

To make it perhaps plainer to some of you, let us remind you that even in your finite Mental Images there is evident many forms of life. You may think of a moving army of thousands of men. And yet the only "I" in these men is your own "I." These characters in your mind move and live and have their being, and yet there is nothing in them except "You!" The characters of Shakespeare, Dickens, Thackeray, Balzac, and the rest, were such strong Mental Images that not only their creators were carried away by their power, and apparent ability, but even you who read of them, many years after, perhaps, feel the apparent reality, and weep, or smile, or grow angry over their actions. And, yet there was no Hamlet, outside of Shakespeare's mind; no Micawber outside of Dickens; no Pere Goriot outside of Balzac.

These illustrations are but finite examples of the Infinite, but still they will give you an idea of the truth that we are trying to unfold in your mind. But you must not imagine that You and I, and all others, and things, are but mere "imaginations," like *our* created characters—that would be a most unhappy belief. The mental creations held by You and I, and other finite minds, are but *finite creations of finite minds*, while WE, ourselves, are the finite creations of an INFINITE MIND. While our, and Dickens', and Balzac's, and Shakespeare's creations live and move and have their being, they have no other "I" than our Finite Minds, while we, the characters in the Divine Drama, Story, or Epic, have for our "I"—our Real Self—the ABSOLUTE REALITY. They have merely a background of our finite personalities, and minds, before which they may desport themselves. until, alas! the very background fades away to dust, and both background and shadows disappear. But, we have behind our personalities the Eternal Background of Reality, which changeth not, neither doth it Disappear. Shadows on a screen though our Personalities may be, yet the Screen is Real and Eternal. Take away the finite screen and the shadows disappear—but our Screen remains forever.

We *are* Mental Images in the Infinite Mind—the Infinite Mind holds us safe—we cannot be lost—we cannot be hurt—we can never disappear, unless we be absorbed in the Infinite Mind itself, and then we STILL ARE! The Infinite Mind never forgets—it never can overlook us—it is aware of our presence, and being, always. We are safe—we are secure—we ARE! Just as we could not be created from Nothing—so we cannot be converted into Nothing. We are in the All—and there is no outside.

At the dawn of the Brahmic Day, The Absolute begins the creation of a new Universe, or the recreation of one, just as you may care to state it. The highest Yogi Teachings inform us that the information relating to this event (which is, of course, beyond the personal knowledge of man as we know him) has been passed down to the race from teachers, who have received it from still higher teachers, and so on, and on and on, higher and higher, until it is believed to have originated with some of those wonderfully developed souls which have visited the earth from higher planes of Being, of which there are many. In these lessons we are making no claims of this sort, but pass on the teachings to you, believing that their truth will appeal to those who are ready for them, without any attempt to attribute to them an authority such as just mentioned. Our reference to this high source of the teachings was made because of its general acceptance in the Eastern countries, and by occultists generally.

The Yogi teachings inform us that, in the Beginning, The Absolute formed a Mental Image, or Thought-Form, of an Universal Mind—that is, of an Universal Principle of Mind. And here the distinction is made between this Universal Mind Principle, or Universal Mind-Stuff, as some have called it, and the Infinite Mind itself. The Infinite Mind is something infinitely above this creation of the Universal Mind Principle, the latter being as much an "emanation" as is Matter. Let there be no mistake about this. The Infinite Mind is Spirit—the Universal Mind Principle is "Mind-Stuff" of which all Finite Mind is a part. This Universal Mind Principle was the first conception of The Absolute, in the process of the creation of the Universe. It was the "Stuff" from which all Finite Mind forms, and is formed. It is the Universal Mental Energy. Know it as such—but do not confound it with Spirit, which we have called Infinite Mind, because we had no other term. There is a subtle difference here, which is most important to a careful understanding of the subject.

The Yogi teachings inform us that from this Mental Principle there was developed the Universal Principle of Force or Energy. And that from this Universal Force Principle there developed the Universal Principle of Matter. The Sanscrit terms for these Three Principles are as follows: *Chitta*, or the Universal Mind Substance, or Principle; *Prana*, or the Universal Energy Principle; and *Akasa*, or the Universal Principle of Matter. We have spoken of these Three Principles, or Three Great Manifestations, in our "Advanced Course" of lessons, which followed our "Fourteen Lessons," several years ago, but it becomes necessary for us to refer to them again at this place in connection with the present presentation of the subject. As was stated in the lessons just mentioned, these Three Manifestations, or Principles, are really one, and shade into each other. This matter has been fully touched upon in the concluding lessons of the aforesaid "Advanced Course," to which we must refer you for further details, in order to avoid repetition here. You will find a wonderful correspondence between these centuries-old Yogi teachings, and the latest conceptions of Modern Science.

Well, to return to the main path once more, the Teachings inform us that The Absolute "thought" into being—that is, held the Mental Image, or Thought-Form, of—*Chitta*, or Universal Mind Principle. This *Chitta* was finite, of course, and was bound and governed by the Laws of Finite Mind, imposed upon it by the Will of The Absolute. Everything that is Finite is governed by Laws imposed by the great LAW which we call The Absolute. Then began the Great INVOLUTION which was necessary before Evolution was possible. The word "Involve," you know, means "to wrap up; to cover; to hide; etc.;" and the word "Evolve" means "to unwrap; to unfold; to un-roll; etc." Before a thing can be "evolved," or "unfolded," it must first have been "involved" or "folded-in, or wrapped up, etc." Everything must be "involved" before it can be "evolved;" remember this, please—it is true on all planes, mental, physical, and spiritual. A thing must be "put in" before it may be "taken out." This truth, if remembered and applied to metaphysical problems, will throw the clearest light upon the darkest problems. Make it your own.

Therefore before the process of Evolution from the gross forms of Matter up to the higher, and then on to the Mental, from higher to higher, and then on the Spiritual plane—that Evolution which we see being performed before our sight today—before that

Evolution became possible there was a necessary Involution, or "wrapping-up." The Spirit of the Absolute first "involved" itself in its Mental Image; Thought-Form, or Creation, of the Mind Principle, just as you may "involve" yourself in an earnest thought in deep meditation. Did you never "lose yourself" in thought, or "forget yourself" in an idea? Have you not spoken of yourself as having been "wrapped in thought?" Well, then you can see something of what is here meant, at least so far as the process of "involution" is concerned. You involve yourself in your meditations—the Absolute involves Itself in Its Mental Creations—but, remember the one is Finite, and the other Infinite, and the results are correspondingly weak or strong.

Obeying the laws imposed upon it, the Mental Principle then involved itself in the Energy Principle, or *Prana*, and the Universal Energy sprang into existence. Then, in obedience to the same Laws, the *Prana* involved itself in the *Akasa*, or Universal Matter Principle. Of course each "involving" practically "created" the "wrapper," "sheath" of the lower Principle. Do you see this? Each, therefore, depends upon the Principle higher than itself, which becomes its "Parent Principle," as the Yogis express it. And in this process of Involution the extreme form of Matter was reached before the process of Evolution became possible. The extreme form of gross Matter is not known to us today, on this planet, for we have passed beyond it. But the teachings inform us that such forms were as much grosser that the grossest Matter that we know today, as the latter is gross in comparison with the most ethereal vapors known to Modern Science. The human mind cannot grasp this extreme of the scale, any more than it can the extreme high degree of manifestation.

At this point we must call your attention to certain occult teachings, widely disseminated, which the highest Yogi teachers discountenance, and contradict. We allude to the teaching that in the process of Involution there was a "degeneration" or "devolution" from higher to lower forms of life, until the gross state of Matter was reached. Such a teaching is horrible, when considered in detail. It would mean that The Absolute deliberately created high forms of life, arch-angels, and higher than these—gods in fact—and then caused them to "devolve" until the lowest state was reached. This would mean the exact opposite of Evolution, and would mean a "going down" in accordance with the Divine Will, just as Evolution is a "going up" in accordance with the Divine Will.

This is contrary to man's best instincts, and the advanced Yogi teachings inform us that it is but an illusion or error that men have created by endeavoring to solve spiritual mysteries by purely intellectual processes. The true teaching is that the process of Involution was accomplished by a Principle involving itself in the lower Principle created within itself, and so on until the lowest plane was reached. Note the difference—"Principles as Principles" did this, and not as Individual Forms of Life or Being. There was no more a "devolution" in this process than there was in The Absolute involving itself in the Mental Image of the Mind Principle. There was no "devolution" or "going down"—only an "involution" or "wrapping up," of Principle, within Principle—the Individual Life not having as yet appeared, and not being possible of appearance until the Evolutionary process began.

We trust that we have made this point clear to you, for it is an important matter. If the Absolute first made higher beings, and then caused them to "devolute" into lower and lower forms, then the whole process would be a cruel, purposeless thing, worthy only of some of the base conceptions of Deity conceived of by men in their ignorance. No! the whole effort of the Divine Will seems to be in the direction of "raising up" Individual Egos to higher and still higher forms. And in order to produce such Egos the process of "Involution" of Principles seems to have been caused, and the subsequent wonderful Evolutionary process instituted. What that "Reason" is, is Unknowable, as we have said over and over again. We cannot pry into the Infinite Mind of the Absolute, but we may form certain conclusions by observing and studying the Laws of the Universe, which seem to be moving in certain directions. From the manifested Will of the Divine One, we may at least hazard an idea as to its purposes. And these purposes seem to be always in an "upward" lifting and evolution. Even the coming of the "Night of Brahm" is no exception to this statement, as we shall see in future lessons.

From the starting of the process of Involution from the Mental Principle, down to the extreme downward point of the grossest Manifestation of Matter, there were many stages. From the highest degree of the Finite Mind, down to lower and still lower degrees; then on to the plane of Force and Energy, from higher to lower degrees of Principle within Principle; then on to the plane of Matter, the Involutionary urge proceeded to work. When the plane of Matter was reached, it, of course, showed its highest degree of manifested Matter—the most subtle form of Ether, or *Akasa*. Then down, down, down, went the degrees of Matter, until the grossest possible form was reached, and then there was a moment's pause, before the Evolutionary process, or upward-movement, began. The impulse of the Original Will, or Thought, had exhausted its downward urge, and now began the upward urge or tendency. But here was manifested a new feature.

This new feature was "The Tendency toward Individualization." During the downward trend the movement was *en masse*, that is, by Principle as *Principle*, without any "splitting up" into portions, or centers. But with the first upward movement there was evidenced a tendency toward creating Centers of Energy, or Units of activity, which then manifested itself, as the evolutionary movement continued, from electrons to atoms; from atoms to man. The gross matter was used as material for the formation of finer and more complex forms; and these in turn combined, and formed higher, and so on, and on. And the forms of Energy operated in the same way. And the manifestations of centers of Mind or consciousness in the same way. But all in connection. Matter, Energy and Mind formed a Trinity of Principles, and worked in connection. And the work was always in the direction of causing higher and higher "forms" to arise—higher and higher Units—higher and higher Centers. But in every form, center or unit, there was manifested the Three Principles, Mind, Energy, and Matter. And within each was the ever present Spirit. For Spirit *must* be in All—just as All must be in Spirit.

And, so this Evolutionary process has continued ever since, and must continue for aeons yet. The Absolute is raising itself up into Itself higher and higher Egos, and is providing them with higher and higher sheaths in which to manifest. And, as we shall see in these lessons, as we progress, this evolution is not only along the physical lines, but also along the mental. And it concerns itself not only with "bodies," but with "souls," which also evolve, from time to time, and bodies are given these souls in order that they may work out their evolution. And the whole end and aim of it all seems to be that Egos may reach the stage where they are conscious of the Real Self—of the Spirit within them, and its relation to the Spirit of the Absolute, and then go on and on and on, to planes of life and being, and activities of which even the most advanced of the race may only dream.

As some of the Ancient Yogi Teachers have said: "Men are evolving into super-men; and super-men into gods; and gods into super-gods; and super-gods into Something still higher; until from the lowest bit of matter enclosing life, unto the highest being—yea, even unto The Absolute—there is an Infinite Ladder of Being—and yet the One Spirit pervades all; is in all, as the all is in It."

The Creative Will, of which we have spoken in these lessons, is in full operation all through Life. The Natural Laws are laws of Life imposed by The Absolute in his Mental Image. They are the Natural Laws of this Universe, just as other Universes have other Laws. But The Absolute Itself has no Laws affecting It—It, in Itself *is* LAW.

And these Laws of Life, and Nature, along its varying planes, Material, of Energy; and Mental; are also, in the Divine Mind, else they would not be at all, even in appearance. And when they are transcended, or apparently defied by some man of advanced development, it is only because such a man is able to rise above the plane upon which such laws are operative. But even this transcending is, in itself, in accordance with some higher law.

And so, we see that All, high and low—good and bad—simple or complex—all are contained Within the Mind of the One. Gods, angels, adepts, sages, heavens, planes,—all, everything—is within the Universe, and the Universe is Within the Mind of the One. And all is proceeding in accordance with Law. And all is moving upward and onward, along the lines of Evolution. All is Well. We are held firmly in The Mind of the One.

And, just as the tendency was from the general Principle toward the particular Individual Soul, so is there a Reconciliation later on, for the Individual soul, as it develops and unfolds, loses its sense of Separateness, and begins to feel its identity with the One Spirit, and moves along the lines of unfoldment, until it becomes in Conscious Union with God. Spiritual Evolution does not mean the "growth of the Spirit," for the Spirit cannot grow—it is already Perfect. The term means the unfoldment of the Individual Mind, until it can recognize the Spirit Within. Let us close this lesson with the

CENTRAL THOUGHT.

There is but ONE. That ONE is Spirit. In the Infinite Mind of that ONE SPIRIT there arose the Mental Image or Thought-Form of this Universe. Beginning with the Thought of the Principle in Mind; and passing on to the Principle of Energy; and then on to the Principle of Matter; proceeded the Involutionary Process of Creation. Then, upward began the Evolutionary Process, and Individual Centers or Units were formed. And the tendency, and evolutionary urge is ever in the direction of "unfolding" within the Ego of the Realization of the Indwelling Spirit. As we throw off sheath after sheath, we approach nearer and nearer to the SPIRIT within us, which is the One Spirit pervading all things. This is the Meaning of Life—the Secret of Evolution. All the Universe is contained Within the Mind of The One. There is Nothing outside of that Infinite Mind. There is no Outside, for the One is All in All; Space, Time, and Laws, being but Mental Images in that Mind, as are likewise all shapes and forms, and phenomena. And as the Ego unfolds into a realization of Itself—Its Real Self—so does its Wisdom and Power expand. It thus enters into a greater and greater degree of its Inheritance. Within the Mind of the One, is All there is. And I, and Thou, and All Things are HERE within that Infinite Mind. We are always "held in Mind" by The Absolute—are always safe here. There is nothing to harm us, in Reality, for our Real Self is the Real Self of the Infinite Mind. All is Within the Mind of the One. Even the tiniest atom is under the Law, and protected by the Law. And the LAW is All there Is. And in that Law we may rest Content and Unafraid. May this Realization be YOURS.

PEACE BE WITH YOU ALL.

THE SEVENTH LESSON

COSMIC EVOLUTION.

We have now reached a most interesting point in this course of lessons, and a period of fascinating study lies before us from now until the close of the course. We have acquainted ourselves with the fundamental principles, and will now proceed to witness these principles in active operation. We have studied the Yogi Teachings concerning the Truth underlying all things, and shall now pass on to a consideration of the process of Cosmic Evolution; the Cyclic Laws; the Law of Spiritual Evolution, or Reincarnation; the Law of Spiritual Cause and Effect, or *Karma*; etc. In this lesson we begin the story of the upward progress of the Universe, and its forms, shapes, and forces, from the point of the "moment's pause" following the ceasing of the process of Involution—the point at which Cosmic Evolution begins. Our progress is now steadily upward, so far as the evolution of Individual Centres is concerned. We shall see the principles returning to the Principle—the centres returning to the great Centre from which they emanated during the process of Involution. We shall study the long, gradual, but steady ascent of Man, in his journey toward god-hood. We shall see the Building of an Universe, and the Growth of the Soul.

In our last lesson we have seen that at the dawn of a Brahmic Day, the Absolute begins the creation of a new Universe. The Teachings inform us that in the beginning, the Absolute forms a Mental Image, or Thought-Form of an Universal Mind Principle, or Universal Mind-Stuff, as some of the teachers express it. Then this Universal Mind Principle creates within itself the Universal Energy Principle. Then this Universal Energy Principle creates within itself the Universal Matter Principle. Thus, Energy is a product of Mind; and Matter a product of Energy.

The Teachings then further inform us that from the rare, tenuous, subtle form of Matter in which the Universal Matter Principle first appeared, there was produced forms of Matter less rare; and so by easy stages, and degrees, there appeared grosser and still grosser forms of matter, until finally there could be no further involution into grosser forms, and the Involutionary Process ceased. Then ensued the "moment's pause" of which the Yogi teachers tell us. At that point Matter existed as much grosser that the grossest form of Matter now known to us, as the latter is when compared to the most subtle vapors known to science. It is impossible to describe these lower forms of matter, for they have ages since disappeared from view, and we would have no words with which to describe them. We can understand the situation only by comparisons similar to the above.

Succeeding the moment's pause, there began the Evolutionary Process, or Cosmic Evolution, which has gone on ever since, and which will go on for ages to come. From the grossest forms of Matter there evolved forms a little more refined, and so on and on. From the simple elementarv forms, evolved more complex and intricate forms. And from these forms combinations began to be formed. And the urge was ever upward.

But remember this, that all of this Evolutionary Process is but a Returning Home. It is the Ascent after the Descent. It is not a Creation but an Unfoldment. The Descent was made by principles as principles—the Ascent is being made by Individualized Centres evolved from the principles. Matter manifests finer and finer forms, and exhibits a greater and greater subservience to Energy or Force. And Energy or Force shows a greater and greater degree of "mind" in it. But, remember this, that there is Mind in even the grossest form of Matter. This must be so, for what springs from a thing must contain the elements of its cause.

And the Cosmic Evolution continues, and must continue for aeons of time. Higher and higher forms of Mind are being manifested, and still higher and higher forms will appear in the scale, as the process continues. The evolution is not only along material lines, but has passed on to the mental planes, and is now operating along the spiritual lines as well. And the end, and aim seems to be that each Ego, after the experiences of many lives, may unfold and develop to a point where it may become conscious of its Real Self, and realize its identity with the One Life, and the Spirit.

At this point we may be confronted with the objection of the student of material science, who will ask why we begin our consideration of Cosmic Evolution at a point in which matter has reached the limit of its lowest vibrations, manifesting in the grossest possible form of matter. These students may point to the fact that Science begins its consideration of evolution with the *nebulae*, or faint cloudlike, vaporous matter, from which the planets were formed. But there is only an apparent contradiction here. The *nebulae* were part of the Process of Involution, and Science is right when it holds that the gross forms were produced from the finer. But the process of change from finer to grosser was *Involution*, not Evolution. Do you see the difference? Evolution begins at the point when the stage of Unfoldment commenced. When the gross forms begin to yield to the new upward urge, and unfold into finer forms—then begins Evolution.

We shall pass over the period of Evolution in which Matter was evolving into finer and still finer forms, until at last it reached a degree of vibration capable of supporting that which we call "life." Of course there is "life" in all matter—even in the atom, as we have shown in previous lessons. But when we speak of "life," as we now do, we mean what are generally called "living forms." The Yogi Teachings inform us that the lowest forms of what we call "life" were evolved from forms of high crystal life, which indeed they very much resemble. We have spoken of this resemblance, in the previous lessons of this series. And, so we shall begin at the point where "living forms" began.

Speaking now of our own planet, the Earth, we find matter emerging from the molten state in which it manifested for ages. Gradually cooling and stratifying, the Earth contained none of those forms that we call living forms. The temperature of the Earth in that period is estimated at about 15,000 times hotter than boiling water, which would, of course, render impossible the existence of any of the present known forms of life. But the Yogi Teachings inform us that even in the molten mass there were elementary forms that were to become the ancestral forms of the later living forms. These elementary forms were composed of a vaporous, peculiar form of matter, of minute size,—little more than the atoms, in fact, and yet, just a little more advanced. From these elementary forms, there gradually evolved, as the Earth cooled and solidified, other forms, and so on until at last the first "living form" manifested.

As the globe cooled at the poles, there was gradually created a tropical climate, in which the temperature was sufficiently cool to support certain rudimentary forms of life. In the rocks in the far northern latitudes, there are found abundant traces of fossils, which goes to prove the correctness of the Yogi Teachings of the origin of life at the north pole, from which the living forms gradually spread south toward the equator, as the Earth's surface cooled.

The elementary evolving life forms were of a very simple structure, and were but a degree above the crystals. They were composed of identically the same substance as the crystals, *the only difference being that they displayed a greater degree of mind.* For that matter, even the highest physical form known to us today is composed of simple chemical materials. And these chemical materials are obtained, either directly or indirectly, from the air, water, or earth. The principal materials composing the physical bodies of plants, animals, and man, are oxygen, carbon, hydrogen, nitrogen, with a still smaller proportion of sulphur and phosphorus, and traces of a few other elements. The material part of all living things is alike—the difference lies in the degree of Mind controlling the matter in which it is embodied.

Of these physical materials, carbon is the most important to the living forms. It seems to possess properties capable of drawing to it the other elements, and forcing them into service. From carbon proceeds what is called "protoplasm," the material of which the cells of animal and vegetable life is composed. From protoplasm the almost infinite varieties of living forms have been built up by the process of Evolution, working gradually and by easy stages. Every living form is made up, or composed, of a multitude of single cells, and their combinations. And every form originates in a single cell which rapidly multiplies and reproduces itself until the form of the amoeba; the plant; the animal; the man, is completed. All living forms are but a single cell multiplied. And every cell is composed of protoplasm. Therefore we must look for the beginning of life in the grade of matter called protoplasm. In this both modern Science and the Yogi Teachings agree fully.

In investigating protoplasm we are made to realize the wonderful qualities of its principal constituent—Carbon. Carbon is the wonder worker of the elements. Manifesting in various forms, as the diamond, graphite, coal, protoplasm—is it not entitled to respect? The Yogi Teachings inform vis that in Carbon we have that form of matter which was evolved as the physical basis of life. If any of you doubt that inorganic matter may be transformed into living forms, let us refer you to the plant life, in which you may see the plants building up cells every day from the inorganic, chemical or mineral substances, in the earth, air, and water. Nature performs every day the miracle of transforming chemicals and minerals into living plant cells. And when animal or man eats these plant cells, so produced, they become transformed into animal cells of which the body is built up. What it took Nature ages to do in the beginning, is now performed in a few hours, or minutes.

The Yogi Teachings, again on all-fours with modern Science, inform us that living forms had their beginning in water. In the slimy bed of the polar seas the simple cell-forms appeared, having their origin in the transitional stages before mentioned. The first living forms were a lowly form of plant life, consisting of a single cell. From these forms were evolved forms composed of groups of cells, and so proceeded the work of evolution, from the lower form to the higher, ever in an upward path.

As we have said, the single cell is the physical centre, or parent, of every living form. It contains what is known as the *nucleus*, or kernel, which seems to be more highly organized than the rest of the material of the cell—it may be considered as the "brain" of the cell, if you wish to use your imagination a little. The single cell reproduces itself by growth and division, or separation. Each cell manifests the functions of life, whether it be a single-celled creature, or a cell which with billions of others, goes to make up a higher form. It feels, feeds, grows, and reproduces itself. In the single-celled creature, the one cell performs all of the functions, of course. But as the forms become more complex, the many cells composing a form perform certain functions which are allotted to it, the division of labor resulting in a higher manifestation. This is true not only in the case of animal forms, but also in the case of plant forms. The cells in the bone, muscle, nerve-tissue and blood of the animal differ according to their offices; and the same is true in the cells in the sap, stem, root, leaf, seed and flower of the plant.

As we have said, the cells multiply by division, after a period of growth. The cell grows by material taken into its substance, as food. When sufficient food has been partaken, and enough new material accumulated to cause the cell to attain a certain size, then it divides, or separates into two cells, the division being equal, and the point of cleavage being at the kernel or nucleus. As the two parts separate, the protoplasm *of* each groups itself around its nucleus, and two living forms exist where there was but one a moment before. And then each of the two cells proceed to grow rapidly, and then separate, and so on to the end, each cell multiplying into millions, as time passes.

Ascending in the scale, we next find the living forms composed of cell-groups. These cell-groups are formed by single cells dividing, and then subdividing, but instead of passing on their way they group themselves in clusters, or masses. There are millions of forms of these cell-group creatures, among which we find the sponges, polyps, etc.

In the early forms of life it is difficult to distinguish between the animal and the plant forms, in fact the early forms partake of the qualities of both. But as we advance in the scale a little there is seen a decided "branching out," and one large branch is formed of the evolving plant forms, and the other of the evolving animal forms. The plant-branch begins with the sea-weeds, and passes on to the fungi, lichens, mosses, ferns, pines and palm-ferns, grasses, etc., then to the trees, shrubs and herbs. The animal-branch begins with the *monera*, or single-cell forms, which are little more than a drop of sticky, glue-like protoplasm. Then it passes on to the *amoebae*, which begins to show a slight difference in its parts. Then on the *foraminifera*, which secretes a shell of lime from the water. Then on a step higher to the *polycystina*, which secretes a shell, or skeleton of flint-like material from the water. Then come the sponges. Then the coral-animals, anemones and jelly-fish. Then come the sea-lilies, star-fish, etc. Then the various families of worms. Then the crabs, spiders, centipedes, insects. Then come the mollusca, which include the oysters, clams and other shell-fish; snails, cuttle-fish, sea-squirts, etc. All of the above families of animal-forms are what are known as "invertebrates," that is, without a backbone.

Then we come to the "vertebrates," or animals having a backbone. First we see the fish family with its thousands of forms. Then come the amphibia, which include the toads, frogs, etc. Then come the reptiles, which include the serpents, lizards, crocodiles, turtles, etc. Then come the great family of birds, with its wonderful variety of forms, sizes, and characteristics. Then come the mammals, the name of which comes from the Latin word meaning "the breast," the characteristic of which group comes from the fact that they nourish their young by milk, or similar fluid, secreted by the mother. The mammals are the highest form of the vertebrates.

First among the mammals we find the aplacentals, or those which bring forth immature young, which are grouped into two divisions, *i.e.*, (1) the *monotremes*, or one-vented animals, in which group belong the duck-bills, spiny ant-eaters, etc.; and (2) the *marsupials*, or pouched animals, in which group belong the kangaroo, opossum, etc.

The next highest form among the mammals are known as the *placentals*, or those which bring forth mature young. In this class are found the ant-eaters, sloth, manatee, the whale and porpoise, the horse, cow, sheep, and other hoofed animals; the elephant, seal, the dog, wolf, lion, tiger, and all flesh eating animals; the hares, rats, mice, and ail other gnawing animals; the bats, moles, and other insect-feeders; then come the great family of apes, from the small monkeys up to the orang-outang, chimpanzee, and other forms nearly approaching man. And then comes the highest, Man, from the Kaffir, Bush-man,

Cave-man, and Digger Indian, up through the many stages until the highest forms of our own race are reached.

From the Monera to Man is a long path, containing many stages, but it is a path including all the intermediate forms. The Yogi Teachings hold to the theory of evolution, as maintained by modern Science, but it goes still further, for it holds not only that the physical forms are subject to the evolutionary process, but that also the "souls" embodied in these forms are subject to the evolutionary process. In other words the Yogi Teachings hold that there is a twin-process of evolution under way, the main object of which is to develop "souls," but which also finds it necessary to evolve higher and higher forms of physical bodies for these constantly advancing souls to occupy.

Let us take a hasty glance at the ascending forms of animal life, as they rise in the evolutionary scale. By so doing we can witness the growth of the soul, within them, as manifested by the higher and higher physical forms which are used as channels of expression by the souls within. Let us first study soul-evolution from the outer viewpoint, before we proceed to examine it from the inner. By so doing we will have a fuller idea of the process than if we ignored the outer and proceed at once to the inner. Despise not the outer form, for it has always been, and is now, the Temple of the Soul, which the latter is remodelling and rebuilding in order to accommodate its constantly increasing needs and demands.

Let us begin with the *Protozoa*, or one-celled forms—the lowest form of animal life. The lowest form of this lowest class is that remarkable creature that we have mentioned in previous lessons—the *Moneron*. This creature lives in water, the natural element in which organic life is believed to have had its beginning. It is a very tiny, shapeless, colorless, slimy, sticky mass—something like a tiny drop of glue—alike all over and in its mass, and without organs or parts of any kind. Some have claimed that below the field of the microscope there may be something like elementary organs in the Moneron, but so far as the human eye may discover there is no evidence of anything of the kind. It has no organs or parts with which to perform particular functions, as is the case with the higher forms of life. These functions, as you know, may be classed into three groups, *i.e.*, nutrition, reproduction, and relation—that is, the function of feeding, the function of reproducing its kind, and the function of receiving and responding to the impressions of the outside world. All of these three classes of functions the Moneron performs—but *with any part of its body, or with all of it.*

Every part, or the whole, of the Moneron absorbs food and oxygen—it is all mouth and lungs. Every part, or the whole, digests the food—it is all stomach. Every part, or the whole, performs the reproductive function—it is all reproductive organism. Every part of it senses the impressions from outside, and responds to it—it is all organs of sense, and organs of motion. It envelops its prey as a drop of glue surrounds a particle of sand, and then absorbs the substance of the prey into its own substance. It moves by prolonging any part of itself outward in a sort of tail-like appendage, which it uses as a "foot," or "finger" with which to propel itself; draw itself to, or push itself away from an object. This prolongation is called a *pseudopod*, or "false-foot." When it gets through using the "false-foot" for the particular purpose, it simply draws back into itself that portion which had been protruded for the purpose.

It performs the functions of digestion, assimilation, elimination, etc., perfectly, just as the higher forms of life—but it has no organs for the functions, and performs them severally, and collectively with any, or all parts of its body. What the higher animals perform with intricate organs and parts—heart, stomach, lungs, liver, kidneys, etc., etc.—this tiny creature performs *without organs*, and with its entire body, or any part thereof. The function of reproduction is startlingly simple in the case of the Moneron. It simply divides itself in two parts, and that is all there is to it. There is no male or female sex in its case—it combines both within itself. The reproductive process is even far more simple than the "budding" of plants. You may turn one of these wonderful creatures inside out, and still it goes on the even tenor of its way, in no manner disturbed or affected. It is simply a "living drop of glue," which eats, digests, receives impressions and responds thereto, and reproduces itself. This tiny glue-drop performs virtually the same life functions as do the higher complex forms of living things. Which is the greater "miracle"—the Moneron or Man?

A slight step upward from the Moneron brings us to the *Amoeba*. The name of this new creature is derived from the Greek word meaning "change," and has been bestowed because the creature is constantly changing its shape. This continual change of shape is caused by a continuous prolongation and drawing-in of its pseudopods, or "false-feet," which also gives the creature the appearance of a "many-fingered" organism. This creature shows the first step toward "parts," for it has something like a membrane or "skin" at its surface, and a "nucleus" at its centre, and also an expanding and contracting cavity within its substance, which it uses for holding, digesting and distributing its food, and also for storing and distributing its oxygen—an elementary combination of stomach and lungs! So you see that the amoeba has taken a step upward from the moneron, and is beginning to appreciate the convenience of parts and organs. It is interesting to note, in this connection, that while the ordinary cells of the higher animal body resemble the *monera* in many ways, still the white corpuscles in the blood of man and the animals bear a startling resemblance to the *amoebae* so far as regards size, general structure, and movements, and are in fact known to Science as "amoeboids." The white corpuscles change their shape, take in food in an intelligent manner, and live a comparatively independent life, their movements showing independent "thought" and "will."

Some of the amoebae (the diatoms, for instance) secrete solid matter from the water, and build therefrom shells or houses, which serve to protect them from their enemies. These shells are full of tiny holes, through which the pseudopods are extended in their search for food, and for purposes of movement. Some of these shells are composed of secreted lime, and others of a flinty substance, the "selection" of these substances from the ether mineral particles in the water, evidencing a degree cf "thought," and mind, even in these lowly creatures. The skeletons of these tiny creatures form vast deposits of chalk and similar substances.

Next higher in the scale are the *Infusoria*. These creatures differ from the amoebae inasmuch as instead of pseudopods, they have developed tiny vibrating filaments, or thread-like appendages, which are used for drawing in their prey and for moving about. These filaments are permanent, and are not temporary like the pseudopods of the monera or amoebae—they are the *first signs of permanent hands and feet*. These creatures have also discovered the possibilities of organs and parts, to a still greater degree than have their cousins the amoebae, and have evolved something like a mouth-opening (very rudimentary) and also a short gullet through which they pass their food and oxygen—*they have developed the first signs of a throat, wind-pipe and food-passage.*

Next come the family of Sponges, the soft skeletons of which form the useful article of everyday use. There are many forms who weave a home of far more delicacy and beauty than their more familiar and homely brothers. The sponge creature itself is a slimy, soft creature, which fills in the spaces in its spongy skeleton. It is fastened to one spot, and gathers in its food from the water around it (and oxygen as well), by means of numerous whip-like filaments called *cilia*, which flash through the water driving in the food and oxygen to the inner positions of its body. The water thus drawn in, as well as the refuse from the food, is then driven out in the same manner. It is interesting to note that in the organisms of the higher animals, including man, there are numerous *cilia* performing offices in connection with nutrition, etc. When Nature perfects an instrument, it is very apt to retain it, even in the higher forms, although in the latter its importance may be dwarfed by higher ones.

The next step in the ascending scale of life-forms is occupied by the *polyps*, which are found in water, fastened to floating matter. The polyps fasten themselves to this floating matter, with their mouths downward, from the latter dangling certain tentacles, or thin, long arms. These tentacles contain small thread-like coils in contact with a poisonous fluid, and enclosed in a cell. When the tentacles come in contact with the prey of the creature, or with anything that is sensed as a possible enemy, they contract around the object and the little cells burst and the tiny thread-like coils are released and twist themselves like a loop around the object, poisoning it with the secreted fluid. Some of the polyps secrete flint-like tubes, which they inhabit, and from the ends of which they emerge like flowers. From these parent polyps emerge clusters of young, resembling buds. These bud-like young afterwards become what are known as jelly-fishes, etc., which in turn reproduce themselves—but here is a wonder—the jelly-fish lay eggs, which when hatched produce stationary polyps like their grandparent, and not moving creatures like their parents. The jelly-fishes have a comparatively complex organism. They have an intricate system of canal-like passages with which to convey their food and oxygen to the various parts. They also have something like muscles, which contract and enable the creature to "swim." They also possess a "nervous system," and, most wonderful of all, they have *rudimentary eyes and ears*. Their tentacles, like those of the parent-polyp, secrete the poisonous fluid which is discharged into prey or enemy.

Akin to the polyps are the sea-anemones, with their beautiful colors, and still more complex structure and organism, the tentacles of which resemble the petals of a flower. Varying slightly from these are the coral-creatures, which form in colonies and the skeletons of which form the coral trees and branches, and other forms, with which we are familiar.

Passing on to the next highest family of life-forms, we see the spiny-bodied sea-creatures, such as the sea-urchin, star-fish, etc., which possess a thick, hard skin, covered by spines or prickly projections. These creatures abound in numerous species. The star-fish has rays projecting from a common centre, which gives it its name, while the sea-urchin resembles a ball. The sea-lilies, with their stems and flowers (so-called) belong to this family, as do also the sea-cucumbers, whose name is obtained from their shape and general appearance, but which are animals possessing a comparatively complex organism, one of the features of which is a stomach which may be discarded at will and replaced by a new one. These creatures have a well defined nervous system, and have eyes, and some of them even rudimentary eyelids.

Ascending the scale of life-forms, we next observe the great family of the *Annulosa*, or jointed creatures, which comprises the various families of the worm, the crab, the spider, the ant, etc. In this great family are grouped nearly four-fifths of the known life-forms. Their bodies are well formed and they have nervous systems running along the body and consisting of two thin threads, knotted at different points into ganglia or masses of nerve cells similar to those possessed by the higher animals. They possess eyes and other sense organs, in some cases highly developed. They possess organs, corresponding to the heart, and have a well-developed digestive apparatus. Note this advance in the nutritive organism: the *moneron* takes its food at any point of its body; the *amoeba* takes its food by means of its "false-feet," and drives it through its body by a rhythmic movement of its substance; the *polyp* distributes its food to its various parts by means of the water which it absorbs with the food; the *sea-urchin and star-fish* distribute their food by canals in their bodies which open directly into the water; in the higher forms of the *annulosa*, the food is distributed by a fluid resembling blood, which carries the nourishment to every part and organ, and which carries away the waste matter, the blood being propelled through the body by a rudimentary heart. The oxygen is distributed by each of these forms in a corresponding way, the higher forms having rudimentary lungs and respiratory organs. Step by step the life-forms are perfected, and the organs necessary to perform certain definite functions are evolved from rudimentary to perfected forms.

The families of worms are the humblest members of the great family of the Annulosa. Next come the creatures called Rotifers, which are very minute. Then come the Crustacea, so called from their crustlike shell. This group includes the crabs, lobsters, etc., and closely resembles the insects. In fact, some of the best authorities believe that the insects and the crustacea spring from the same parent form, and some of the Yogi authorities hold to this belief, while others do not attempt to pass upon it, deeming it immaterial, inasmuch as all life-forms have a common origin. The western scientists pay great attention to outward details, while the Oriental mind is apt to pass over these details as of slight importance, preferring to seek the cause back of the outward form. On one point both the Yogi teachers and the scientists absolutely agree, and that is that the family of insect life had its origin in some aquatic creature. Both hold that the wings of the insect have been evolved from organs primarily used for breathing purposes by the ancestor when it took short aerial flights, the need for means of flight afterwards acting to develop these rudimentary organs into perfected wings. There need be no more wonder expressed at this change than in the case of the transformation of the insect from grub to chrysalis, and then to insect. In fact this process is a reproduction of the stages through which the life-form passed during the long ages between sea-creature and land-insect.

We need not take up much of your time in speaking of the wonderful complex organism of some of the insect family, which are next on the scale above the crustacea. The wonders of spider-life—the almost human life of the ants—the spirit of the beehive—and all the rest of the wonders of insect life are familiar to all of our readers. A study of some good book on the life of the higher forms of the insect family will prove of value to anyone, for it will open his or her eyes to the wonderful manifestation of life and mind among these creatures. Remember the remark of Darwin, that the brain of the ant, although not much larger than a pin point, "is one of the most marvelous atoms of matter in the world, perhaps more so than the brain of man."

Closely allied to the crustacea is the sub-family of the *mollusca*, which includes the oyster, clams, and similar creatures; also the snails, cuttle-fish, slugs, nautilus, sea-squirts, etc., etc. Some are protected by a hard shell, while others have a gristly outer skin, serving as an armor, while others still are naked. Those having shells secrete the material for their construction from the water. Some of them are fixed to rocks, etc., while others roam at will. Strange as it may appear at first sight, some of the higher forms of the mollusca show signs of a rudimentary vertebra, and science has hazarded the opinion that the sea-squirts and similar creatures were descended from some ancestor from whom also descended the vertebrate animals, of which man is the highest form known today on this planet. We shall mention this connection in our next lesson, where we will take up the story of "The Ascent of Man" from the lowly vertebrate forms.

And now, in closing this lesson, we must remind the reader that we are *not* teaching Evolution as it is conceived by modern science. We are viewing it from the opposite viewpoint of the Yogi Teaching. Modern Science teaches that Mind is a by-product of the evolving material forms—while the Yogi Teachings hold that there was Mind *involved* in the lowest form, and that that Mind constantly pressing forward for unfoldment *compelled* the gradual evolution, or unfoldment of the slowly advancing degrees of organization and function. Science teaches that "function precedes organization," that is, that a form performs certain functions, imperfectly and crudely, before it evolves the organs suitable for the functioning. For instance the lower forms digested food before they evolved stomachs—the latter coming to meet the need. But the Yogi Teachings go further and claim that "desire precedes function," that is, that the lowly life form "desires" to have digestive apparatus, in order to proceed in the evolutionary scale, before it begins the functioning that brings about the more complex organism. There is ever the "urge" of the Mind which craves unfoldment, and which the creature feels as a dim desire, which grows stronger and stronger as time goes on. Some yield more readily to the urge, and such become the parents of possible higher forms. "Many are called, but few are chosen," and so matters move along slowly from generation to generation, a few forms serving to carry on the evolutionary urge to their descendants. But is always the Evolutionary Urge of the imprisoned Mind striving to cast aside its sheaths and to have more perfect machinery with which, and through which, to manifest and express itself? This is the difference between the "Evolution" of Modern Science and the "Unfoldment" of the Yogi Teachings. The one is all material, with mind as a mere by-product, while the other is all Mind, with matter as a tool and instrument of expression and manifestation.

As we have said in this lesson—and as we shall point out to you in detail in future lessons—accompanying this evolution of bodies there is an evolution of "souls" producing the former. This evolution of souls is a basic principle of the Yogi Teachings, but it is first necessary that you acquaint yourselves with the evolution of bodies and forms, before you may fully grasp the higher teachings.

Our next lesson will be entitled "The Ascent of Man," in which the rise of man—that is, his body—from the lowly forms of the vertebrates is shown. In the same lesson we shall begin our consideration of the "evolution of souls." We trust that the students are carefully studying the details of each lesson, for every lesson has its part in the grand whole of the Teachings.

THE EIGHTH LESSON

THE ASCENT OF MAN.

In our last lesson we led you by successive steps from the beginnings of Life in living forms up to the creatures closely resembling the family of vertebrates—the highest family of living forms on this planet. In this present lesson we take up the story of the "Ascent of Man" from the lowly vertebrate forms.

The large sub-family of forms called "The Vertebrates" are distinguished from the Invertebrates by reason of the former possessing an *internal* bony skeleton, the most important feature of which is the vertebra or spinal column. The vertebrates, be it remembered, possess practically the same organs as the lower forms of life, but differ from them most materially by the possession of the *internal* skeleton, the lower forms having an *external* or outside *skeleton*, which latter is merely a hardening of the skin.

The flexibility of the vertebra creates a wonderful strength of structure, combined with an ease of movement peculiar to the vertebrates, and which renders them the natural forms of life capable of rapid development and evolution. By means of this strength, and ease, these forms are enabled to move rapidly in pursuit of their prey, and away from their pursuers, and also to resist outside pressure or attack. They are protected in a way similar to the invertebrates having shells, and yet have the additional advantage of easy movement. Differing in shape and appearance as do the numerous members of the sub-family of vertebrates, still their structure is easily seen to spring from a single form—all are modifications of some common pattern, the differences arising from the necessities of the life of the animal, as manifested through the desire and necessities of the species.

Science shows the direct relationship between the Vertebrates, and the Invertebrates by means of several connecting-links, the most noticeable of which is the Lancelot, a creature resembling the fish-form, and yet also closely resembling the lower (invertebrate) forms of life. This creature has no head, and but one eye. It is semi-transparent, and possesses *cilia* for forcing in the water containing its food. It has something like gills, and a gullet like the lower forms. It has no heart, the blood being circulated by means of contracting vessels or parts. Strictly speaking, it has no back-bone, or vertebra, but still Science has been compelled to class it among the vertebrates because is has a gristly cartilage where the back-bone is found in the higher forms. This gristle may be called an "elementary spine." It has a nervous system consisting of a single cord which spreads into a broadened end near the creature's mouth, and which may therefore be regarded as "something like a brain." This creature is really a developed form of

Invertebrate, shaped like a Vertebrate, and showing signs of a rudimentary spine and nervous system of the latter. It is a "connecting-link."

The lowest forms of the true Vertebrates are the great families of Fishes. These Fish families include fishes of high and low degree, some of the higher forms being as different from the lowest as they (the highest) are different from the Reptile family. It is not necessary to go into detail regarding the nature of the fish families, for every student is more or less familiar with them.

Some peculiar forms of fish show a shading into the Reptile family, in fact they seem to belong nearly as much to the latter as to their own general family. Some species of fish known as the *Dipnoi* or "double-breathers," have a remarkable dual system of breathing. That is, they have gills for breathing while in the water, and also have a primitive or elementary "lung" in the shape of an air-bladder, or "sound," which they use for breathing on land. The Mud-fish of South America, and also other forms in Australia and other places, have a modification of fins which are practically "limbs," which they actually use for traveling on land from pond to pond. Some of these fish have been known to travel enormous distances in search of new pools of water, or new streams, having been driven from their original homes by droughts, or perhaps by instincts similar to the migrating instinct of birds. Eels are *fish* (although many commonly forget this fact) and many of their species are able to leave the water and travel on land from pond to pond, their breathing being performed by a peculiar modification of the gills. The climbing perch of India are able to live out of water, and have modified gills for breathing purposes, and modified fins for climbing and walking. So you see that without leaving the fish family proper, we have examples of land living creatures which are akin to "connecting links."

But there are real "connecting-links"' between the Fish and the Reptiles. Passing over the many queer forms which serve as links between the two families, we have but to consider our common frog's history for a striking example. The Tadpole has gills, has no limbs, uses its tail like a fish's fin, eats plants, etc. Passing through several interesting stages the Tadpole reaches a stage in which it is a frog with a tail—then it sheds its tail and is a full fledged Frog, with four legs; web-feet; no tail; and feeding on animals. The Frog is amphibious, that is, able to live on land or in water—and yet it is compelled to come to the surface of the water for air to supply its lungs. Some of the amphibious animals possess both lungs and gills, even when matured; but the higher vertebrates living in the water breathe through lungs which are evolved from the air-bladder of fishes, which in turn have been evolved from the primitive gullet of the lower forms. There are fishes known which are warm-blooded. Students will kindly remember that the Whale is not a fish, but an aquatic animal—a mammal, in fact, bringing forth its young alive, and suckling it from its breasts.

So we readily see that it is but a step, and a short step at that, between the land-traveling and climbing fishes and the lower forms of Reptiles. The Frog shows us the process of evolution between the two families, its life history reproducing the gradual evolution which may have required ages to perfect in the case of the species. You will remember that the embryo stages of all creatures reproduce the various stages of evolution through which the species has passed—this is true in Man as well as in the Frog.

We need not tarry long in considering the Reptile family of living forms. In its varieties of serpents, lizards, crocodiles, turtles, etc., we have studied and observed its forms. We see the limbless snakes; the lizards with active limbs; the huge, clumsy, slow crocodiles and alligators—the armor-bearing turtles and tortoises—all belonging to the one great family of Reptiles, and nearly all of them being degenerate descendants of the mighty Reptile forms of the geological Age of Reptiles, in which flourished the mighty forms of the giant reptiles—the monsters of land and water. Amidst the dense vegetation of that pre-historic age, surrounded by the most favorable conditions, these mighty creatures flourished and lived, their fossilized skeleton forms evidencing to us how far their descendants have fallen, owing to less favorable conditions, and the development of other life-forms more in harmony with their changed environment.

Next comes the great family of Birds. The Birds ascended from the Reptiles. This is the Eastern Teaching, and this is the teaching of Western Science It was formerly taught in the text-books that the line of ascent was along the family of winged reptiles which existed in the Age of Reptiles, in the early days of the Earth. But the later writers on the subject, in the Western world, have contradicted this. It is now taught that these ancient winged-reptiles were featherless, and more closely resembled the Bat family than birds. (You will remember that a Bat is neither a reptile nor a bird—it is a mammal, bringing forth its young alive, and suckling them at its breast. The Bat is more like a mouse, and its wings are simply membrane stretched between its fingers, its feet, and its tail.)

The line of ascent from Reptile to Bird was along the forms of the Reptiles that walked on land. There are close anatomical and physiological relations and correspondences between the two families (Reptiles and Birds) which we need not refer to here. And, of course, many modifications have occurred since the "branching-out." The scales of the reptiles, and the feathers of the birds, are known to be but modifications of the original outer skin, as are also the hair, claws, hoofs, nails, etc., of all animals. Even teeth arose in this way, strange as it may now seem—they are all secreted from the skin. What a wonderful field for thought—this gradual evolution from the filmy outer covering of the lowest living forms to the beautiful feathers, beaks, and claws of the bird!

The evolving of wings meant much to the ascending forms of life. The Reptiles were compelled to live in a narrow circle of territory, while the Birds were able to travel over the earth in wide flights. And travel always develops the faculties of observation, memory, etc., and cultivates the senses of seeing, hearing, etc. And the creature is compelled to exercise its evolving "thinking" faculties to a greater extent. And so the Birds were compelled by necessity of their travels to develop a greater degree of thinking organism. The result is that among birds we find many instances of intelligent thought, which cannot be dismissed as "mere instinct." Naturalists place the Crow at the head of the family of Birds, in point of intelligence, and those who have watched these creatures and studied the mental processes, will agree that this is a just decision. It has been proven that Crows are capable of counting up to several figures, and in other ways they display a wonderful degree of almost human sagacity.

Next above the Bird family comes the highest form of all—the Mammals. But before we begin our consideration of these high forms, let us take a hasty glance at the "connecting-links" between the Birds and the Mammals. The lowest forms of the Mammals resemble Birds in many ways. Some of them are toothless, and many of them have the same primitive intestinal arrangements possessed by the birds, from which arises their name, *Monotremes*. These *Monotremes* may be called half-bird and half-mammal. One of the most characteristic of their family is the *Ornithorhynchus*, or Duck-bill, which the early naturalists first thought was a fraud of the taxidermists, or bird-stuffers, and then, when finally convinced, deemed it a "freak-of-nature." But it is not a freak creature, but a "connecting-link" between the two great families of creatures. This animal presents a startling appearance to the observer who witnesses it for the first time. It resembles a beaver, having a soft furry coat, but also has a horny, flat bill like a duck, its feet being webbed, but also furnished with claws projecting over the edge of the web-foot. It lays eggs in an underground nest—two eggs at a time, which are like the eggs of birds, inasmuch as they contain not only the protoplasm from which the embryo is formed, but also the "yolk." on which the embryo feeds until hatched. After the young Duck-bill is hatched, it feeds from teatless glands in the mother's body, the milk being furnished by the mother by a peculiar process. Consider this *miracle—an animal which lays eggs and then when her young are hatched nourishes them with milk*. The milk-glands in the mother are elementary "breasts."

The above-mentioned animal is found in Australia, the land of many strange forms and "connecting-links," which have survived there while in other parts of the globe they have vanished gradually from existence, crowded out by the more perfectly evolved forms. Darwin has called these surviving forms "living fossils." In that same land is also found the *Echidna* or spiny ant-eater, which lays an egg and then hatches it in her pouch, after which she nourishes it on milk, in a manner similar to that of the Duck-bill. This animal, like the Duck-bill, is a Monotreme.

Scientists are divided in theories as to whether the Monotremes are actually descended directly from the Reptiles or Birds, or whether there was a common ancestor from which Reptiles and Birds and Mammals branched off. But this is not important, for the relationship between Reptiles, Birds and Mammals is clearly proven. And the Monotremes are certainly one of the surviving forms of the intermediate stages.

The next higher step in the ascent of Mammal life above the Monotreme is occupied by the Marsupials, or *milk-giving, pouched animals*, of which family the opossum and kangaroo are well known members. The characteristic feature of this family of creatures is the possession of an external pouch in the female, in which the young are kept and nourished until they can take care of themselves as the young of other animals are able to do. The young of the Marsupials are brought forth, or born, in an imperfect condition, and undeveloped in size and strength. There are fossil remains of Marsupials showing that in past ages creatures of this kind existed which were as large as elephants.

In the more common form of Mammals the young are brought forth fully formed, they having received "nourishment, before birth, from the mother's body, through the *placenta*, the appendage which connects the fetus with the parent. The Placental Mammals were the best equipped of all the life-forms for survival and development, for the reason that the young were nourished during their critical period, and the care that the mammal must of necessity give to her young operated in the direction of affording a special protection far superior to that of the other forms. This and other causes acted to place the Placentals in the "Royal line" from which Man was evolved.

The following families of Placental Mammals are recognized by Science, each having its own structural peculiarities:

The *Edentata*, or Toothless creatures, among which are the sloths, ant-eaters, armadillos, etc. These animals seem to be closer to the Monotremes than they are to the Marsupials;

The *Sirenia*, so called by reason of their fanciful resemblance to the sirens of mythology, among which are the sea-cows, manatees, dugongs, etc., which are fish-like in structure and appearance, the fore-limbs being shaped like paddles, or fins, and the hind-limbs being absent or rudimentary;

The *Cetacea*, or Whale Family, including whales, Porpoises, dolphins, etc., which are quite fish-like in appearance and structure, their forms being adapted for life in the sea, although they are, of course, Mammals, bringing forth matured young which are suckled at the breast;

The *Ungulata*, or Hoofed Animals, which comprise many varied forms, such as the horse, the tapir, the rhinoceros, the swine, the hippopotamus, the camel, the deer, the sheep, the cow, etc., etc.;

The *Hyracoidea*, which is a small family, the principal member of which is the coney, or rock rabbit, which has teeth resembling those of the hoofed animals, in some ways, and those of the gnawing animals in the others.

The *Proboscidea*, or Trunked Animals, which family is represented in this age only by the families of elephants, which have a peculiar appendage called a "trunk," which they use as an additional limb;

The *Carnivora*, or Flesh-eaters, represented by numerous and various forms, such as the seal, the bear, the weasel, the wolf, the dog, the lion, the tiger, the leopard, etc. The wolf and similar forms belong to the sub-family of dogs; while the lion, tiger, etc., belong to the sub-family of cats;

The *Rodentia*, or Gnawers, comprising the rat, the hare, the beaver, the squirrel, the mouse, etc., etc.;

The *Insectivora*, or Insect Feeders, comprising the mole, the shrew, the hedgehog, etc.;

The *Chiroptera*, or Finger-Winged Animals, comprising the great family of Bats, etc., which are very highly developed animals;

The *Lemuroidea*, or Lemurs, the name of which is derived from the Latin word meaning a "ghost," by reason of the Lemur's habits of roaming about at night. The Lemur is a nocturnal animal, somewhat resembling the Monkey in general appearance, but with a long, bushy tail and sharp muzzle like a fox. It is akin to a small fox having hands and feet like a monkey, the feet being used to grasp like a hand, as is the case with the true Monkey family. These creatures are classed by some naturalists among the Monkeys by reason of being "four-handed," while others are disposed to consider as still more important their marked relationship with, and affinity to, the marsupials, gnawers and insect-feeders. On the whole, these creatures are strangely organized and come very near to being a "connecting-link" between other forms. One of the Lemurs is what is known as the *colugo*, or "flying lemur," which resembles a squirrel in many particulars, and yet has a membranous web extending from its hands, which enables it to make flying leaps over great distances. This last named variety seems to furnish a link between the insect-feeders and the Primates;

The *Primates*, which is a large family comprising the various forms of monkeys, baboons, man-apes, such as the gibbon, gorilla, chimpanzee, orang-outang, etc., all of which have big jaws, small brains, and a stooping posture. This family also includes MAN, with his big brain and erect posture, and his many races depending upon shape of skull, color of skin, character of hair, etc.

In considering the Ascent of Man (physical) from the lowly forms of the Monera, etc., up to his present high position, the student is struck with the continuity of the ascent, development and unfoldment. While there are many "missing-links," owing to the disappearance of the forms which formed the connection, still there is sufficient proof left in the existing forms to satisfy the fair-minded inquirer. The facts of embryology alone are sufficient proof of the ascent of Man from the lowly forms. Each and every man today has passed through all the forms of the ascent within a few months, from single cell to the new-born, fully formed infant.

Embryology teaches us that the eggs from which all animal forms evolve are all practically alike so far as one can ascertain by microscopic examination, no matter how diverse may be the forms which will evolve from them, and this resemblance is maintained even when the embryo of the higher forms begins to manifest traces of its future form. Von Baer, the German scientist, was the first to note this remarkable and suggestive fact. He stated it in the following words: "In my possession are two little embryos, preserved in alcohol, whose names I have omitted to attach, and at present I am unable to state to what class they belong. They may be lizards, or small birds, or very young mammals, so complete is the similarity in the mode of the formation of the head and trunk in these animals. The extremities, however, are still absent in these embryos. But even if they had existed in the earliest stage of their development, we should learn nothing, for the feet of lizards and mammals, the wings and feet of birds, no less than the hands and feet of man, all arise from the same fundamental form."

As has been said by Prof. Clodd, "the embryos of all living creatures epitomize during development the series of changes through which the ancestral forms passed if their ascent from the simple to the complex; the higher structures passing through the same stages as the lower structures up to the point when they are marked off from them, yet never becoming in detail the form which they represent for the time being. For example, the embryo of man has at the outset gill-like slits on each side of the neck, like a fish. These give place to a membrane like that which supersedes gills in the development of birds and reptiles; the heart is at first a simple pulsating chamber like that in worms; the backbone is prolonged into a movable tail; the great toe is extended, or opposable, like our thumbs, and like the toes of apes; the body three months before birth is covered all over with hair except on the palms and soles. At birth the head is relatively larger, and the arms and legs relatively longer than in the adult; the nose is bridgeless; both features, with others which need not be detailed, being distinctly ape-like. Thus does the egg from which man springs, a structure only one hundred and twenty-fifth of an inch in size, compress into a few weeks the results of millions of years, and set before us the history of his development from fish-like and reptilian forms, and of his more immediate descent from a hairy, tailed quadruped. That which is individual or peculiar to him, the physical and mental character inherited, is left to the slower development which follows birth."

This, then, in brief is the Western theory of Evolution—the Physical Ascent of Man. We have given it as fully as might be in the small space at our disposal in these lessons on the Yogi Philosophy. Why? Because we wish to prove to the Western mind, in the Western way, that Western Science corroborates the Ancient Yogi Teachings of the Unfoldment of Living Forms, from Monad to Man. The Eastern teachers scorn to "prove" anything to their pupils, who sit at the feet of teachers and accept as truth that which is taught them, and which has been handed down from the dim ages long past. But this method will never do for the Western student—he must have it "proven" to him by physical facts and instances, not by keen, subtle, intellectual reasoning alone. The Eastern student wishes to be "told"—the Western student wishes to be "shown." Herein lies the racial differences of method of imparting knowledge. And so we have recognized this fact and have heaped up proof after proof from the pages of Western Science, in order to prove to you the reasonableness, from the Western point of view, of the doctrine of Physical Unfoldment as taught for ages past by the Yogi *gurus* to their *chelas*. You have now the Eastern Teachings on the subject, together with the testimony of Western Science to the reasonableness of the idea.

But, alas! Western Science, while performing a marvelous work in piling up fact after fact to support its newly-discovered theory of Evolution, in a way utterly unknown to the Oriental thinker who seeks after principles by mental concentration—*within* rather than without—while actually proving by physical facts the *mental* conceptions of the Oriental Teachings, still misses the vital point of the subject-thought. In its materialistic tendencies it has failed to recognize *the mental cause of the physical unfoldment*. It is true that Lamark, the real Western discoverer of Evolution, taught that Desire and Mental Craving, was the real force behind Evolution, but his ideas were jeered at by his contemporaries, and are not regarded seriously by the majority of Evolutionists even today. And yet he was nearer to the truth than Darwin or any other Western Evolutionist. And time will show that Science has overlooked his genius, which alone throws the true light upon the subject.

In order to see just this difference between the Darwinian school and the Yogi Teachings let us examine into what causes the Western Evolutionists give for the fact of Evolution itself. We shall do this briefly.

The Darwinians start out to explain the causes of the "Origin of Species," with the statement that "no two individuals of the same species are exactly alike; each tends to vary." This is a self-evident fact, and is very properly used as a starting point for Variation. The next step is then stated as "variations are transmitted, and therefore tend to become permanent," which also is self-evident, and tends to prove the reasonableness of the gradual evolution of species. The next step in the argument is "as man produces new species and forms, by breeding, culture, etc., so has Nature in a longer time produced the same effect, in the same way." This also is reasonable, although it tends to personify Nature, and to give it a *mind* before the evolutionists admit "mind" was evolved.

It will be as well to quote Darwin himself on this point. He says; "As man can produce, and certainly has produced, a great result by his methodical and unconscious means of selection, what may not natural selection effect? Man can act only on external and visible characters, while Nature, if I may be allowed to personify the natural preservation or survival of the fittest, cares nothing for appearances except in so far as they are useful to any being. She can act on every internal organ, on every shade of constitutional difference, on the whole machinery of life. Man selects only for his own good; Nature only for the good of the being which she tends. Every selected character is fully exercised by her, as is implied by the fact of their selection. Man keeps the natives of many climates in the same country; he seldom exercises each selected character in some peculiar and fitting manner; he feeds a long-beaked and a short-beaked pigeon on the same food; he does not exercise a long-backed or long-legged quadruped in any peculiar manner; he exposes sheep with long hair and short wool in the same climate. He does not allow the most vigorous males to struggle for the females. He does not rigidly destroy all inferior animals, but protects during each varying season, so far as lies in his power, all his productions. He often begins his selection by some half-monstrous form, or at least by some modification prominent enough to catch the eye or to be plainly useful to him. Under Nature the slightest differences of structure or constitution may- well turn the nicely balanced scale in the struggle for life, and so be preserved. How fleeting are the wishes and efforts of man! how short his time! and consequently how poor will be his results, compared with those accumulated by nature during whole geological periods! Can we wonder, then, that Nature's productions should be far 'truer' in character than man's productions; that they should be infinitely better adapted to the most complex conditions of life, and should plainly bear the stamp of far higher workmanship?"

Darwin's theory of survival of the fittest is begun by the statement of the fact that the number of organisms that survive are very small compared with the number that are born. To quote his own words, "There is no exception to the rule that every organic being naturally increases at so high a rate that, if not destroyed, the earth would soon be covered by the progeny of a single pair. Even slow-breeding man has doubled in twenty-five years, and at this rate in less than a thousand years there would literally not be standing room for the progeny." It has been computed that if the offspring of the elephant, which is believed to be the slowest breeding animal known, were to survive, there would be about 20,000,000 elephants on the earth in 750 years. The roe of a single cod contains eight or nine millions of eggs, and if each egg were to hatch, and the fish survive, the sea would shortly become a solid mass of codfish. The house fly is said to have 20,000,000 descendants in a season, counting several generations of progeny, from its several broods. And some scientist has computed that the *aphis*, or plant-louse, breeds so rapidly, and in such enormous quantity, that the tenth generation of one set of parents would be so large that it would contain more ponderable animal matter than would the population of China, which is estimated at 500,000,000! And this without counting the progeny preceding the tenth generation!

The result of the above conditions is very plain. There must ensue a Struggle for Existence, which necessitates the Survival of the Fittest. The weak are crushed out by the strong; the swift out-distance the slow. The individual forms or species best adapted to their environment and best equipped for the struggle, be the equipment physical or mental, survive those less well equipped or less well adapted to environment. Animals evolving variations in structure that give them even a slight advantage over others not so favored, naturally have a better chance to survive. And this, briefly, is what Evolutionists call "The Survival of the Fittest."

As appertaining to the Struggle for Existence, color and mimicry are important factors. Grant Allen, in his work on Darwin, says concerning this, and also as illustrating "Natural Selection": "In the desert with its monotonous sandy coloring, a black insect or a white insect, still more a red insect or a blue insect, would be immediately detected and devoured by its natural enemies, the birds and the lizards. But any greyish or yellowish insects would be less likely to attract attention at first sight, and would be overlooked as long as there were any more conspicuous individuals of their own kind about for the birds and lizards to feed on. Hence, in a very short time the desert would be depopulated of all but the greyest and yellowest insects; and among these the birds would pick out those which differed most markedly in hue and shade from the sand around them. But those which happened to vary most in the direction of a sandy or spotty color would be more likely to survive, and to become the parents of future generations. Thus, in the course of long ages, all the insects which inhabit deserts have become sand-colored, because the less sandy were perpetually picked out for destruction by their ever-watchful foes, while the most sandy escaped, and multiplied and replenished the earth with their own likes."

Prof. Clodd, remarking upon this fact, adds: "Thus, then, is explained the tawny color of the larger animals that inhabit the desert; the stripes upon the tiger, which parallel with the vertical stems of bamboo, conceal him as he stealthily nears his prey; the brilliant green of tropical birds; the leaf-like form and colors of certain insects; the dried, twig-like form of many caterpillars; the bark-like appearance of tree-frogs; the harmony of the ptarmigan's summer plumage with the lichen-colored stones upon which it sits; the dusky color of creatures that haunt the night; the bluish transparency of animals which live on the surface of the sea; the gravel-like color of flat-fish that live at the bottom; and the gorgeous tints of those that swim among the coral reefs."

All this does not run contrary to the Yogi Philosophy, although the latter would regard these things as but the secondary cause for the variation and survival of species, etc. The Oriental teachings are that it is the *desire* of the animal that *causes* it to assume the colors and shapes in accordance with its environment, the desire of course operating along sub-conscious lines of physical manifestation. The mental influence, which is the real cause of the phenomena, and which is taught as such by the Yogis, is almost lost sight of by the Western Evolutionists, who are apt to regard Mind as a "by-product" of matter. On the contrary, *the Yogis regard Matter as the product of Mind.* But there is no conflict here as far as regards the law of the Survival of the Fittest. The insects that *most desired* to become sand-colored became so, and were thus protected, while their less "desireful" brethren were exterminated. The Western scientist explains the outward phenomena, but does not look for the *cause* behind it, which is taught by the Oriental sages.

The doctrine of "Sexual Selection" is another of the leading tenets of the Darwinists. Briefly, it may be expressed as the theory that in the rivalry and struggle of the males for the females the strongest males win the day, and thus transmit their particular qualities to their offspring. Along the same lines is that of the attraction exerted by bright colors in the plumage of the males of birds, etc., which give them an advantage in the eyes of the females, and thus, naturally, the bright colors are perpetuated.

This, then, is the brief outline of the Story of Man's Physical Evolution, as stated by Western Science, and compared with the Yogi Teachings. The student should compare the two ideas, that he may harmonize and reconcile them. It must be remembered, however, that Darwin did *not* teach that Man descended from the monkeys, or apes, as we know them now. The teaching of Western Evolution is that the apes, and higher forms of monkey life descended from some common ancestral form, which same ancestor was also the ancestor of Man. In other words, Man and Apes are the different branches that emerged from the common trunk ages ago. Other forms doubtless emerged from the same trunk, and perished because less adapted to their environments. The Apes were best adapted to their own environments, and Man was best adapted to his. The weaker branches failed.

One must remember that the most savage races known to us today are practically as far different from the highest American, European or Hindu types of Man as from the highest Apes. Indeed, it would seem far easier for a high Ape to evolve into a Kaffir,

Hottentot, or Digger Indian, than for the latter to evolve into an Emerson, Shakespeare, or Hindu Sage. As Huxley has shown, the brain-structure of Man compared with that of the Chimpanzee shows differences but slight when compared with the difference between that of the Chimpanzee and that of the Lemur. The same authority informs us that in the important feature of the deeper brain furrows, and intricate convolutions, the chasm between the highest civilized man and the lowest savage is far greater than between the lowest savage and the highest man-like ape. Darwin, describing the Fuegians, who are among the very lowest forms of savages, says: "Their very signs and expressions are less intelligible to us than those of the domesticated animal. They are men who do not possess the instinct of those animals, nor yet appear to boast of human reason, or at least of arts consequent upon that reason."

Professor Clodd, in describing the "primitive man," says: "Doubtless he was lower than the lowest of the savages of today—a powerful, cunning biped, with keen sense organs always sharper, in virtue of constant exercise, in the savage than in the civilized man (who supplements them by science), strong instincts, uncontrolled and fitful emotions, small faculty of wonder, and nascent reasoning power; unable to forecast tomorrow, or to comprehend yesterday, living from hand to mouth on the wild products of Nature, clothed in skin and bark, or daubed with clay, and finding shelter in trees and caves; ignorant of the simplest arts, save to chip a stone missile, and perhaps to produce fire; strong in his needs of life and vague sense of right to it and to what he could get, but slowly impelled by common perils and passions to form ties, loose and haphazard at the outset, with his kind, the power of combination with them depending on sounds, signs and gestures."

Such was the ancestral man. Those who are interested in him are referred to the two wonderful tales of the cave-man written in the form of stories by two great modern novelists. The books referred to are (1) "*The Story of Ab*," by Stanley Waterloo, and (2) "*Before Adam*," by Jack London. They may be obtained from any bookseller. Both are works of fiction, with the scientific facts cleverly interwoven into them.

And now in conclusion before we pass on the subject of "Spiritual Evolution," which will form the subject of our next lesson, we would again call your attention to the vital difference between the Western and the Eastern Teachings. The Western holds to a mechanical theory of life, which works without the necessity of antecedent Mind, the latter appearing as a "product" at a certain stage. The Eastern holds *that Mind is back of, under, and antecedent to all the work of Evolution*—the *cause*, not the effect or product. The Western claims that Mind was produced by the struggle of Matter to produce higher forms of itself. *The Eastern claims that the whole process of Evolution is caused by Mind striving, struggling and pressing forward toward expressing itself more fully—to liberate itself from the confining and retarding Matter—the struggle resulting in an Unfoldment which causes sheath after sheath of the confining material bonds to be thrown off and discarded, in the effort to release the confined Spirit which is behind even the Mind. The Yogi Teachings are that the Evolutionary Urge is the pressure of the confined Spirit striving to free itself from the fetters and bonds which sorely oppress it.*

The struggle and pain of Evolution is the parturition-pangs of the Spiritual deliverance from the womb of Matter. Like all birth it is attended by pain and suffering, but the end justifies it all. And as the human mother forgets her past suffering in the joy of witnessing the face, and form, and life, of her loved child, so will the soul forget the pain of the Spiritual birth by reason of the beauty and nobility of that which will be born to and from it.

Let us study well the story of Physical Evolution, but let us not lose ourselves in it, for it is but the preliminary to the story of the Unfoldment of the Soul.

Let us not despise the tale of the Body of Man—for it is the story of the Temple of the Spirit which has been built up from the most humble beginnings, until it has reached the present high stage. And yet even this is but the beginning, for the work will go on, and on, and on, in the spirit of those beautiful lines of Holmes:

> "Build thee more stately mansions, oh, my soul!
> As the swift seasons roll!
> Leave thy low-vaulted past!
> Let each new temple, nobler than the last,
> Shut thee from heaven with a dome more vast,
> Till thou at last *art free*,
> Leaving thine outgrown shell by life's unresting sea."

THE NINTH LESSON

METEMPSYCHOSIS.

As we have said in our last lesson, while the Yogi Teachings throw an important light upon the Western theory of Evolution, still there is a vital difference between the Western scientific teachings on the subject and the Eastern theories and teachings. The Western idea is that the process is a mechanical, material one, and that "mind" is a "by-product" of Matter in its evolution. But the Eastern Teachings hold that Mind is under, back of, and antecedent to all the work of Evolution, and that Matter is a "by-product" of Mind, rather than the reverse.

The Eastern Teachings hold that Evolution is caused by Mind striving, struggling, and pressing forward toward fuller and fuller expression, using Matter as a material, and yet always struggling to free itself from the confining and retarding influence of the latter. The struggle results in an Unfoldment, causing sheath after sheath of the confining material bonds to be thrown off and discarded, as the Spirit presses upon the Mind, and the Mind moulds and shapes the Matter. Evolution is but the process of birth of the Individualized Spirit, from the web of Matter in which it has been confined. And the pains and struggles are but incidents of the spiritual parturition.

In this and following lessons we shall consider the "Spiritual Evolution, of the race—that is the Unfoldment of Individualized Spirit—just as we did the subject Physical Evolution in the last two lessons.

We have seen that preceding Spiritual Evolution, there was a Spiritual Involution. The Yogi Philosophy holds that in the Beginning, the Absolute meditated upon the subject of Creation, and formed a Mental Image, or Thought-Form, of an Universal Mind—that is, of an Universal Principle of Mind. This Universal Principle of Mind is the Great Ocean of "Mind-Stuff" from which all the phenomenal Universe is evolved. From this Universal Principle of Mind, proceeded the Universal Principle of Force or Energy. And from the latter, proceeded the Universal Principle of Matter.

The Universal Principle of Mind was bound by Laws imposed upon it by the mental-conception of the Absolute—the Cosmic Laws of Nature. And these laws were the compelling causes of the Great Involution. For before Evolution was possible, Involution was necessary. We have explained that the word "involve" means "to wrap up; to cover; to hide, etc." Before a thing can be "evolved," that is "unfolded," it must first be "involved," that is "wrapped up." A thing must be *put in*, before it may be *taken out.*

Following the laws of Involution imposed upon it, the Universal Mental Principle involved itself in the Universal Energy Principle; and then in obedience to the same laws, the latter involved itself in the Universal Material Principle. Each stage of Involution, or *wrapping-up*, created for itself (out of the higher principle which in being involved) the wrapper or sheath which is to be used to wrap-up the higher principle. And the higher forms of the Material Principle formed sheaths of lower forms, until forms of Matter were produced far more gross than any known to us now, for they have disappeared in the Evolutionary ascent. Down, down, down went the process of Involution, until the lowest point was reached. Then ensued a moment's pause, preceding the beginning of the Evolutionary Unfoldment.

Then began the Great Evolution. But, as we have told you, the Upward movement was distinguished by the "Tendency toward Individualization." That is, while the Involuntary Process was accomplished by Principles as Principles, the Upward Movement was begun by a tendency toward "splitting up," and the creation of "individual forms," and the effort to perfect them and build upon them higher and still higher succeeding forms, until a stage was reached in which the Temple of the Spirit was worthy of being occupied by Man, the self-conscious expression of the Spirit. For the coming of Man was the first step of a higher form of Evolution—the Spiritual Evolution. Up to this time there had been simply an Evolution of Bodies, but now there came the Evolution of Souls.

And this Evolution of Souls becomes possible only by the process of Metempsychosis (pronounced *me-temp-si-ko-sis*) which is more commonly known as Reincarnation, or Re-embodiment.

It becomes necessary at this point to call your attention to the general subject of Metempsychosis, for the reason that the public mind is most confused regarding this important subject. It has the most vague ideas regarding the true teachings, and has somehow acquired the impression that the teachings are that human souls are re-born into the bodies of dogs, and other animals. The wildest ideas on this subject are held by some people. And, not only is this so, but even a number of those who hold to the doctrine of Reincarnation, in some of its forms, hold that their individual souls were once the individual souls of animals, from which state they have evolved to the present condition. This last is a perversion of the highest Yogi Teachings, and we trust to make same plain in these lessons. But, first we must take a look at the general subject of Metempsychosis, that we may see the important part it has played in the field of human thought and belief.

While to many the idea of Metempsychosis may seem new and unfamiliar, still it is one of the oldest conceptions of the race, and in ages past was the accepted belief of the whole of the civilized race of man of the period. And even today, it is accepted as Truth by the majority of the race

The almost universal acceptance of the idea by the East with its teeming life, counterbalances its comparative non-reception by the Western people of the day. From the early days of written or legendary history, Metempsychosis has been the accepted belief of many of the most intelligent of the race. It is found underlying the magnificent civilization of ancient Egypt, and from thence it traveled to the Western world being held as the highest truth by such teachers as Pythagoras, Empedocles, Plato, Virgil and Ovid. Plato's Dialogues are full of this teaching. The Hindus have always held to it. The Persians, inspired by their learned Magi, accepted it implicitly. The ancient Druids, and Priests of Gaul, as well as the ancient inhabitants of Germany, held to it. Traces of it may be found in the remains of the Aztec, Peruvian and Mexican civilizations.

The Eleusinian Mysteries of Greece, the Roman Mysteries, and the Inner Doctrines of the Cabbala of the Hebrews all taught the Truths of Metempsychosis. The early Christian Fathers; the Gnostic and Manichaeans and other sects of the Early Christian people, all held to the doctrine. The modern German philosophers have treated it with the greatest respect, if indeed they did not at least partially accept it. Many modern writers have considered it gravely, and with respect. The following quotations will give an idea of "how the wind is blowing" in the West:

"Of all the theories respecting the origin of the soul, Metempsychosis seems to me the most plausible and therefore the one most likely to throw light on the question of a life to come."—*Frederick H. Hedge.*

"It would be curious if we should find science and philosophy taking up again the old theory of metempsychosis, remodelling' it to suit our present modes of religious and scientific thought, and launching it again on the wide ocean of human belief. But stranger things have happened in the history of human opinions."—*James Freeman Clarke.*

"If we could legitimately determine any question of belief by the number of its adherents, the —— would apply to metempsychosis more fitly than to any other. I think it is quite as likely to be revived and to come to the front as any rival theory."—*Prof. Wm. Knight.*

"It seems to me, a firm and well-grounded faith in the doctrine of Christian metempsychosis might help to regenerate the world. For it would be a faith not hedged around with many of the difficulties and objections which beset other forms of doctrine, and it offers distinct and pungent motives for trying to lead a more Christian life, and for loving and helping our brother-man."—*Prof. Francis Bowen.*

"The doctrine of Metempsychosis may almost claim to be a natural or innate belief in the human mind, if we may judge from its wide diffusion among the nations of the earth, and its prevalence throughout the historical ages."—*Prof. Francis Bowen.*

"When Christianity first swept over Europe, the inner thought of its leaders was deeply tinctured with this truth. The Church tried ineffectually to eradicate it, but in various sects it kept sprouting forth beyond the time of Erigina and Bonaventura, its mediaeval advocates. Every great intuitional soul, as Paracelsus, Boehme, and Swedenborg, has adhered to it. The Italian luminaries, Giordano Bruno and Campanella. embraced it. The best of German philosophy is enriched by it. In Schopenhauer, Lessing, Hegel, Leibnitz, Herder, and Fichte, the younger, it is earnestly advocated. The anthropological systems of Kant and Schelling furnish points of contact with it. The younger Helmont, in *De Revolutione Animarum*, adduces in two hundred problems all the arguments which may be urged in favor of the return of souls into human bodies according to Jewish ideas. Of

English thinkers, the Cambridge Platonists defended it with much learning and acuteness, most conspicuously Henry More; and in Cudsworth and Hume it ranks as the most rational theory of immortality. Glanvil's *Lux Orientalis* devotes a curious treatise to it. It captivated the minds of Fourier and Leroux. Andre Pezzani's book on *The Plurality of the Soul's Lives* works out the system on the Roman Catholic idea of expiation."—E.D. WALKER, in "*Re-Incarnation, a Study of Forgotten Truth.*"

And in the latter part of the Nineteenth Century, and this the early part of the Twentieth Century, the general public has been made familiar with the idea of Metempsychosis, under the name of Re-incarnation, by means of the great volume of literature issued by The Theosophical Society and its allied following. No longer is the thought a novelty to the Western thinker, and many have found within themselves a corroborative sense of its truth. In fact, to many the mere mention of the idea has been sufficient to awaken faint shadowy memories of past lives, and, to such, many heretofore unaccountable traits of character, tastes, inclinations, sympathies, dislikes, etc., have been explained.

The Western world has been made familiar with the idea of the re-birth of souls into new bodies, under the term of "Re-incarnation," which means "a re-entry into flesh," the word "incarnate" being derived from the words "*in*," and "*carnis*," meaning flesh—the English word meaning "to clothe with flesh," etc. The word Metempsychosis, which we use in this lesson, is concerned rather with the "passage of the soul" from one tenement to another, the "fleshly" idea being merely incidental.

The doctrine of Metempsychosis, or Re-incarnation, together with its accompanying doctrine, Karma, or Spiritual Cause and Effect, is one of the great foundation stones of the Yogi Philosophy, as indeed it is of the entire system of systems of Oriental Philosophy and Thought. Unless one understands Metempsychosis he will never be able to understand the Eastern Teachings, for he will be without the Key. You who have read the *Bhagavad Gita*, that wonderful Hindu Epic, will remember how the thread of Re-Birth runs through it all. You remember the words of *Krishna* to *Arjuna*: "As the soul, wearing this material body, experienceth the stages of infancy, youth, manhood, and old age, even so shall it, in due time, pass on to another body, and in other incarnations shall it again live, and move and play its part." "These bodies, which act as enveloping coverings for the souls occupying them, are but finite things—things of the moment—and not the Real Man at all. They perish as all finite things perish—let them perish." "As a man throweth away his old garments, replacing them with new and brighter ones, even so the Dweller of the body, having quitted its old mortal frame, entereth into others which are new and freshly prepared for it. Weapons pierce not the Real Man, nor doth the fire burn him; the water affecteth him not, nor the wind drieth him nor bloweth him away. For he is impregnable and impervious to these things of the world of change—he is eternal, permanent, unchangeable, and unalterable—Real."

This view of life gives to the one who holds to it, an entirely different mental attitude. He no longer identifies himself with the particular body that he may be occupying, nor with any other body for that matter. He learns to regard his body just as he would a garment which he is wearing, useful to him for certain purposes, but which will in time be discarded and thrown aside for a better one, and one better adapted to his new requirements and needs. So firmly is this idea embedded in the consciousness of the Hindus, that they will often say "My body is tired," or "My body is hungry," or "My body is full of energy," rather than that "I am" this or that thing. And this consciousness, once attained, gives to one a sense of strength, security and power unknown to him who regards his body as himself. The first step for the student who wishes to grasp the idea of Metempsychosis, and who wishes to awaken in his consciousness a certainty of its truth, is to familiarize himself with the idea of his "I" being a thing independent and a part from his body, although using the latter as an abiding place and a useful shelter and instrument for the time being.

Many writers on the subject of Metempsychosis have devoted much time, labor and argument to prove the reasonableness of the doctrine upon purely speculative, philosophical, or metaphysical grounds. And while we believe that such efforts are praiseworthy for the reason that many persons must be first convinced in that way, still we feel that one must really *feel* the truth of the doctrine from something within his own consciousness, before he will really *believe* it to be truth. One may convince himself of the logical necessity of the doctrine of Metempsychosis, but at the same time he may drop the matter with a shrug of the shoulders and a "still, who knows?" But when one begins to feel within himself the awakening consciousness of a "something in the past," not to speak of the flashes of memory, and feeling of former acquaintance with the subject, then, and then only, does he begin to *believe.*

Many people have had "peculiar experiences" that are accountable only upon the hypothesis of Metempsychosis. Who has not experienced the consciousness of having *felt the thing before—having thought it some time in the dim past? Who has not witnessed new scenes that appear old, very old? Who has not met persons for the first time, whose presence awakened memories of a past lying far back in the misty ages of long ago? Who has not been seized at times with the consciousness of a mighty "oldness" of soul? Who has not heard music, often entirely new compositions, which somehow awakens memories of similar strains, scenes, places, faces, voices, lands, associations and events, sounding dimly on the strings of memory as the breezes of the harmony floats over them? Who has not gazed at some old painting, or piece of statuary, with the sense of having seen it all before? Who has not lived through events, which brought with them a certainty of being merely a repetition of some shadowy occurrences away back in lives lived long ago? Who has not felt the influence of the mountain, the sea, the desert, coming to them when they are far from such scenes—coming so vividly as to cause the actual scene of the present to fade into comparative unreality. Who has not had these experiences—we ask?*

Writers, poets, and others who carry messages to the world, have testified to these things—and nearly every man or woman who hears the message recognizes it as something having correspondence in his or her own life. Sir Walter Scott tells us in his diary: "I cannot, I am sure, tell if it is worth marking down, that yesterday, at dinner time, I was strangely haunted by what I would call the sense of preexistence, viz., a confused idea that nothing that passed was said for the first time; that the same topics had been discussed and the same persons had stated the same opinions on them. The sensation was so strong as to resemble what is called the mirage in the desert and a calenture on board ship." The same writer, in one of his novels, "Guy Mannering," makes one of his characters say: "Why is it that some scenes awaken thoughts which belong as it were, to dreams of early and shadowy recollections, such as old Brahmin moonshine would have ascribed to a state of previous existence. How often do we find ourselves in society which we have never before met, and yet feel impressed with a mysterious and ill-defined consciousness that neither the scene nor the speakers nor the subject are entirely new; nay, feel as if we could anticipate that part of the conversation which has not yet taken place."

Bulwer speaks of "that strange kind of inner and spiritual memory which so often recalls to us places and persons we have never seen before, and which Platonists would resolve to be the unquenched consciousness of a former life." And again, he says: "How strange is it that at times a feeling comes over us as we gaze upon certain places, which associates the scene either with some dim remembered and dreamlike images of the Past, or with a prophetic and fearful omen of the Future. Every one has known a similar strange and indistinct feeling at certain times and places, and with a similar inability to trace the cause." Poe has written these words on the subject: "We walk about, amid the destinies of our world existence, accompanied by dim but ever present memories of a Destiny more vast—very distant in the bygone time and infinitely awful. We live out a youth peculiarly haunted by such dreams, yet never mistaking them for dreams. As memories we know them. During our youth the distinctness is too clear to deceive us even for a moment. But the doubt of manhood dispels these feelings as illusions."

Home relates an interesting incident in his life, which had a marked effect upon his beliefs, thereafter. He relates that upon an occasion when he visited a strange house in London he was shown into a room to wait. He says: "On looking around, to my astonishment everything appeared perfectly familiar to me. I seemed to recognize every object. I said to myself, 'What is this? I have never been here before, and yet I have seen all this, and if so, then there must be a very peculiar knot in that shutter.'" He proceeded to examine the shutter, and much to his amazement the knot was there.

We have recently heard of a similar case, told by an old lady who formerly lived in the far West of the United States. She states that upon one occasion a party was wandering on the desert in her part of the country, and found themselves out of water. As that part of the desert was unfamiliar even to the guides, the prospect for water looked very poor indeed. After a fruitless search of several hours, one of the party, a perfect stranger to that part of the country, suddenly pressed his hand to his head, and acted in a dazed manner, crying out "I know that a water-hole is over to the right—this way," and away he started with the party after him. After a half-hour's journey they reached an old hidden water-hole that was unknown even to the oldest man in the party. The stranger said that he did not understand the matter, but that he had somehow experienced a sensation of *having been there before*, and knowing just where the water-hole was located. An old Indian who was questioned about the matter, afterward, stated that the place had been well known to his people who formerly travelled much on that part of the desert; and that they had legends relating to the "hidden water-hole," running back for many generations. In this case, it was remarked that the water-hole was situated in such a peculiar and unusual manner, as to render it almost undiscoverable even to people familiar with the characteristics of that part of the country. The old lady who related the story, had it direct from the lips of one of the party, who regarded it as "something queer," but who had never even heard of Metempsychosis.

A correspondent of an English magazine writes as follows: "A gentleman of high intellectual attainments, now deceased, once told me that he had dreamed of being in a strange city, so vividly that he remembered the streets, houses and public buildings as distinctly as those of any place he ever visited. A few weeks later he was induced to visit a panorama in Leicester Square, when he was startled by seeing the city of which he had dreamed. The likeness was perfect, except that one additional church appeared in the picture. He was so struck by the circumstance that he spoke to the exhibitor, assuming for the purpose the air of a traveller acquainted with the place, when he was informed that the church was a recent erection." The fact of the addition of the church, seems to place the incident within the rule of awakened memories of scenes known in a past life, for clairvoyance, astral travel, etc., would show the scene as it was at the time of the dream, not as it had been years before.

Charles Dickens mentions a remarkable impression in his work "Pictures from Italy." "In the foreground was a group of silent peasant girls, leaning over the parapet of the little bridge, looking now up at the sky, now down into the water; in the distance a deep dell; the shadow of an approaching night on everything. If I had been murdered there in some former life I could not have seemed to remember the place more thoroughly, or with more emphatic chilling of the blood; and the real remembrance of it acquired in that minute is so strengthened by the imaginary recollection that I hardly think I could forget it."

We have recently met two people in America who had very vivid memories of incidents in their past life. One of these, a lady, has a perfect horror of large bodies of water, such as the Great Lakes, or the Ocean, although she was born and has lived the greater part of her life inland, far removed from any great body of water, She has a distinct recollection of falling from a large canoe-shape vessel, of peculiar lines, and drowning. She was quite overcome upon her first visit to the Field Museum in Chicago, where there were exhibited a number of models of queer vessels used by primitive people. She pointed out one similar in shape, and lines, to the one she remembers as having fallen from in some past life.

The second case mentioned is that of a married couple who met each other in a country foreign to both, on their travels. They fell in love with each other, and both have felt that their marriage was a reunion rather than a new attachment. The husband one day shortly after their marriage told his wife in a rather shamed-faced way that he had occasional flashes of memory of having held in his arms, in the dim past, a woman whose face he could not recall, but who wore a strange necklace, he describing the details of the latter. The wife said nothing, but after her husband had left for his office, she went to the attic and unpacked an old trunk containing some odds and ends, relics, heirlooms, etc., and drew from it an old necklace of peculiar pattern that her grandfather had brought back from India, where he had lived in his younger days, and which had been in the family ever since. She laid the necklace on the table, so that her husband would see it upon his return. The moment his eyes fell upon it, he turned white as death, and gasped "My God! *that's the necklace!*"

A writer in a Western journal gives the following story of a Southern woman. "When I was in Heidelberg, Germany, attending a convention of Mystics, in company with some friends I paid my first visit to the ruined Heidelberg Castle. As I approached it I was impressed with the existence of a peculiar room in an inaccessible portion of the building. A paper and pencil were provided me, and I drew a diagram of the room even to its peculiar floor. My diagram and description were perfect, when we afterwards visited the room. In some way, not yet clear to me, I have been connected with that apartment. Still another impression came to me with regard to a book, which I was made to feel was in the old library of the Heidelberg University. I not only knew what the book was, but even felt that a certain name of an old German professor would be found written in it. Communicating this feeling to one of the Mystics at the convention, a search was made for the volume, but it was not found. Still the impression clung to me, and another effort was made to find the book; this time we were rewarded for our pains. Sure enough, there on the margin of one of the leaves was the very name I had been given in such a strange manner. Other things at the same time went to convince me that I was in possession of the soul of a person who had known Heidelberg two or three centuries ago."

A contributor to an old magazine relates, among other instances, the following regarding a friend who remembers having died in India during the youth of some former life. He states: "He sees the bronzed attendants gathered about his cradle in their white dresses: they are fanning him. And as they gaze he passes into unconsciousness. Much of his description concerned points of which he knew nothing from any other source, but all was true to the life, and enabled me to fix on India as the scene which he recalled."

While comparatively few among the Western races are able to remember more than fragments of their past lives, in India it is quite common for a man well developed spiritually to clearly remember the incidents and details of former incarnations, and the evidence of the awakening of such power causes little more than passing interest among his people. There is, as we shall see later, a movement toward conscious Metempsychosis, and many of the race are just moving on to that plane. In India the highly developed individuals grow into a clear recollection of their past lives when they reach the age of puberty, and when their brains are developed sufficiently to grasp the knowledge locked up in the depths of the soul. In the meantime the individual's memory of the past is locked away in the recesses of his mind, just as are many facts and incidents of his present life so locked away, to be remembered only when some one mentions the subject, or some circumstance serves to supply the associative link to the apparently forgotten matter.

Regarding the faculty of memory in our present lives, we would quote the following from the pen of Prof. William Knight, printed in the Fortnightly Review. He says: "Memory of the details of the past is absolutely impossible. The power of the conservative faculty, though relatively great, is extremely limited. We forget the larger portion of experience soon after we have passed through it, and we should be able to recall the particulars of our past years, filling all the missing links of consciousness since we entered on the present life, before we were in a position to remember our ante-natal experience. Birth must necessarily be preceded by crossing the river of oblivion, while the capacity for fresh acquisition survives, and the garnered wealth of old experience determines the amount and character of the new."

Another startling evidence of the proof of Metempsychosis is afforded us in the cases of "infant prodigies," etc., which defy any other explanation. Take the cases of the manifestation of musical talent in certain children at an early age, for instance. Take the case of Mozart who at the age of four was able to not only perform difficult pieces on the piano, but actually composed original works of merit. Not only did he manifest the highest faculty of sound and note, but also an instinctive ability to compose and arrange music, which ability was superior to that of many men who had devoted years of their life to study and practice. The laws of harmony—the science of commingling tones, was to him not the work of years, but a faculty born in him. There are many similar cases of record.

Heredity does not explain these instances of genius, for in many of the recorded cases, none of the ancestors manifested any talent or ability. From whom did Shakespeare inherit his genius? From whom did Plato derive his wonderful thought? From what ancestor did Abraham Lincoln inherit his character—coming from a line of plain, poor, hard-working people, and possessing all of the physical attributes and characteristics of his ancestry, he, nevertheless, manifested a mind which placed him among the foremost of his race. Does not Metempsychosis give us the only possible key? Is it not reasonable to suppose that the abilities displayed by the infant genius, and the talent of the men who spring from obscure origin, have their root in the experiences of a previous life?

Then take the cases of children at school. Children of even the same family manifest different degrees of receptivity to certain studies. Some "take to" one thing, and some to another. Some find arithmetic so easy that they almost absorb it intuitively, while grammar is a hard task for them; while their brothers and sisters find the exact reverse to be true. How many have found that when they would take up some new study, it is almost like recalling something already learned. Do you student, who are now reading these lines take your own case. Does not all this Teaching seem to you like the repetition of some lesson learned long ago? Is it not like remembering something already learned, rather than the learning of some new truth? Were you not attracted to these studies, in the first place, by a feeling that you had known it all before, somewhere, somehow? Does not your mind leap ahead of the lesson, and see what is coming next, long before you have turned the pages? These inward evidences of the fact of pre-existence are so strong that they outweigh the most skillful appeal to the intellect.

This intuitive knowledge of the truth of Metempsychosis explains why the belief in it is sweeping over the Western world at such a rapid rate. The mere mention of the idea, to many people who have never before heard of it, is sufficient to cause them to recognize its truth. And though they may not understand the laws of its operation, yet deep down in their consciousness they find a something that convinces them of its truth. In spite of the objections that are urged against the teaching, it is making steady headway and progress.

The progress of the belief in Metempsychosis however has been greatly retarded by the many theories and dogmas attached to it by some of the teachers. Not to speak of the degrading ideas of re-birth into the bodies of animals, etc., which have polluted the spring of Truth, there are to be found many other features of teaching and theory which repel people, and cause them to try to kill out of the minds the glimmer of Truth that they find there. The human soul instinctively revolts against the teaching that it is bound to the wheel or re-birth, *willy-nilly*, compulsorily, without choice—compelled to live in body after body until great cycles are past. The soul, perhaps already sick of earth-life, and longing to pass on to higher planes of existence, fights against such teaching. And it does well to so fight, for the truth is nearer to its hearts desire. There is no soul longing that does not carry with it the prophecy of its own fulfillment, and so it is in this case. It is true that the soul of one filled with earthly desires, and craving for material things, will by the very force of those desires be drawn back to earthly re-birth in a body best suited for the gratification of the longings, desires and cravings that it finds within itself. But it is likewise true that the earth-sick soul is not compiled to return unless its own desires bring it back. Desire is the key note of Metempsychosis, although up to a certain stage it may operate unconsciously. The sum of the desires of a soul regulate its re-birth. Those who have become sickened of all that earth has for them at this stage of its evolution, may, and do, rest in states of existence far removed from earth scenes, until the race progresses far enough to afford the resting soul the opportunities and environments that it so earnestly craves.

And more than this, when Man reaches a certain stage, the process of Metempsychosis no longer remains unconscious, but he enters into a conscious knowing, willing passage from one life to another. And when that stage is reached a full memory of the past lives is unfolded, and life to such a soul becomes as the life of a day, succeeded by a night, and then the awakening into another day with full knowledge and recollection of the events of the day before. We are in merely the babyhood of the race now, and the fuller life of the conscious soul lies before us. Yea, even now it is being entered into by the few of the race that have progressed sufficiently far on the Path. And you, student, who feel within you that craving for conscious re-birth and future spiritual evolution, and the distaste for, and horror of, a further blind, unconscious re-plunge into the earth-life—know you, that this longing on your part is but an indication of what lies before you. It is the strange, subtle, awakening of the nature within you, which betokens the higher state. Just as the young person feels within his or her body strange emotions, longings and stirrings, which betoken the passage from the child state into that of manhood or womanhood, so do these spiritual longings, desires and cravings betoken the passage from unconscious re-birth into conscious knowing Metempsychosis, when you have passed from the scene of your present labors.

In our next lesson we shall consider the history of the race as its souls passed on from the savage tribes to the man of to-day. It is the history of the race—the history of the individual—your own history, student—the record of that through which you have passed to become that which you now are. And as you have climbed step after step up the arduous path, so will you, hereafter climb still higher paths, but no longer in unconsciousness, but with your spiritual eyes wide open to the Rays of Truth pouring forth from the great Central Sun—the Absolute.

Concluding this lesson, we would quote two selections from the American poet, Whitman, whose strange genius was undoubtedly the result of vague memories springing from a previous life, and which burst into utterances often not more than half understood by the mind that gave them birth. Whitman says:

"Facing West from California's shores,
Inquiring, tireless, seeking what is yet unfound,
A, a child, very old, over waves, toward the house of
maternity, the land of migrations, look afar,
Look off the shores of my Western sea, the circle
almost circled:
For starting Westward from Hindustan, from the
vales of Kashmere,
From Asia, from the north, from God, the sage, and
the hero,
From the south, from the flowery peninsulas and
spice islands,
Long having wandered since, round the earth having
wandered,
Now I face home again, very pleased and joyous.
(But where is what I started for so long ago?
And why is it yet unfound?)"

* * * * *

"I know I am deathless.

I know that this orbit of mine cannot be swept by a
carpenter's compass;
And whether I come to my own to-day, or in ten
thousand or ten million years,

I can cheerfully take it now or with equal cheerfulness
can wait."

* * * * *

"As to you, Life, I reckon you are the leavings of
many deaths.
No doubt I have died myself ten thousand times before."

* * * * *

> "Births have brought us richness and variety, and other births have brought us richness and variety."

* * * * *

And this quotation from the American poet N.P. Willis:

"But what a mystery this erring mind?
It wakes within a frame of various powers
A stranger in a new and wondrous world.
It brings an instinct from some other sphere,
For its fine senses are familiar all,
And with the unconscious habit of a dream
It calls and they obey. The priceless sight
Springs to its curious organ, and the ear
Learns strangely to detect the articulate air
In its unseen divisions, and the tongue
Gets its miraculous lesson with the rest,
And in the midst of an obedient throng
Of well trained ministers, the mind goes forth
To search the secrets of its new found home."

THE TENTH LESSON

SPIRITUAL EVOLUTION.

One of the things that repel many persons who have had their attention directed to the subject of Metempsychosis for the first time, is the idea that they have evolved *as a soul* from individual lowly forms, for instance that they have at one time been an individual plant, and then an individual animal form, and then an individual higher animal form, and so on until now they are the particular individual human form contemplating the subject. This idea, which has been taught by many teachers, is repellent to the average mind, for obvious reasons, and naturally so, for it has no foundation in truth.

While this lesson is principally concerned with the subject of the Spiritual Evolution of the human soul, since it became a human soul, still it may be as well to mention the previous phase of evolution, briefly, in order to prevent misconception, and to dispel previously acquired error.

The atom, although it possesses life and a certain degree of mind, and acts as an individual temporarily, has no permanent individuality that reincarnates. When the atom is evolved it becomes a centre of energy in the great atomic principle, and when it is finally dissolved it resolves itself back into its original state, and its life as an individual atom ceases, although the experience it has gained becomes the property of the entire principle. It is as if a body of water were to be resolved into millions of tiny dew-drops for a time, and each dew-drop was then to acquire certain outside material in solution. In that case, each dew-drop when it again returned to the body of water, would carry with it its foreign material, which would become the property of the whole. And subsequently formed dew-drops would carry in their substance a particle of the foreign matter brought back home by the previous generation of dewdrops, and would thus be a little different from their predecessors. And this process, continuing for many generations of dew-drops, would ultimately cause the greatest changes in the composition of the successive generations.

This, in short, is the story of the change and improving forms of life. From the atoms into the elements; from the lower elements into those forming protoplasm; from the protoplasm to the lower forms of animal life; from these lower forms on to higher forms—this is the story. But it is all a counterpart of the dew-drop and the body of water, *until the human soul is evolved.*

The plants and the lower forms of animal life are not permanent individual souls, but each family is a *group-soul* corresponding to the body of water from which the dew-drop arose. From these family group-souls gradually break off minor groups, representing species, and so on into sub-species. At last when the forms reach the plane of man, the group-soul breaks itself up into *permanent individual souls*, and true Metempsychosis begins. That is, *each individual human soul becomes a permanent individual entity*, destined to evolve and perfect itself along the lines of spiritual evolution.

And from this point begins our story of Spiritual Evolution.

The story of Man, the Individual, begins amidst humble surroundings. Primitive man, but little above the level of the lower animals in point of intelligence, has nevertheless that distinguishing mark of Individuality—"Self-Consciousness," which is the demarkation between Beast and Man. And even the lowest of the lowest races had at least a "trace" of this Self-Consciousness, which made of them individuals, and caused the fragment of the race-soul to separate itself from the general principle animating the race, and to fasten its "I" conscious upon itself, rather than upon the underlying race-soul, along instinctive lines. Do you know just what this Self-Consciousness is, and how it differs from the Physical Consciousness of the lower animals? Perhaps we had better pause a moment to consider it at this place.

The lower animals are of course conscious of the bodies, and their wants, feelings, emotions, desires, etc., and their actions are in response to the animating impulses coming from this plane of consciousness. But it stops there. They "know," but they do not "know that they know"; that is, they have not yet arrived at a state in which they can think of themselves as "I," and to reason upon their thoughts and mental operations. It is like the consciousness of a very young child, which feels and knows its sensations and wants, but is unable to think of itself as "I," and to turn the mental gaze inward. In another book of these series we have used the illustration of the horse which has been left standing out in the cold sleet and rain, and which undoubtedly feels and knows the unpleasant sensations arising therefrom, and longs to get away from the unpleasant environment. But, still, he is unable to analyze his mental states and wonder whether his master will come out to him soon, or think how cruel it is to keep him out of his warm comfortable stable; or wonder whether he will be taken out in the cold rain again tomorrow; or feel envious of other horses who are indoors; or wonder why he is kept out cold nights, etc., etc. In short, the horse is unable to think as would a reasoning man under just the same circumstances. He is aware of the discomfort, just as would be the man; and he would run away home, if he were able, just as would the man. But he is not able to pity himself, nor to think about his personality, as would a man—he is not able to wonder whether life is worth the living, etc., as would a man. He "knows" but is not able to reflect upon the "knowing."

In the above illustration, the principal point is that the horse does not "know himself" as an entity, while even the most primitive man is able to so recognize himself as an "I." If the horse were able to think in words, he would think "feel," "cold," "hurt," etc., but he would be unable to think "*I* feel; *I* am cold; *I* am hurt," etc. The thought "I" would be missing.

It is true that the "I" consciousness of the primitive man was slight, and was but a degree above the Physical Consciousness of the higher apes, but nevertheless it had sprung into being, never again to be lost. The primitive man was like a child a few years old—he was able to say "I," and to think "I." *He had become an individual soul.*

And this individual soul inhabited and animated a body but little removed from that of an ape. But this new consciousness began to mould that rude body and the ascent was begun. Each generation showed a physical improvement over that of the preceding one, according to the lines of physical evolution, and as the developing soul demanded more perfect and developed bodies the bodies were evolved to meet the demand, for the mental demand has ever been the cause of the physical form.

The soul of the primitive man reincarnated almost immediately after the death of the physical body, because the experiences gained were mostly along the lines of the physical, the mental planes being scarcely brought into play, while the higher and spiritual faculties were almost entirely obscured from sight. Life after life the soul of the primitive man lived out in rapid succession. But in each new embodiment there was a slight advance over that of the previous one. Experience, or rather the result of experiences, were carried over, and profited by. New lessons were learned and unlearned, improved upon or discarded. And the race grew and unfolded.

After a time the number of advancing souls which had outstripped their fellows in progress became sufficiently large for sub-races to be formed, and so the branching off process began. In this way the various races and types were formed, and the progress of Mankind gained headway. At this point we may as well consider the history of the Races of Mankind, that we may see how the great tide-wave of Soul has ever pressed onward, marking higher and still higher stages of progress, and also how the various minor waves of the great wave pushed in and then receded, only to be followed by still higher waves. The story is most interesting.

The Yogi Teachings inform us that the Grand Cycle of Man's Life on the Earth is composed of Seven Cycles, of which we are now living in the third-seventh part of the Fifth Cycle. These Cycles may be spoken of as the Great Earth Periods, separated from each other by some great natural cataclysm which destroyed the works of the previous races of men, and which started afresh the progress called "civilization," which, as all students know, manifests a rise and fall like unto that of the tides.

Man in the First Cycle emerged from a gross animal-like state into a condition somewhat advanced. It was a slow progress, but nevertheless a distinct series of advances were made by the more progressive souls who passed over on to the Second Cycle, embodying themselves as the ruling races in the same, their less progressive brothers incarnating in the lower tribes of the Second Cycle. It must be remembered that the souls which do not advance during a Cycle reincarnate in the next Cycle among the lower races. So that even in this Fifth Cycle we have remnants of the previous cycles, the lives of the members of which give us an idea of what life in the earlier cycles must have been.

The Yogi Teachings give us but little information regarding the people of the First and Second Cycles, because of the low state of these ages. The tale, if told, would be the story of the Cave-dweller, and Stone-age people; the Fire-peoples, and all the rest of savage, barbarian crew; there was but little trace of anything like that which we call "civilization," although in the latter periods of the Second Cycle the foundations for the coming civilizations were firmly laid.

After the cataclysm which destroyed the works of Man of the Second Cycle, and left the survivors scattered or disorganized, awaiting the touch of the organizing urge which followed shortly afterward, there dawned the first period of the Third Cycle. The scene of the life of the Third Cycle was laid in what is known to Occultists as Lemuria. Lemuria was a mighty continent situated in what is now known as the Pacific Ocean, and parts of the Indian Ocean. It included Australia, Australasia, and other portions of the Pacific islands, which are in fact surviving portions of the great continent of Lemuria, its highest points, the lower portion having sunk beneath the seas ages and ages ago.

Life in Lemuria is described as being principally concerned with the physical senses, and sensual enjoyment, only a few developed souls having broken through the fetters of materiality and reached the beginnings of the mental and spiritual planes of life. Some few indeed made great progress and were saved from the general wreck, in order to become the leaven which would lighten the mass of mankind during the next Cycle. These developed souls were the teachers of the new races, and were looked upon by the latter as gods and supernatural beings, and legends and traditions concerning them are still existent among the ancient peoples of our present day. Many of the myths of the ancient peoples arose in this way.

The Yogi traditions hold that just prior to the great cataclysm which destroyed the races of the Second Cycle, there was a body of the Chosen Ones which migrated from Lemuria to certain islands of the sea which are now part of the main land of India. These people formed the nucleus of the Occult Teachings of the Lemurians, and developed into the Fount of Truth which has been flowing ever since throughout the successive periods and cycles.

When Lemuria passed away, there arose from the depths of the ocean the continent which was to be the scene of the life and civilization of the Fourth Cycle—the continent of Atlantis. Atlantis was situated in a portion of what is now known as the Atlantic Ocean, beginning at what is now known as the Caribbean Sea and extending over to the region of what is now known as Africa. What are now known as Cuba and the West Indies were among the highest points of the continent, and now stand like monuments to its departed greatness.

The civilization of Atlantis was remarkable, and its people attained heights which seem almost incredible to even those who are familiar with the highest achievements of man in our own times. The Chosen Ones preserved from the cataclysm which destroyed Lemuria, and who lived to a remarkably old age, had stored up within their minds the wisdom and learning of the races that had been destroyed, and they thus gave the Atlanteans an enormous starting-advantage. They soon attained great advancement along all the lines of human endeavor. They perfected mechanical inventions and appliances, reaching far ahead of even our present attainments. In the field of electricity especially they reached the stages that our present races will reach in about two or three hundred years from now. Along the lines of Occult Attainment their progress was far beyond the dreams of the average man of our own race, and in fact from this arose one of the causes of their downfall, for they prostituted the power to base and selfish uses, and Black Magic.

And, so the decline of Atlantis began. But the end did not come at once, or suddenly, but gradually. The continent, and its surrounding islands gradually sank beneath the waves of the Atlantic Ocean, the process occupying over 10,000 years. The Greeks and Romans of our own Cycle had traditions regarding the sinking of the continent, but their knowledge referred only to the disappearance of the small remainder—certain islands—the continent itself having disappeared thousands of years before their time. It is recorded that the Egyptian priests had traditions that the continent itself had disappeared nine thousand years before their time. As was the case with the Chosen Ones of Lemuria, so was it with the Elect of Atlantis, who were taken away from the doomed land some time prior to its destruction. The few advanced people left their homes and migrated to portions of what are now South America and Central America, but which were then islands of the sea. These people have left their traces of their civilization and works, which our antiquaries are discovering to-day.

When the Fifth Cycle dawned (our own cycle, remember) these brave and advanced souls acted as the race-teachers and became as "gods" to those who came afterward. The races were very prolific, and multiplied very rapidly under the most favorable conditions. The souls of the Atlanteans were pressing forward for embodiment, and human forms were born to supply the demand. And now begins the history of our own Cycle—the Fifth Cycle.

But before we begin a consideration of the Fifth Cycle, let us consider for a moment a few points about the laws operating to cause these great changes.

In the first place, each Cycle has a different theatre for its work and action. The continent of Lemuria was not in existence during the Second Cycle, and arose from the ocean bed only when its appointed time came. And, likewise the continent of Atlantis reposed beneath the waves while the Lemurian races manifested during the Third Cycle, rising by means of a convulsion of the earth's surface to play its part during its own period—the Fourth Cycle—only to sink again beneath the waves to make way for the birth of the Fifth Cycle with its races. By means of these cataclysms the races of each Cycle were wiped out when the time came, the few Elect or Chosen ones, that is those who have manifested the right to live on, being carried away to some favorable environment where they became as leaven to the mass—as "gods" to the new races that quickly appear.

It must be remembered, however, that these Chosen Ones are not the only ones saved from the destruction that overtakes the majority of the race. On the contrary a few survivors are preserved, although driven away from their former homes, and reduced to "first principles of living" in order to become the parents of the new races. The new races springing from the fittest of these survivors quickly form sub-races, being composed of the better adapted souls seeking reincarnation, while the less fit sink into barbarism, and show evidences of decay, although a remnant drags on for thousands of years, being composed of the souls of those who have not advanced sufficiently to take a part in the life of the new races. These "left-overs" are in evidence in our own times in the cases of the Australian savages, and some of the African tribes, as well as among the Digger Indians and others of similar grade of intelligence.

In order to understand the advance of each race it must be remembered that the more advanced souls, after passing out of the body, have a much longer period of rest in the higher planes, and consequently do not present themselves for reincarnation until a period quite late when compared with the hasty reincarnation of the less advanced souls who are hurried back to rebirth by reason of the strong earthly attachments and desires. In this way it happens that the earlier races of each Cycle are more primitive folk than those who follow them as the years roll by. The soul of an earth-bound person reincarnates in a few years, and sometimes in a few days, while the soul of an advanced man may repose and rest on the higher planes for centuries—nay, even for thousands of years, until the earth has reached a stage in which the appropriate environment may be afforded it.

Observers, unconnected with Occultism, have noted certain laws which seem to regulate the rise and fall of nations—the procession of ruling races. They do not understand the law of Metempsychosis that alone gives the key to the problem, but nevertheless they have not failed to record the existence of the laws themselves. In order to show that these laws are recognized by persons who are not at all influenced by the Occult Teachings, we take the liberty of quoting from Draper's "History of the Intellectual Development of Europe."

Dr. Draper writes as follows: "We are, as we often say, the creatures of circumstances. In that expression there is a higher philosophy than might at first appear. From this more accurate point of view we should therefore consider the course of these events, recognizing the principle that the affairs of men pass forward in a determinate way, expanding and unfolding themselves. And hence we see that the things of which we have spoken as if they were matters of choice, were in reality forced upon their apparent authors by the necessity of the times. But in truth they should be considered as the presentation of a certain phase of life which nations in their onward course sooner or later assume. To the individual, how well we know that a sober moderation of action, an appropriate gravity of demeanor, belonging to the mature period of life, change from the wanton willfulness of youth, which may be ushered in, or its beginnings marked by many accidental incidents; in one perhaps by domestic bereavements, in another by the loss of fortune, in a third by ill-health. We are correct enough in imputing to such trials the change of character; but we never deceive ourselves by supposing that it would have failed to take place had these incidents not occurred. There runs an irresistible destiny in the midst of these vicissitudes. There are analogies between the life of a nation, and that of an individual, who, though he may be in one respect the maker of his own fortunes, for happiness or for misery, for good or for evil, though he remains here or goes there as his inclinations prompt, though he does this or abstains from that as he chooses, is nevertheless held fast by an inexorable fate—a fate which brought him into the world involuntarily, so far as he was concerned, which presses him forward through a definite career, the stages of which are absolutely invariable,—infancy, childhood, youth, maturity, old age, with all their characteristic actions and passions,—and which removes him from the scene at the appointed time, in most cases against his will. So also is it with nations; the voluntary is only the outward semblance, covering but hardly hiding the predetermined. Over the events of life we may have control, but none whatever over the law of its progress. There is a geometry that applies to nations an equation of their curve of advance. That no mortal man can touch."

This remarkable passage, just quoted, shows how the close observers of history note the rise and fall of the tides of human race progress, although ignorant of the real underlying causing energy or force. A study of the Occult Teachings alone gives one the hidden secret of human actions and throws the bright light of Truth upon the dark corners of phenomena.

At the beginning of the Fifth Cycle (which is the present one), there were not only the beginnings of the new races which always spring up at the beginning of each new cycle and which are the foundations for the coming races which take advantage of the fresh conditions and opportunities for growth and development—but there were also the descendants of the Elect Saved from the destruction of Atlantis by having been led away and colonized far from the scene of danger. The new races were the descendant of the scattered survivors of the Atlantean peoples, that is, the common run of people of the time. But the Elect few were very superior people, and imparted to their descendants their knowledge and wisdom. So that we see at the beginning of the Fifth Cycle hordes of new, primitive people in certain lands, and in other places advanced nations like the ancestors of the Ancient Egyptians, Persians, Chaldeans, Hindus, etc.

These advanced races were old souls—advanced souls—the progressed and developed souls of Ancient Lemuria and Atlantis, who lived their lives and who are now either on higher planes of life, or else are among us to-day taking a leading part in the world's affairs, striving mightily to save the present races from the misfortunes which overtook their predecessors.

The descendants of the people were the Assyrians and Babylonians. In due time the primitive new races developed and the great Roman, Grecian, and Carthaginian peoples appeared. Then came the rise of other peoples and nations down to the present time. Each race or nation has its rise, its height of attainment, and its decline. When a nation begins to decline it is because its more advanced souls have passed on, and only the less progressive souls are left. The history of all nations show the truth of the Occult the term. Men are forsaking old ideals, creeds and dogmas, and are running hither and thither seeking something they feel to be necessary, but of the nature of which they know nothing. They are feeling the hunger for Peace—the thirst for Knowledge—and they are seeking satisfaction in all directions.

This is not only the inevitable working of the Law of Evolution, but is also a manifestation of the power and love of the great souls that have passed on to higher planes of existence, and who have become as angels and arch-angels. These beings are filled with the love of the race, and are setting into motion influences that are being manifest in many directions, the tendency of which are to bring the race to a realization of its higher power, faculties, and destiny.

As we have said in other places, one of the greatest difficulties in the way of the seeker after Truth in his consideration of the question of Spiritual Evolution is the feeling that rebirth is being forced upon him, without any say on his part, and against his desires. But this is far from being correct. It is true that the whole process is according to the Great Law, but that Law operates through the force of Desire and Attraction. The soul is attracted toward rebirth by reason of its desire or rather the essence of its desires. It is reborn only because it has within itself the desire for further experience, and opportunity for unfoldment. And it is reborn into certain environments solely because it has within itself unsatisfied desires for those environments, etc. The process is just as regular and scientific as is the attraction of one atom of matter for another.

Each soul has within itself certain elements of desire and attraction, and it attracts to itself certain conditions and experiences, and is in turn attracted by these things. This is the law of life, in the body and out of it. And there is no injustice in the law it is the essence of justice itself, for it gives to each just what is required to fill the indwelling desires, or else the conditions and experiences designed to burn out the desires which are holding one back, and the destruction of which will make possible future advancement.

For instance, if one is bound by the inordinate desire for material wealth, the Law of Karma will attract him to a rebirth in conditions in which he will be surrounded by wealth and luxury until he becomes sickened with them and will find his heart filled with the desire to flee from them and toward higher and more satisfying things. Of course the Law of Karma acts in other ways, as we shall see in our next lesson—it deals with one's debts and obligations, also. The Law of Karma is closely connected with Metempsychosis, and one must be considered in connection with the other, always.

Not only is it true that man's rebirths are in strict accordance with the law of Attraction and Desire, but it is also true that after he attains a certain stage of spiritual unfoldment he enters into the conscious stage of rebirth, and thereafter he is reborn consciously and with full foreknowledge. Many are now entering into this stage of development, and have a partial consciousness of their past lives, which also implies that they have had at least a partial consciousness of approaching rebirth, for the two phases of consciousness run together.

Those individuals of a race who have outstripped their fellows in spiritual unfoldment, are still bound by the Karma of the particular race to which they belong, up to a certain point. And as the entire race, or at least a large proportion of it, must move forward as a whole, such individuals must needs wait also. But they are not compelled to suffer a tiresome round of continued rebirths amid environments and conditions which they have outgrown. On the contrary, the advanced individual soul is allowed to wait until the race reaches its own stage of advancement, when it again joins in the upward movement, in full consciousness, however. In the interim he may pass his well earned rest either on some of the higher planes of rest, or else in conscious temporary sojourn in other material spheres helping in the great work as a Teacher and worker for Good and Spiritual Evolution among those who need such help. In fact there are in the world to-day, individual souls which have reached similar stages on other planets, and who are spending their rest period here amidst the comparatively lower Earth conditions, striving to lift up the Earth souls to greater heights.

So long as people allow themselves to become attached to material objects, so long will they be reborn in conditions in which these objects bind them fast. It is only when the soul frees itself from these entangling obstructions that it is born in conditions of freedom. Some outgrow these material attachments by right thinking and reasoning, while others seem to be compelled to live them out, and thus outlive them, before they are free. At last when the soul realizes that these things are merely incidents of the lower personality, and have naught to do with the real individuality, then, and then only, do they fall from it like a wornout cloak, and are left behind while it bounds forward on The Path fresh from the lighter weight being carried.

The Yogi Philosophy teaches that Man will live forever, ascending from higher to higher planes, and then on and on and on. Death is but the physical symbol of a period of Soul Rest, similar to sleep of the tired body, and is just as much to be welcomed and greeted with thanks. Life is continuous, and its object is development, unfoldment and growth. We are in Eternity now as much as we ever shall be. Our souls may exist out of the body as well as in it, although bodily incarnation is necessary at this stage of our development. As we progress on to higher planes of life, we shall incarnate in bodies far more ethereal than those now used by us, just as in the past we used bodies almost incredibly grosser and coarser than those we call our own to-day. Life is far more than a thing of three-score and ten years—it is really a succession of such lives, on an ascending scale, that which we call our personal self to-day being merely the essence of the experiences of countless lives in the past.

The Soul is working steadily upward, from higher to higher, from gross to finer forms and manifestations. And it will steadily work for ages to come, always progressing, always advancing, always unfolding. The Universe contains many worlds for the Soul to inhabit, and then after it has passed on to other Universes, there will still be Infinitude before it. The destiny of the Soul of Man is of wondrous promise and possibilities—the mind to-day cannot begin to even dream of what is before the Soul. Those who have already advanced many steps beyond you—those Elder Brethren—are constantly extending to you aid in many directions. They are extending to you the Unseen Hand, which lifts you over many a hard place and dangerous crossing—but you recognize it not except in a vague way. There are now in existence, on planes infinitely higher than your own, intelligences of transcendent glory and magnificence—but they were once Men even as you are to-day. They have so far progressed upon the Path that they have become as angels and archangels when compared with you. And, blessed thought, even as these exalted ones were once even as you, so shall you, in due course of Spiritual Evolution, become even as these mighty ones.

The Yogi Philosophy teaches that You who are reading these lines have lived many lives previous to the present one. You have lived in the lower forms, and have worked your way arduously along the Path until now you are reaching the stage of Spiritual Consciousness in which the past and future will begin to appear plain to you for the first time. You have lived as the cave-man—the cliff-dweller—the savage—the barbarian. You have been the warrior—the priest—the Medieval scholar and occultist—the prince—the pauper. You have lived in Lemuria—in Atlantis—in India—in Persia—in Egypt—in ancient Rome and Greece—and are now playing your part in the Western civilization, associating with many with whom you have had relations in your past lives.

In closing this lesson, let us quote from a previous writing from the same pen that writes this lesson:

"Toward what goal is all this Spiritual Evolution tending? What does it all mean? From the low planes of life to the highest—all are on The Path. To what state or place does The Path lead? Let us attempt to answer by asking you to imagine a series of millions of circles, one within the other. Each circle means a stage of Life. The outer circles are filled with life in its lowest and most material stages—each circle nearer the Centre holds higher and higher forms—until Men (or what were once Men) become as gods. Still on, and on, and on. does the form of life grow higher, until the human mind cannot grasp the idea. But what is the Centre? The MIND of the entire Spiritual Body—the ABSOLUTE! And we are traveling toward that Centre!"

And again from the same source:

"But beyond your plane, and beyond mine, are plane after plane, connected with our earth, the splendors of which man cannot conceive. And there are likewise many planes around the other planets of our chain—and there are millions of other worlds—and there are chains of universes just as there are chains of planets—and then greater groups of these chains—and so on greater and grander beyond the power of man to imagine—on and on and on and on—higher and higher—to inconceivable heights. An infinity of infinities of worlds are before us. Our world and our planetary system and our system of suns, and our system of solar systems, are but as grains of sand on the beach of the mighty ocean. But then you cry, 'But what am I—poor mortal thing—lost among all this inconceivable greatness?' The answer comes that You are that most precious thing—a living soul. And if you were destroyed the whole system of universes would crumble, for you are as necessary as the greatest part of it—it cannot do without you—you cannot be lost or destroyed—you are a part of it all, and are eternal. 'But,' you ask, 'beyond all of this of which you have told me, what is there—what is the Centre of it All?' Your Teacher's face takes on a rapt expression—a light not of earth beams forth from his countenance. '*THE ABSOLUTE*!' he replies.

THE ELEVENTH LESSON.

THE LAW OF KARMA.

"Karma" is a Sanscrit term for that great Law known to Western thinkers as Spiritual Cause and Effect, or Causation. It relates to the complicated affinities for either good or evil that have been acquired by the soul throughout its many incarnations. These affinities manifest as characteristics enduring from one incarnation to another, being added to here, softened or altered there, but always pressing forward for expression and manifestation. And, so, it follows that what each one of us is in this life depends upon is what we have been and how we have acted in our past lives.

Throughout the operations of the Law of Karma the manifestation of Perfect Justice is apparent. We are not punished *for* our sins, as the current beliefs have it, but instead we are punished *by* our sins. We are not rewarded *for* our good acts, but we received our reward *through and by* characteristics, qualities, affinities, etc., acquired by reason of our having performed these good acts in previous lives. We are our own judges and executioners. In our present lives we are storing up good or bad Karma which will stick to us closely, and which will demand expression and manifestation in lives to come. When we fasten around ourselves the evil of bad Karma, we have taken to shelter a monster which will gnaw into our very vitals until we shake him off by developing opposite qualities. And when we draw to ourselves the good Karma of Duty well performed, kindness well expressed, and Good Deeds freely performed without hope of reward, then do we weave for ourselves the beautiful garments which we are destined to wear upon the occasion of our future lives.

The Yogi Teachings relating to the Law of Karma do not teach us that Sin is an offense against the Power which brought us into being, so much as it is an offense against ourselves. We cannot injure the Absolute, nor harm It in any way. But we may harm each other, and in so doing harm ourselves. The Yogis teach that Sin is largely a matter of ignorance and misunderstanding of our true nature, and that the lesson must be well learned until we are able to see the folly and error of our former course, and thus are able to remedy our past errors and to avoid their recurrence. By Karma the effects arising from our sins cling to us, until we become sick and weary of them, and seek their cause in our hearts. When we have discovered the evil cause of these effects, we learn to hate it and tear it from us as a foul thing, and are thence evermore relieved of it.

The Yogis view the sinning soul as the parent does the child who will persist in playing with forbidden things. The parent cautions the child against playing with the stove, but still the child persists in its disobedience, and sooner or later receives a burn for its meddling. The burn is not a *punishment* for the disobedience (although it may seem so to it) but comes in obedience to a natural law which is invariable. To child finds out that stoves and burns are connected, and begins to see some sense and reason in the admonitions of the parent. The love of the parent sought to save the child the pain of the burn, and yet the child-nature persisted in experimenting, and was taught the lesson. But the lesson once thoroughly learned, it is not necessary to forbid the child the stove, for it has learned the danger for itself and thereafter avoids it.

And thus it is with the human soul passing on from one life to another. It learns new lessons, gathers new experiences, and learns to recognize the pain that invariably comes from Wrong Action, and the Happiness that invariably comes from Right Action. As it progresses it learns how hurtful certain courses of action are, and like the burnt child it avoids them thereafter.

If we will but stop to consider for a moment the relative degrees of temptation to us and to others, we may see the operations of past Karma in former lives. Why is it that this thing is "no temptation" to you, while it is the greatest temptation to another. Why is it that certain things do not seem to have any attraction for him, and yet they attract you so much that you have to use all of your will power to resist them? It is because of the Karma in your past lives. The things that do not now tempt you, have been outlived in some former life, and you have profited by your own experiences, or those of others, or else through some teaching given you by one who had been attracted to you by your unfolding consciousness of Truth.

We are profiting to-day by the lessons of our past lives. If we have learned them well we are receiving the benefit, while if we have turned our backs on the words of wisdom offered us, or have refused to learn the lesson perfectly, we are compelled to sit on the same old school-benches and hear the same old lesson repeated until it is fairly driven into our consciousness. We wonder why it is that other persons can perform certain evil acts that seem so repulsive to us, and are apt to pride ourselves upon our superior virtue. But those who know, realize that their unfortunate brethren have not paid sufficient attention to the lesson of the past, and are having it repeated to them in a more drastic form this time. They know that the virtuous ones are simply reaping the benefit of their own application in the past, but that their lesson is not over, and that unless they advance and hold fast to that which they have attained, as well, they will be outstripped by many of those whose failure they are now viewing with wonder and scorn.

It is hard for us to fully realize that we are what we are because of our past experiences. It is difficult for us to value the experiences that we are now going through, because we do not fully appreciate the value of bitter experiences once lived out and outlived. Let us look back over the experiences of this present life, for instance. How many bitter episodes are there which we wish had never happened, and how we wish we could tear them out of our consciousness. But we do not realize that from these same bitter experiences came knowledge and wisdom that we would not part with under any circumstances. And yet if we were to tear away from us the cause of these benefits, we would tear away the benefits also, and would find ourselves back just where we were before the experience happened to us. What we would like to do is to hold on to the benefits that came from the experience—-the knowledge and wisdom that were picked from the tree of pain. But we cannot separate the effect from the cause in this way, and must learn to look back upon these bitter experiences as the causes from which our present knowledge, wisdom and attainment proceeded. Then may we cease to hate these things, and to see that good may come from evil, under the workings of the Law.

And when we are able to do this, we shall be able to regard the painful experiences of our present day as the inevitable outcome of causes away back in our past, but which will work surely toward increased knowledge, wisdom and attainment, if we will but see the Good underlying the working of the Law. When we fall in with the working of the Law of Karma we recognize its pain not as an injustice or punishment, but as the beneficent operation of a Law which, although apparently working Evil, has for its end and aim Ultimate Good.

Many object to the teachings of the Law of Karma by saying that the experiences of each life not being remembered, must be useless and without value. This is a very foolish position to take concerning the matter. These experiences although not fully remembered, are not lost to us at all—they are made a part of the material of which our minds are composed. They exist in the form of feelings, characteristics, inclinations, likes and dislikes, affinities, attractions, repulsions, etc., etc., and are as much in evidence as are the experiences of yesterday which are fresh in our memory. Look back over your present life, and try to remember the experiences of the past years. You will find that you remember but few of the events of your life. The pressing and constant experiences of each of the days that you have lived have been, for the most part, forgotten. Though these experiences may have seemed very vivid and real to you when they occurred, still they have faded into nothingness now, and they are to all intents and purposes *lost* to you. But *are* they lost? Not at all. You are what you are because of the results of these experiences. Your character has been moulded and shaped, little by little, by these apparently forgotten pains, pleasures, sorrows and happinesses. This trial strengthened you along certain lines; that one changed your point of view and made you see things with a broader sweep of vision. This grief caused you to feel the pain of others; that disappointment spurred you on to new endeavors. And each and every one of them left a permanent mark upon your personality—upon your character. All men are what they are by reason of what they have lived through and out. And though these happenings, scenes, circumstances, occurrences, experiences, have faded from the memory, their effects are indelibly imprinted upon the fabric of the character, and the man of to-day is different from what he would have been had the happening or experience not entered into his life.

And this same rule applies to the characteristics brought over from past incarnations. You have not the memory of the experiences, but you have the fruit in the shape of "characteristics," tastes, inclinations, etc. You have a tendency toward certain things, and a distaste for others. Certain things attract, while others repel you. All of these things are the result of your experiences in former incarnations. Your very taste and inclination toward occult studies which has caused you to read these lessons is your legacy from some former life in which some one spoke a word or two to you regarding the subject, and attracted your interest and desire. You learned some little about the subject then—perhaps much—and developed a desire for more knowledge along these lines, which manifesting in your present life has brought you in contact with further instruction. The same inclination will lead to further advancement in this life, and still greater opportunities in future incarnations. Nearly every one who reads these lines has felt that much of this occult instruction imparted is but a "re-learning" of something previously known, although many of the things taught have never been heard before in this life. You pick up a book and read something, and know at once that it is so, because in some vague way you have a consciousness of having studied and worked out the problem in some past period of your lives. All this is the working of the Law of Karma, which caused you to attract that for which you have an affinity, and which also causes others to be attracted to you.

Many are the reunions of people who have been related to each other in previous lives. The old loves, and old hates work out their Karmic results in our lives. We are bound to those whom we have loved, and also to those whom we may have injured. The story must be worked out to the end, although a knowledge of the Law undoubtedly relieves one of many entangling attachments and Karmic relationships, by pointing out the nature of the relation, and enabling one to free himself mentally from the bond, which process tends to dissolve much of the Karmic entanglements.

Life is a great school for the learning of lessons. It has many grades, many classes, many scales of progress. And the lessons must be learned whether we will or no. If we refuse or neglect to learn the lesson we are sent back to accomplish the task, again and again, until the lesson is finally learned. Nothing once learned is ever forgotten entirely. There is an indelible imprint of the lesson in our character, which manifests as predispositions, tastes, inclinations, etc. All that goes to make up that which we call "Character" is the workings of the Law of Karma. There is no such thing as Chance. Nothing ever "happens." All is regulated by the Law of Cause and Effect or Karma. As a man sows so shall he reap, in a literal sense. You are what you are to-day, by reason of what you were in your last life. And in your next life you will be what you are making of yourself to-day. You are your own judge, and executioner—your own bestower of rewards. But the Love of the Absolute is ever working to lead you upward to the Light, and to open your soul to that knowledge that, in the words of the Yogis, "burns up Karma," and enables you to throw off the burden of Cause and Effect that you have been carrying around with you, and which has weighted you down.

In the Fourteen Lessons we quoted from Mr. Berry Benson, a writer in the *Century Magazine* for May, 1894. The quotation fits so beautifully into this place, that we venture to reproduce it here once more, with your permission. It reads as follows:

"A little boy went to school. He was very little. All that he knew he had drawn in with his mother's milk. His teacher (who was God) placed him in the lowest class, and gave him these lessons to learn: Thou shalt not kill. Thou shalt do no hurt to any living thing. Thou shalt not steal. So the man did not kill; but he was cruel, and he stole. At the end of the day (when his beard was gray—when the night was come) his teacher (who was God) said: Thou hast learned not to kill, but the other lessons thou hast not learned. Come back tomorrow.

"On the morrow he came back a little boy. And his teacher (who was God) put him in a class a little higher, and gave him these lessons to learn: Thou shalt do no hurt to any living thing. Thou shalt not steal. Thou shalt not cheat. So the man did no hurt to any living thing; but he stole and cheated. And at the end of the day (when his beard was gray—when the night was come) his teacher (who was God) said: Thou hast learned to be merciful. But the other lessons thou hast not learned. Come back tomorrow.

"Again, on the morrow, he came back, a little boy. And his teacher (who was God) put him in a class yet a little higher, and gave him these lessons to learn: Thou shalt not steal. Thou shalt not cheat. Thou shalt not covet. So the man did not steal; but he cheated and he coveted. And at the end of the day (when his beard was gray—when the night was come) his teacher (who was God) said: Thou hast learned not to steal. But the other lessons thou hast not learned. Come back, my child, tomorrow.

"This is what I have read in the faces of men and women, in the book of the world, and in the scroll of the heavens, which is writ with stars."

Under the operation of the Law of Karma every man is master of his own destiny—he rewards himself—he punishes himself—he builds, tears down and develops his character, always, however, under the brooding influence of the Absolute which is Love Infinite and which is constantly exerting the upward spiritual urge, which is drawing the soul toward its ultimate haven of rest. Man must, and does, work out his own salvation and destiny, but the upward urge is always there—never tiring—never despairing—knowing always that Ultimate Victory belongs to the soul.

Under the Law of Karma every action, yea, every thought as well, has its Karmic effect upon the future incarnations of the soul. And, not exactly in the nature of punishment or rewards, in the general acceptation of the term, but as the invariable operation of the Law of Cause and Effect. The thoughts of a person are like seeds which seek to press forward into growth, bud, blossom and fruit. Some spring into growth in this life, while others are carried over into future lives. The actions of this life may represent only the partial growth of the thought seed, and future lives may be necessary for its full blossoming and fruition. Of course, the individual who understands the Truth, and who has mentally divorced himself from the fruits of his actions—who has robbed material Desire of its vital force by seeing it as it is, and not as a part of his Real Self—his seed-thoughts do not spring into blossom and fruit in future lives, for he has killed their germ. The Yogis express this thought by the illustration of the baked-seeds. They show their pupils that while ordinary seeds sprout, blossom and bear fruit, still if one bakes the seeds their vitality is gone, and while they may serve the purposes of a nourishing meal still they can never cause sprout, blossom or fruit. Then the pupil is instructed in the nature of Desire, and shown how desires invariably spring into plant, blossom and fruit, the life of the person being the soil in which they flourish. But Desires understood, and set off from the Real Man, are akin to baked-seeds—they have been subjected to the heat of spiritual wisdom and are thus robbed of their vitality, and are unable to bear fruit. In this way the understood and mastered Desire bears no Karmic fruit of future action.

The Yogis teach that there are two great principles at work in the matter of Karmic Law affecting the conditions of rebirth. The first principle is that whereby the prevailing desires, aspirations, likes, and dislikes, loves and hates, attractions and repulsions, etc., press the soul into conditions in which these characteristics may have a favorable and congenial soil for development. The second principle is that which may be spoken of as the urge of the unfolding Spirit, which is always urging forward toward fuller expression, and the breaking down of confining sheaths, and which thus exerts a pressure upon the soul awaiting reincarnation which causes it to seek higher environments and conditions than its desires and aspiration, as well as its general characteristics, would demand. These two apparently conflicting (and yet actually harmonious) principles acting and reacting upon each other, determine the conditions of rebirth, and have a very material effect upon the Karmic Law. One's life is largely a conflict between these two forces, the one tending to hold the soul to the present conditions resulting from past lives, and the other ever at work seeking to uplift and elevate it to greater heights.

The desires and characteristics brought over from the past lives, of course, seek fuller expression and manifestation upon the lines of the past lives. These tendencies simply wish to be let alone and to grow according to their own laws of development and manifestation. But the unfolding Spirit, knowing that the soul's best interests are along the lines of spiritual unfoldment and growth, brings a steady pressure to bear, life after life, upon the soul, causing it to gradually kill out the lower desires and characteristics, and to develop qualities which tend to lead it upward instead of allowing it to remain on its present level, there to bring to blossom and fruit many low thoughts and desires. Absolute Justice reigns over the operations of the Law of Karma, but back of that and superior even to its might is found the Infinite Love of the absolute which tends to Redeem the race. It is that love that is back of all the upward tendencies of the soul, and which we all feel within our inner selves in our best moments. The light of the Spirit (Love) is ever there.

Our relationship to others in past lives has its effect upon the working of the Law of Karma. If in the past we have formed attachments for other individuals, either through love or hate; either by kindness or cruelty; these attachments manifest in our present life, for these persons are bound to us, and we to them, by the bonds of Karma, until the attachment is worn out. Such people will in the present life have certain relationships to us, the object of which is the working out of the problems in which we are mutually concerned, the adjustment of relationship, the "squaring up" of accounts, the development of both. We are apt to be placed in a position to receive hurts from those whom we have hurt in past lives, and this not through the idea of revenge, but by the inexorable working out of the Law of Compensation in Karmic adjustments. And when we are helped, comforted and receive favors from those who we helped in past lives, it is not merely a reward, but the operation of the same law of Justice. The person who hurts us in this way may have no desire to do so, and may even be distressed because he is used as an instrument in this way, but the Karmic Law places him in a position where he unwittingly and without desire acts so that you receive pain through him. Have you not felt yourselves hurting another, although you had no desire and intention of so doing, and, in fact, were sorely distressed because you could not prevent the pain? This Is the operation of Karma. Have you not found yourself placed where you unexpectedly were made the bestower of favors upon some almost unknown persons? This is Karma. The Wheel turns slowly, but it makes the complete circle.

Karma is the companion law to Metempsychosis. The two are inextricably connected, and their operations are closely interwoven. Constant and unvarying in operation, Karma manifests upon and in worlds, planets, races, nations, families and persons Everywhere in space is the great law in operation in some form. The so-called mechanical operations called Causation are as much a phase of Karma as is the highest phases manifest on the higher planes of life, far beyond our own. And through it all is ever the urge toward perfection—the upward movement of all life. The Yogi teachings regard the Universe as a mighty whole, and the Law of Karma as the one great law operating and manifesting through that whole.

How different is the workings of this mighty Law from the many ideas advanced by man to account for the happenings of life. Mere Chance is no explanation, for the careful thinker must inevitably come to the conclusion that in an Universe governed by law, there can be no room for Chance. And to suppose that all rewards and punishments are bestowed by a personal deity, in answer to prayers, supplications, good behavior, offerings, etc., is to fall back into the childhood stage of the race thought. The Yogis teach that the sorrow, suffering and affliction witnessed on all sides of us, as well as the joy, happiness and blessings also in evidence, are not caused by the will or whim of some capricious deity to reward his friends and punish his enemies—but by the working of an invariable Law which metes out to each his measure of good and ill according to his Karmic attachments and relationships.

Those who are suffering, and who see no cause for their pain, are apt to complain and rebel when they see others of no apparent merit enjoying the good things of life which have been denied their apparently more worthy brethren. The churches have no answer except "It is God's will," and that "the Divine motive must not be questioned." These answers seem like mockery, particularly when the idea of Divine Justice is associated with the teaching. There is no other answer compatible with Divine Justice other than the Law of Karma, which makes each person responsible for his or her happiness or misery. And there is nothing so stimulating to one as to know that he has within himself the means to create for himself newer and better conditions of life and environment. We are what we are to-day by reason of what we were in our yesterdays. We will be in our tomorrows that which we have started into operation to-day. As we sow in this life, so shall we reap in the next—we are now reaping that which we have sown in the past. St. Paul voiced a world truth when he said: "Brethren, be not deceived. God is not mocked, for whatsoever a man soweth that shall he also reap."

The teachers divide the operation of Karma into three general classes, as follows: (1) The Karmic manifestations which are now under way in our lives, producing results which are the effects of causes set into motion in our past lives. This is the most common form, and best known phase of Karmic manifestation.

(2) The Karma which we are now acquiring and storing up by reason of our actions, deeds, thoughts and mental and spiritual relationships. This stored up Karma will spring into operation in future lives, when the body and environments appropriate for its manifestation presents itself or is secured; or else when other Karma tending to restrict its operations is removed. But one does not necessarily have to wait until a future life in order to set into operation and manifestation the Karma of the present life. For there come times in which there being no obstructing Karma brought over from a past life, the present life Karma may begin to manifest.

(3) The Karma brought over from past incarnations, which is not able to manifest at the present time owing to the opposition presented by other Karma of an opposite nature, serves to hold the first in check. It is a well known physical law, which likewise manifests on the mental plane, that two opposing forces result in neutralization, that is, both of the forces are held in check. Of course, though, a more powerful Karma may manage to operate, while a weaker is held in check by it.

Not only have individuals their own Karma, but families, races, nations and worlds have their collective Karma. In the cases of races, if the race Karma generated in the past be favorable on the whole, the race flourishes and its influence widens. If on the contrary its collective Karma be bad, the race gradually disappears from the face of the earth, the souls constituting it separating according to their Karmic attractions, some going to this race and some to another. Nations are bound by their Karma, as any student of history may perceive if he studies closely the tides of national progress or decline.

The Karma of a nation is made up of the collective Karma of the individuals composing it, so far as their thoughts and acts have to do with the national spirit and acts. Nations as nations cease to exist, but the souls of the individuals composing them still live on and make their influence felt in new races, scenes and environments. The ancient Egyptians, Persians, Medes, Chaldeans, Romans, Grecians and many other ancient races have disappeared, but their reincarnating souls are with us to-day. The modern revival of Occultism is caused by an influx of the souls of these old peoples pouring in on the Western worlds.

The following quotation from *The Secret Doctrine*, that remarkable piece of occult literature, will be interesting at this point:

> "Nor would the ways of Karma be inscrutable were men to work in union and harmony instead of disunion and strife. For our ignorance of those ways—which one portion of mankind calls the ways of Providence, dark and intricate, while another sees in them the action of blind fatalism, and a third simple Chance with neither gods nor devils to guide them—would surely disappear if we would but attribute all these to their correct cause. With right knowledge, or at any rate with a confident conviction that our neighbors will no more work harm to us than we would think of harming them, two-thirds of the world's evil would vanish into thin air. Were no man to hurt his brother, Karma-Nemesis would have neither cause to work for, nor weapons to act through … We cut these numerous windings in our destinies daily with our own hands, while we imagine that we are pursuing a track on the royal road of respectability and duty, and then complain of those ways being so intricate and so dark. We stand bewildered before the mystery of our own making and the riddles of life that we will not solve, and then accuse the great Sphinx of devouring us. But verily there is not an accident in our lives, not a misshapen day or a misfortune, that could not be traced back to our own doings in this or another life … Knowledge of Karma gives the conviction that if—
>
> 'Virtue in distress and vice in triumph
> Makes atheists of Mankind,'
>
> it is only because that mankind has ever shut its eyes to the great truth that man is himself his own savior as his own destroyer; that he need not accuse heaven, and the gods, fates and providence, of the apparent

injustice that reigns in the midst of humanity. But let him rather remember that bit of Grecian wisdom which warns man to forbear accusing THAT which 'Just though mysterious, leads us on unerring Through ways unmarked from guilt to punishment'—which are now the ways and the high road on which move onward the great European nations. The Western Aryans have every nation and tribe like their eastern brethren of the fifth race, their Golden and their Iron ages, their period of comparative irresponsibility, or the Satya age of purity, while now several of them have reached their Iron Age, the *Kali Yuga*, an age black with horrors. This state will last … until we begin acting from within instead of ever following impulses from without. Until then the only palliative is union and harmony—a Brotherhood in *actu* and *altruism* not simply in name."

Edwin Arnold, in his wonderful poem, "The Light of Asia," which tells the story of the Buddha, explains the doctrine of Karma from the Buddhist standpoint. We feel that our students should become acquainted with this view, so beautifully expressed, and so we herewith quote the passages referred to:

"Karma—all that total of a soul
  Which is the things it did, the thoughts it had,
The 'self' it wove with woof of viewless time
  Crossed on the warp invisible of acts.

* * * * *

"What hath been bringeth what shall be, and is,
  Worse—better—last for first and first for last;
The angels in the heavens of gladness reap
  Fruits of a holy past.

"The devils in the underworlds wear out
  Deeds that were wicked in an age gone by.
Nothing endures: fair virtues waste with time,
  Foul sins grow purged thereby.

"Who toiled a slave may come anew a prince
  For gentle worthiness and merit won;
Who ruled a king may wander earth in rags
  For things done and undone.

"Before beginning, and without an end,
 As space eternal and as surety sure,
Is fixed a Power divine which moves to good,
 Only its laws endure.

"It will not be contemned of any one:
 Who thwarts it loses, and who serves it gains;
The hidden good it pays with peace and bliss,
 The hidden ill with pains.

"It seeth everywhere and marketh all:
 Do right—it recompenseth! Do one wrong—
The equal retribution must be made,
 Though DHARMA tarry long.

"It knows not wrath nor pardon; utter-true
 Its measures mete, its faultless balance weighs;
Times are as naught, to-morrow it will judge,
 Or after many days.

"By this the slayer's knife did stab himself;
 The unjust judge hath lost his own defender;
The false tongue dooms its lie; the creeping thief
 And spoiler rob, to render.

"Such is the law which moves to righteousness,
 Which none at last can turn aside or stay;
The heart of it is love, the end of it
 Is peace and consummation sweet. Obey!

* * * * *

"The books say well, my brothers! each man's life
 The outcome of his former living is;
The bygone wrongs bring forth sorrow and woes,
 The bygone right breeds bliss.

"That which ye sow ye reap. See yonder fields!
 The sesamum was sesamum, the corn
Was corn. The silence and the darkness knew;
 So is a man's fate born.

"He cometh, reaper of the things he sowed,
  Sesamum, corn, so much cast in past birth;
And so much weed and poison-stuff, which mar
  Him and the aching earth.

"If he shall labor rightly, rooting these,
  And planting wholesome seedlings where they grew,
Fruitful and fair and clean the ground shall be,
  And rich the harvest due.

"If he who liveth, learning whence woe springs,
  Endureth patiently, striving to pay
His utmost debt for ancient evils done
  In love and truth always;

If making none to lack, he thoroughly purge
  The lie and lust of self forth from his blood;
Suffering all meekly, rendering for offence
  Nothing but grace and good:

"If he shall day by day dwell merciful,
  Holy and just and kind and true; and rend
Desire from where it clings with bleeding roots,
  Till love of life have end:

"He—dying—leaveth as the sum of him
  A life-count closed, whose ills are dead and quit,
Whose good is quick and mighty, far and near,
  So that fruits follow it.

"No need hath such to live as ye name life;
  That which began in him when he began
Is finished: he hath wrought the purpose through
  Of what did make him man.

"Never shall yearnings torture him, nor sins
  Stain him, nor ache of earthly joys and woes
Invade his safe eternal peace; nor deaths
  And lives recur. He goes

"Unto NIRVANA. He is one with Life
  Yet lives not. He is blest, ceasing to be.
OM, MANI PADME OM! the dewdrop slips
  Into the shining sea!

"This is the doctrine of the Karma. Learn!
  Only when all the dross of sin is quit,
Only when life dies like a white flame spent.
  Death dies along with it."

And so, friends, this is a brief account of the operations of the Law of Karma. The subject is one of such wide scope that the brief space at our disposal enables us to do little more than to call your attention to the existence of the Law, and some of its general workings. We advise our students to acquaint themselves thoroughly with what has been written on this subject by ourselves and others. In our first series of lessons—the *"Fourteen Lessons"*—the chapter or lesson on Spiritual Cause and Effect was devoted to the subject of Karma. We advise our students to re-study it. We also suggest that Mr. Sinnett's occult story entitled *"Karma"* gives its readers an excellent idea of the actual working of Karma in the everyday lives of people of our own times. We recommend the book to the consideration of our students. It is published at a popular price, and is well worth the consideration of every one interested in this wonderful subject of Reincarnation and Karma.

THE TWELFTH LESSON.

OCCULT MISCELLANY.

In this, the last lesson of this series, we wish to call your attention to a variety of subjects, coming under the general head of the Yogi Philosophy, and yet apparently separated from one another. And so we have entitled this lesson "Occult Miscellany," inasmuch as it is made up of bits of information upon a variety of subjects all connected with the general teaching of the series. The lesson will consist of answers to a number of questions, asked by various students of the courses in Yogi Philosophy coming from our pen. While these answers, of necessity, must be brief, still we will endeavor to condense considerable information into each, so that read as a whole the lesson will give to our students a variety of information upon several important subjects.

QUESTION 1: *"Are there any Brotherhoods of Advanced Occultists in existence, in harmony with the Yogi Teachings? And if so, what information can you give regarding them?"*

ANSWER: Yes, there are a number of Occult Brotherhoods, of varying degrees of advancement, scattered through the various countries of the earth. These Brotherhoods agree in principle with the Yogi Teachings, although the methods of interpretation may vary somewhat. There is but one TRUTH, which becomes apparent to all deep students of Occultism, and therefore all true Occultists have a glimpse of that Truth, and upon this glimpse is founded their philosophies and teachings. These Occult Brotherhoods vary in their nature. In some, the members are grouped together in retired portions of the earth, dwelling in the community life. In others the headquarters are in the large cities of the earth, their membership being composed of residents of those cities, with outlying branches. Others have no meeting places, their work being managed from headquarters, their members being scattered all over the face of the earth, the communication being kept up by personal correspondence and privately printed and circulated literature. Admission to these true Occult Brotherhoods is difficult. They seek their members, not the members them. No amount of money, or influence, or energy can gain entrance to these societies. They seek to impart information and instruction only to those who are prepared to receive it—to those who have reached that stage of spiritual unfoldment that will enable them to grasp and assimilate the teachings of the Inner Circles. While this is true, it is also true that these Societies or Brotherhoods are engaged in disseminating Occult Knowledge, suited to the minds of the public, through various channels, and cloaked in various disguises of name, authority and style. Their idea is to gradually open the mind of the public to the great truths underlying and back of all of these various fragmentary teachings. And they recognize the fact that one mind may be reached in a certain way, and another mind in a second way, and so on. And, accordingly, they wrap their teachings in covers likely to attract the attention of various people, and to cause them to investigate the contents. But, under and back of all of these various teachings, is the great fundamental TRUTH. It has often been asked of us how one might distinguish the real Brotherhoods from the spurious ones which have assumed the name and general style of the true societies, for the purpose of exploiting the public, and making money from their interest in the great occult truths. Answering this, we would say that the true Occult Brotherhoods and Societies *never sell their knowledge.* It is given free as water to those who seek for it, and is never sold for money. The true adept would as soon think of selling his soul as selling Spiritual Knowledge for gain. While money plays its proper place in the world, and the laborer is worthy of his hire; and while the Masters recognize the propriety of the sale of books on Occultism (providing the price is reasonable and not in excess of the general market price of books) and while they also recognize the propriety of having people pay their part of the expenses of maintaining organizations, magazines, lecturers, instructors, etc., still the idea stops there—it does not extend to the selling of the Inner Secrets of Occultism for silver or gold. Therefore if you are solicited to become a member of any so-called Brotherhood or Occult Society for a consideration of money, you will know at once that the organization is not a true Occult Society, for it has violated one of the cardinal principles at the start. Remember the old occult maxim:

"When the Pupil is ready, the Master appears"—and so it is with the Brotherhoods and Societies—if it is necessary for your growth, development, and attainment, to be connected with one of these organizations then, when the time comes—when you are ready—you will receive your call, and then will know for a certainty that those who call are the true messengers of Truth.

QUESTION II: "*Are there any exalted human beings called Masters, or Adepts, or are the tales regarding them mere fables, etc?*"

ANSWER: Of a truth there are certain highly developed, advanced and exalted souls in the flesh, known as Masters and Adepts, although many of the tales told concerning them are myths, or pure fiction originating in the minds of some modern sensational writers. And, moreover, these souls are members of the Great Lodge, an organization composed of these almost super-human beings—these great souls that have advanced so very far on THE PATH. Before beginning to speak of them, let us answer a question often asked by Western people, and that is, "Why do not these people appear to the world, and show their powers?" Each of you may answer that question from your own experiences. Have you ever been foolish enough to open your soul to the crowd, and have it reveal the sacred Truth that rests there? Have you ever attempted to impart the highest teachings known to you, to persons who had not attained sufficient spiritual development to even understand the meaning of your words? Have you ever committed the folly of throwing spiritual pearls to material swine? If you have had these experiences, you may begin to faintly imagine the reasons of these illumined souls for keeping away from the crowd—for dwelling away from the multitude. No one who has not suffered the pain of having the vulgar crowd revile the highest spiritual truths to him, can begin to understand the feelings of the spiritually illumined individuals. It is not that they feel that they are better or more exalted than the humblest man—for these feelings of the personality have long since left them. It is because they see the folly of attempting to present the highest truths to a public which is not prepared to understand even the elementary teachings. It is a feeling akin to that of the master of the highest musical conceptions attempting to produce his wonderful compositions before a crowd fit only for the "rag-time" and slangy songs of the day.

Then again, these Masters have no desire to "work miracles" which would only cause the public to become still more superstitious than they now are. When one glances back over the field of religions, and sees how the miraculous acts of some of the great leaders have been prostituted and used as a foundation for the grossest credulity and basest superstition, he may understand the wisdom of the masters in this respect. There is another reason for the non-appearance of the Masters, and that is that there is no occasion for it. The laws of Spiritual Evolution are as regular, constant and fixed as are the laws of Physical Evolution, and any attempt to unduly force matters only results in confusion, and the abortive results soon fade away. The world is not ready for the appearance of the Masters. Their appearance at this time would not be in accordance with The Plan.

The Masters or Adepts are human beings who have passed from lower to higher planes of consciousness, thus gaining wisdom, power and qualities that seem almost miraculous to the man of the ordinary consciousness. A Hindu writer speaking of them has said: "To him who hath traveled far along The Path, sorrow ceases to trouble; fetters cease to bind; obstacles cease to hinder. Such an one is free. For him there is no more fever or sorrow. For him there are no more unconscious re-births. His old Karma is exhausted, and he creates no new Karma. His heart is freed from the desire for future life. No new longings arise within his soul. He is like a lamp which burneth from the oil of the Spirit, and not from the oil of the outer world." Lillie in his work on Buddhism, tells his readers: "Six supernatural faculties were expected of the ascetic before he could claim the grade of *Arhat*. They are constantly alluded to in the *Sutras* as the six supernatural faculties, usually without further specification.... In this transitory body the intelligence of Man is enchained. The ascetic finding himself thus confused, directs his mind to the creation of *Manas*. He represents to himself, in thought, another body created from this material body,—a body with a form, members and organs. This body in relation to the material body is like a sword and the scabbard, or a serpent issuing from a basket in which it is confined. The ascetic then, purified and perfected, begins to practice supernatural faculties. He finds himself able to pass through material obstacles, walls, ramparts, etc.; he is able to throw his phantasmal appearance into many places at once. He acquires the power of hearing the sounds of the unseen world as distinctly as those of the phenomenal world—more distinctly in point of fact. Also by the power of *Manas* he is able to read the most secret thoughts of others, and to tell their characters."

These great Masters are above all petty sectarian distinctions. They may have ascended to their exalted position along the paths of the many religions, or they may have walked the path of no-denomination, sect, or body. They may have mounted to their heights by philosophical reasoning alone, or else by scientific investigation. They are called by many names, according to the viewpoint of the speaker, but at the last they are of but one religion; one philosophy; one belief—TRUTH.

The state of Adeptship is reached only after a long and arduous apprenticeship extending over many lives. Those who have reached the pinnacle were once even as You who read these lines. And some of you—yes, perhaps even You who are now reading these words may have taken the first steps along the narrow path which will lead you to heights equally as exalted as those occupied by even the highest of these great beings of whom we are speaking. Unconsciously to yourself, the urge of the Spirit has set your feet firmly upon The Path, and will push you forward to the end. In order to understand the occult custom that finds its full fruit in the seclusion of the Masters, one needs to be acquainted with the universal habit among true occultists of refraining from public or vulgar displays of occult power. While the inferior occultists often exhibit some of the minor manifestations to the public, it is a fact that the true advanced occultists scrupulously refrain from so doing. In fact, among the highest teachers, it is a condition imposed upon the pupil that he shall refrain from exhibitions of his developing powers among the uninitiated public. "The Neophyte is bound over to the most inviolable secrecy as to everything connected with his entrance and further progress in the schools. In Asia, in the same way, the *chela*, or pupil of occultism, no sooner becomes a *chela* than he ceases to be a witness on behalf of the reality of occult knowledge," says Sinnett in his great work on "Esoteric Buddhism," And he then adds: "I have been astonished to find, since my own connection with the subject, how numerous such *chelas* are. But it is impossible to imagine any human act more improbable than the unauthorized revelation by any such *chela*, to persons in the outer world, that he is one; and so the great esoteric school of philosophy guards its seclusion."

QUESTION III: "*Does the Yogi Philosophy teach that there is a place corresponding to the 'Heavens' of the various religions? Is there any basis for the belief that there is a place resembling 'Heaven'?*"

ANSWER: Yes, the Yogi Philosophy *does* teach that there is a real basis for the popular religious beliefs in "Heaven," and that there are states of being, the knowledge of which has filtered through to the masses in the more or less distorted theories regarding "heavens."

But the Yogis do not teach that these "heavens" are *places* at all. The teaching is that they are *planes of existence*. It is difficult to explain just what is meant by this word "plane." The nearest approach to it in English is the term or word "State." A portion of space may be occupied by several planes at the same time, just as a room may be filled with the rays of the sun, those of a lamp. X-rays, magnetic and electric vibrations and waves, etc., each interpenetrating each other and yet not affecting or interfering with each other.

On the lower planes of the Astral World there are to be found the earth-bound souls which have passed out from their former bodies, but which are attracted to the earthly scenes by strong attractions, which serve to weight them down and to prevent them from ascending to the higher planes. On the higher planes are souls that are less bound by earthly attractions, and who, accordingly, are relieved of the weight resulting therefrom. These planes rise in an ascending scale, each plane being higher and more spiritual than the one lower than itself. And dwelling on each plane are the souls fitted to occupy it, by reason of their degree of spiritual development, or evolution. When the soul first leaves the body it falls into a sleep-like stage, from which it awakens to find itself on the plane for which it is fitted, by reason of its development, attractions, character, etc. The particular plane occupied by each soul is determined by the progress and attainment it has made in its past lives. The souls on the higher planes may, and often do, visit the planes lower in the scale than their own, but those on the lower planes may not visit those higher than their own. Quoting from our own writings on this subject, published several years ago, we repeat: This prohibition regarding the visiting of higher planes is not an arbitrary rule, but a law of nature. If the student will pardon the commonplace comparison, he may get an understanding of it, by imagining a large screen, or series of screens, such as used for sorting coal into sizes. The large coal is caught by the first screen; the next size by the second; and so on until the tiny coal is reached. Now, the large coal cannot get into the receptacle of the smaller sizes, but the small sizes may easily pass through the screen and join the larger sizes, if force be imparted to them. Just so in the Astral World, the soul with the greatest amount of materiality, and gross nature, is stopped by the spiritual screen of a certain plane, and cannot pass on to the higher ones, while other souls have cast off some of the confining and retarding material sheaths, and readily pass on to higher and finer planes. And it may be readily seen that those souls which dwell on the higher planes are able to re-visit the lower and grosser planes, while the souls on the grosser cannot penetrate the higher boundries of their plane, being stopped by the spiritual screen. The comparison is a crude one, but it almost exactly pictures the existing conditions on the spiritual world.

Souls on the upper planes, may, and often do, journey to the lower planes for the purpose of "visiting" the souls of friends who may be dwelling there, and thus affording them comfort and consolation. In fact, the teaching is that in many cases a highly developed soul visits souls on the lower planes in whom it is interested, and actually imparts spiritual teaching and instruction to those souls, so that they may be re-born into much better conditions than would have been the case otherwise. All of the planes have Spiritual Instructors from very high planes, who sacrifice their well-earned rest and happiness on their own planes in order that they may work for the less-developed souls on the lower planes.

As we have said, the soul awakens on the plane to which it is suited. It finds itself in the company of congenial souls, in whose company it is enabled to pursue those things which were dear to its heart when alive. It may be able to make considerable advancement during its sojourn in "heaven," which will result to its benefit when it is reborn on earth. There are countless sub-planes, adapted to the infinite requirements of the advancing souls in every degree of development, and each soul finds an opportunity to develop and enjoy to the fullest the highest of which it is capable, and to also perfect itself and to prepare itself for future development, so that it may be re-born under the very best possible conditions and circumstances in the next earth life. But, alas, even in this higher world, all souls do not live up to the best that is in them, and instead of making the best of their opportunities for development, and growing spiritually, they allow the attractions of their material natures to draw them downward, and too often spend much of their time on the planes beneath them, not to help and assist, but to live the less spiritual lives of their friends on the lower planes. In such cases the soul does not reap the benefit of the sojourn in the "after-life," but is born again according to the attractions of its lower, instead of its higher nature, and is compelled to learn its lesson over again.

The Yogi teachings inform us that the lower planes of the Astral World are inhabited by souls of a very gross and degraded type, undeveloped and animal-like. These low souls live out the tendencies and characteristics of their former earth lives, and reincarnate rapidly in order to pursue their material attractions. Of course, there is slowly working even in these undeveloped souls an upward tendency, but it is so slow as to be almost imperceptible. In time these undeveloped souls grow sick and tired of their materiality, and then comes the chance for a slight advance. Of course these undeveloped souls have no access to the higher planes of the Astral world, but are confined to their own degraded plane and to the sub-planes which separate the Astral World from the material world. They cling as closely as possible to the earthly scenes, and are separated from the material world by only a thin screen (if we may use the word). They suffer the tantalizing condition of being within sight and hearing of their old material scenes and environments, and yet unable to manifest on them. These souls form the low class of "spirits" of which we hear so much in certain circles. They hang around their old scenes of debauchery and sense gratification, and often are able to influence the minds of living persons along the same line and plane of development. For instance, these creatures hover around low saloons and places of ill-repute, influencing the sodden brains of living persons to participate in the illicit gratifications of the lower sensual nature.

Souls on the higher planes are not bound by these earthly and material attractions, and take advantage of their opportunities to improve themselves and develop spiritually. It is a rule of the Astral World that the higher the plane occupied by a soul, the longer the sojourn there between incarnations. A soul on the lowest planes may reincarnate in a very short time, while on the higher planes hundreds and even thousands of years may elapse before the soul is called upon to experience re-birth. But re-birth comes to all who have not passed on to other spheres of life. Sooner or later the soul feels that inward urge toward re-birth and further experience, and becomes drowsy and falls into a state resembling sleep, when it is caught up in the current that is sweeping on toward re-birth, and is gradually carried on to re-birth in conditions chosen by its desires and characteristics, in connection with the operation of the laws of Karma. From the soul-slumber it passes through what may be called a "death" on the Astral plane, when it is re-born on the earth plane. But, remember this, the soul, when it is re-born on earth, does not fully awaken from its Astral sleep. In infancy and in early childhood the soul is but slowly awakening, gradually from year to year, the brain being built to accommodate this growth. The rare instances of precocious children, and infant genius are cases in which the awakening has been more rapid than ordinary. On the other hand, cases are known where the soul does not awaken as rapidly as the average, and the result is that the person does not show signs of full intellectual activity until nearly middle age. Cases are known when men seemed to "wake up" when they were forty years of age, or even later in life, and would then take on a freshened activity and energy, surprising those who had known them before.

On some of the planes of the Astral world the souls dwelling there do not seem to realize that they are "dead," but act and live as if they were in the flesh.

They have a knowledge of the planes beneath them, just as we on earth know of conditions beneath us (spiritually), but they seem to be in almost absolute ignorance of the planes above them, just as many of us on earth cannot comprehend the existence of beings more highly developed spiritually than ourselves. This, of course, is only true of the souls who have not been made acquainted with the meaning and nature of life on the Astral Plane. Those who have acquired this information and knowledge readily understand their condition and profit thereby. It will be seen from this that it is of the greatest importance for persons to become acquainted with the great laws of Occultism in their present earth life, for the reason that when they pass out of the body and enter some one of the Astral Planes they will not be in ignorance of the condition, but will readily grasp the meaning and nature of their surroundings and take advantage of the same in order to develop themselves more rapidly.

It will be seen from what has been written by us here and elsewhere that there are planes after planes on the Astral side of life. All that has been dreamt of Heaven, Purgatory or Hell has its correspondence there, although not in the literal sense in which these things have been taught. For instance, a wicked man dying immersed in his desires and longings of his lower nature, and believing that he will be punished in a future life for sins committed on earth—such a one is very apt to awaken on the lower planes or sub-planes, in conditions corresponding with his former fears. He finds the fire and brimstone awaiting him, although these things are merely figments of his own imagination, and having no existence in reality. Murderers may roam for ages (apparently) pursued by the bleeding corpses of their victims, until such a horror of the crime arises in the mind that at last sinking from exhaustion into the soul-sleep, their souls pass into re-birth with such a horror of bloodshed and crime as to make them entirely different beings in the new life. And, yet the "hell" that they went through existed only in their imaginations. They were their own Devil and Hell. Just as a man in earth life may suffer from *delirium tremens*, so some of these souls on the Astral plane suffer agonies from their delirium arising from their former crimes, and the belief in the punishment therefor which has been inculcated in them through earth teachings. And these mental agonies, although terrible, really are for their benefit, for by reason of them the soul becomes so sickened with the thought and idea of crime that when it is finally re-born it manifests a marked repulsion to it, and flies to the opposite. In this connection we would say that the teaching is that although the depraved soul apparently experiences ages of this torment, yet, in reality, there is but the passage of but a short time, the illusion arising from the self-hypnotization of the soul, just as arises the illusion of the punishment itself.

In the same way the soul often experiences a "heaven" in accordance with its hopes, beliefs and longings of earth-life. The "heaven" that it has longed for and believed in during its earth-life is very apt to be at least partially reproduced on the Astral plane, and the pious soul of any and all religious denominations finds itself in a "heaven" corresponding to that in which it believed during its earth-life. The Mohammedan finds his paradise; the Christian finds his; the Indian finds his—but the impression is merely an illusion created by the Mental Pictures of the soul. But the illusion tends to give pleasure to the soul, and to satisfy certain longings which in time fade away, leaving the soul free to reach out after higher conceptions and ideals. We cannot devote more space to this subject at this time, and must content ourselves with the above statements and explanations. The principal point that we desire to impress upon your minds is the fact that the "heaven-world" is not a place or state of permanent rest and abode for the disembodied soul, but is merely a place or temporary sojourn between incarnations, and thus serves as a place of rest wherein the soul may gather together its forces, energies, desires and attractions preparatory to re-birth. In this answer we have merely limited ourselves to a general statement of the states and conditions of the Astral World, or rather of certain planes of that world. The subject itself requires far more extensive treatment.

QUESTION IV: "*Is Nirvana a state of the total extinction of consciousness; and is it a place, state or condition?*"

ANSWER: The teaching concerning *Nirvana*, the final goal of the soul, has been much misunderstood, and much error has crept into the teaching even among some very worthy teachers. To conceive of *Nirvana* as a state of extinction of consciousness would be to fall into the error of the pessimistic school of philosophy which thinks of life and consciousness as a curse, and regards the return into a total unconsciousness as the thing to be most desired. The true teaching is that *Nirvana* is a state of the fullest consciousness—a state in which the soul is relieved of all the illusion of separateness and relativity, and enters into a state of Universal Consciousness, or Absolute Awareness, in which it is conscious of Infinity, and Eternity—of all places and things and time. *Nirvana* instead of being a state of Nothingness, is a state of "Everythingness." As the soul advances along the Path it becomes more and more aware of its connection with, relation to, and identity with the Whole. As it grows, the Self enlarges and transcends its former limited bounds. It begins to realize that it is more than the tiny separated atom that it had believed itself to be, and it learns to identify itself in a constantly increasing scale with the Universal Life. It feels a sense of Oneness in a fuller degree, and it sets its feet firmly upon the Path toward *Nirvana*. After many weary lives on this and other planets—in this and other Universes—after it has long since left behind it the scale of humanity, and has advanced into god-like states, its consciousness becomes fuller and fuller, and time and space are transcended in a wonderful manner. And at last the goal is attained—the battle is won—and the soul blossoms into a state of Universal Consciousness, in which Time and Place disappear and in which every place is Here; every period of Time is Now; and everything is "I." This is *Nirvana*.

QUESTION V: "*What is that which Occultists call 'an Astral Shell,' or similar name? Is it an entity, or force, or being?*"

ANSWER: When the soul passes out from the body at the moment of death it carries with it the "Astral Body" as well as the higher mental and spiritual principles (see the first three lessons in the "Fourteen Lessons"). The Astral Body is the counterpart of the material or physical body, although it is composed of matter of a much finer and ethereal nature than is the physical body. It is invisible to the ordinary eye, but may be seen clairvoyantly. The Astral Body rises from the physical body like a faint, luminous vapor, and for a time is connected with the dying physical body by a thin, vapory cord or thread, which finally breaks entirely and the separation becomes complete. The Astral Body is some time afterward discarded by the soul as it passes on to the higher planes, as we have described a few pages further back, and the abandoned Astral Body becomes an "Astral Shell," and is subject to a slow disintegration, just as is the physical body. It is no more the soul than is the physical body—it is merely a cast off garment of fine matter. It will be seen readily that it is not an entity, force or being—it is only cast off matter—a sloughed skin. It has no life or intelligence, but floats around on the lower Astral Plane until it finally disintegrates. It has an attraction toward its late physical associate—the physical body—and often returns to the place where the latter is buried, where it is sometimes seen by persons whose astral sight is temporarily awakened, when it is mistaken for a "ghost" or "spirit" of the person. These Astral Shells are often seen floating around over graveyards, battlefields, etc. And sometimes these shells coming in contact with the psychic magnetism of a medium become "galvanized" into life, and manifest signs of intelligence, which, however, really comes from the mind of the medium. At some seances these re-vitalized shells manifest and materialize, and talk in a vague, meaningless manner, the shell receiving its vitality from the body and mind of the medium instead of speaking from any consciousness of its own. This statement is not to be taken as any denial of true "spirit return," but is merely an explanation of certain forms of so-called "spiritualistic phenomena" which is well understood by advanced "spiritualists," although many seekers after psychic phenomena are in ignorance of it.

QUESTION VI: *What is meant by "the Days and Nights of Brahm"; the "Cycles"; the "Chain of Worlds", etc., etc.?*

ANSWER: In Lesson Sixth, of the present series, you will find a brief mention of the "Days and Nights of Brahm"—those vast periods of the In-breathing and Out-breathing of the Creative Principle which is personified in the Hindu conception of *Brahma*. You will see mentioned there that universal philosophical conception of the Universal Rhythm, which manifests in a succession of periods of Universal Activity and Inactivity.

The Yogi Teachings are that all Time is manifested in Cycles. Man calls the most common form of Cyclic Time by the name of "a Day," which is the period of time necessary for the earth's revolution on its axis. Each Day is a reproduction of all previous Days, although the incidents of each day differ from those of the other—all Days are but periods of Time marked off by the revolution of the earth on its axis. And each Night is but the negative side of a Day, the positive side of which is called "day." There is really no such thing as a Day, that which we call a "Day" being simply a record of certain physical changes in the earth's position relating to its own axis.

The second phase of Cyclic Time is called by man by the name "a Month," by which is meant certain changes in the relative positions of the moon and the earth. The true month consists of twenty-eight lunar days. In this Cycle (the Month) there is also a light-time or "day," and a dark-time or "night," the former being the fourteen days of the moon's visibility, and the second being the fourteen days of the moon's invisibility.

The third phase of Cyclic Time is that which we call "a Year," by which is meant the time occupied by the earth in its revolution around the sun. You will notice that the year has its positive and negative periods, also, known as Summer and Winter.

But the Yogis take up the story where the astronomers drop it, at the Year. Beyond the Year there are other and greater phases of Cyclic Time. The Yogis know many cycles of thousands of years in which there are marked periods of Activity and Inactivity. We cannot go into detail regarding these various cycles, but may mention another division common to the Yogi teachings, beginning with the Great Year. The Great Year is composed of 360 earth years. Twelve thousand Great Years constitute what is known as a Great Cycle, which is seen to consist of 4,320,000 earth years. Seventy-one Great Cycles compose what is called a *Manwantara*, at the end of which the earth becomes submerged under the waters, until not a vestige of land is left uncovered. This state lasts for a period equal to 71 Great Cycles. A *Kalpa* is composed of 14 Manwantaras. The largest and grandest Cycle manifested is known as the *Maya-Praylaya*, consisting of 36,000 *Kalpas* when the Absolute withdraws into Itself its entire manifestations, and dwells alone in its awful Infinity and Oneness, this period being succeeded by a period equally long—the two being known as the Days and Nights of Brahm.

You will notice that each of these great Cycles has its "Day" period and its "Night" period—its Period of Activity. and its Period of Inactivity. From Day to Maya-Praylaya, it is a succession of Nights and Days—Creative Activity and Creative Cessation.

The "Chain of Worlds," is that great group of planets in our own solar system, seven in number, over which the Procession of Life passes, in Cycles. From globe to globe the great wave of soul life passes in Cyclic Rhythm. After a race has passed a certain number of incarnations upon one planet, it passes on to another, and learns new lessons, and then on and on until finally it has learned all of the lessons possible on this Universe, when it passes on to another Universe, and so on, from higher to higher until the human mind is unable to even think of the grandeur of the destiny awaiting each human soul on THE PATH. The various works published by the Theosophical organizations go into detail regarding these matters, which require the space of many volumes to adequately express, but we think that we have at last indicated the general nature of the question, pointing out to the student the nature of the subject, and indicating lines for further study and investigation.

CONCLUSION.

And now, dear students, we have reached the end of this series of lessons. You have followed us closely for the past four years, many of you having been with us as students from the start. We feel many ties of spiritual relationship binding you to us, and the parting, although but temporary, gives a little pang to us—a little pull upon our heart strings. We have tried to give to you a plain, practical and simple exposition of the great truths of this world-old philosophy—have endeavored to express in plain simple terms the greatest truths known to man on earth to-day, *the Yogi Philosophy*. And many have written us that our work has not been in vain, and that we have been the means of opening up new worlds of thought to them, and have aided them in casting off the old material sheaths that had bound them for so long, and the discarding of which enabled them to unfold the beautiful blossom of Spirituality. Be this as it may, we have been able merely to give you the most elementary instruction in this world-philosophy, and are painfully conscious of the small portion of the field that we have tilled, when compared with the infinite expanse of Truth still untouched. But such are the limitations of Man—he can speak only of that which lies immediately before him, leaving for others the rest of the work which is remote from his place of abode. There are planes upon planes of this Truth which every soul among you will some day make his or her own. It is yours, and you will be impelled to reach forth and take that which is intended for you. Be not in too much haste—be of great patience—and all will come to you, for it is your own.

"MYSTIC CHRISTIANITY."

We have here to make an announcement that will please our readers, judging from the many letters that we have received during the several years of our work. We will now enter upon a new phase of our work of presenting the great truths underlying life, as taught by the great minds of centuries ago, and carefully transmitted from master to student from that time unto our own. We have concluded our presentation of the mystic teachings underlying the Hindu Philosophies, and shall now pass on to a consideration and presentation of the great Mystic Principles underlying that great and glorious creed of the Western world—the religion, teachings, and philosophy of JESUS THE CHRIST. These teachings, too, as we should remember, are essentially Eastern in their origin, and source, although their effects are more pronounced in the Western world. Underlying the teaching and philosophy of the Christ are to be found the same esoteric principles that underlie the other great systems of philosophies of the East. Covered up though the Truth be by the additions of the Western churches and sects, still it remains there burning brightly as ever, and plainly visible to one who will brush aside the rubbish surrounding the Sacred Flame and who will seek beneath the forms and non-essentials for the Mystic Truths underlying Christianity.

We realize the importance of the work before us, but we shrink not from the task, for we know that when the bright Light of the Spirit, which is found as the centre of the Christian philosophy, is uncovered, there will be great rejoicing from the many who while believing in and realizing the value of the Eastern Teachings, still rightly hold their love, devotion and admiration for Him who was in very Truth the Son of God, and whose mission was to raise the World spiritually from the material quagmire into which it was stumbling.

And now, dear pupils, we must close this series of lessons on the Yogi Philosophy. We must rest ere we so soon engage upon our new and great work. We must each take a little rest, ere we meet again on The Path of Attainment. Each of these temporary partings are milestones upon our Journey of Spiritual Life. Let each find us farther advanced.

And now we send you our wishes of Peace. May The Peace be with you all, now and forever, even unto NIRVANA, which is PEACE itself.

THE HATHA YOGA PRADIPIKA

Translated into English by

PANCHAM SINH

Panini Office, Allahabad

[1914]

TABLE OF CONTENTS.

INTRODUCTION.

There exists at present a good deal of misconception with regard to the practices of the Haṭha Yoga. People easily believe in the stories told by those who themselves heard them second hand, and no attempt is made to find out the truth by a direct reference to any good treatise. It is generally believed that the six practices, (षट्कर्म) in Haṭha Yoga are compulsory on the student and that besides being dirty, they are fraught with danger to the practiser. This is not true, for these practices are necessary only in the existence of impurities in the Nâdis, and not otherwise.

There is the same amount of misunderstanding with regard to the Prâṇâyâma. People put their faith implicitly in the stories told them about the dangers attending the practice, without ever taking the trouble of ascertaining the fact themselves. We have been inspiring and expiring air from our birth, and will continue to do so till death; and this is done without the help of any teacher. Prâṇâyâma is nothing but a properly regulated form of the otherwise irregular and hurried flow of air, without using much force or undue restraint; and if this is accomplished by patiently keeping the flow slow and steady, there can be no danger. It is the impatience for the Siddhis which cause undue pressure on the organs and thereby causes pains in the ears, the eyes, the chest, etc. If the three bandhas (बन्ध) be carefully performed while practising the Prâṇâyâma, there is no possibility of any danger.

There are two classes of students of Yoga: (1) those who study it theoretically; (2) those who combine the theory with practice.

Yoga is of very little use, if studied theoretically. It was never meant for such a study. In its practical form, however, the path of the student is beset with difficulties. The books on Yoga give instructions so far as it is possible to express the methods in words, but all persons, not being careful enough to follow these instructions to the very letter, fail in their object. Such persons require a teacher versed in the practice of Yoga. It is easy to find a teacher who will explain the language of the books, but this is far from being satisfactory. For instance, a Pandit without any knowledge of the science of Materia Medica will explain कंटकारि as कंटकस्यारिः कंटकारिः or an enemy of thorns, *i.e.*, shoes, while it is in reality the name of a medicinal plant, The importance of a practical Yogî as a guide to a student of Yoga cannot be overestimated; and without such a teacher it is next to impossible for him to achieve anything. The methods followed by the founders of the system and followed ever afterwards by their followers, have been wisely and advisedly kept secret; and this is not without a deep meaning. Looking to the gravity of the subject and the practices which have a very close relation with the vital organs of the human body, it is of paramount importance that the instructions should be received by students of ordinary capacity, through a practical teacher only, in order to avoid any possibility of mistake in practice. Speaking broadly, all men are not equally fitted to receive the instructions on equal terms. Man inherits on birth his mental and physical capitals, according to his actions in past births, and has to increase them by manipulation, but there are, even among such, different grades. Hence, one cannot become a Yogî in one incarnation, as says Śri Kṛiṣṇa बहूनांजन्मनामन्ते मामप्रपद्यतिभारत । and again

मनुष्याणां सहस्रेषु कश्चिद्यतति सिद्धये । यततामपिसिद्धानां कश्चिन्मांवेत्ति तत्त्वतः ॥ गीता ॥

There are men who, impelled by the force of their actions of previous births, go headlong and accomplish their liberation in a single attempt; but others have to earn it in their successive births. If the student belongs to one of such souls and being earnest, desires from his heart to get rid of the pains of birth and death, he will find the means too. It is well-known that a true Yogî is above temptations and so to think that he keeps his knowledge secret for selling it to the highest bidder is simply absurd. Yoga is meant for the good of all creatures, and a true Yogî is always desirous of benefitting as many men as possible. But he is not to throw away this precious treasure indiscriminately. He carefully chooses its recipients, and when he finds a true and earnest student, who will not trifle with this knowledge, he never hesitates in placing his valuable treasure at the disposal of the man. What is essential in him is that he should have a real thirst for such knowledge—a thirst which will make him restless till satisfied; the thirst that will make him blind to the world and its enjoyments. He should be, in short, fired with मुमुक्षुत्व or desire for emancipation. To such a one, there is nothing dearer than the accomplishment of this object. A true lover will risk his very life to gain union with his beloved like Tulasîdâs. A true lover will see everywhere, in every direction, in every tree and leaf, in every blade of grass his own beloved. The whole of the world, with all its beauties, is a dreary waste in his eyes, without his beloved. And he will court death, fall into the mouth of a gaping grave, for the sake of his beloved. The student whose heart burns with such intense desire for union with Paraṃâtmâ, is sure to find a teacher, and through him he will surely find Him It is a tried experience that Paraṃâtmâ will try to meet you half way, with the degree of intensity with which you will go to meet Him. Even He Himself will become your guide, direct you on to the road to success, or put you on the track to find a teacher, or lead him to you.

Well has it been said

जिन ढूंढा तिन पाइयां गहरे पानी पैठि । मैं बावरि ढूंढन चली रही किनारे बैठि ॥

It is the half-hearted who fail. They hold their worldly pleasures dearer to their hearts than their God, and therefore He in His turn does not consider them worthy of His favours. Says the Upaniṣad:—

नायमात्मा प्रवचनेन लभ्यो न मेधया न बहुना श्रुतेन । यमेवैष वृणुते तेनलभ्यस्तस्यैष आत्मा विवृणुते तनुस्वाम् ॥

The âtmâ will choose you its abode only if it considers you worthy of such a favour, and not otherwise. It is therefore necessary that one should first make oneself worthy of His acceptance. Having prepared the temple (your heart) well fitted for His installation there, having cleared it of all the impurities which stink and make the place unsuitable for the highest personage to live in, and having decorated it beautifully with objects as befit that Lord of the creation, you need not wait long for Him to adorn this temple of yours which you have taken pains to make it worthy of Him. If you have done all this, He will shine in you in all His glory. In your difficult moments, when you are embarrassed, sit in a contemplative mood, and approach your Parama Guru submissively and refer your difficulties to Him, you are sure to get the proper advice from Him. He is the Guru of the ancients, for He is not limited by Time. He instructed the ancients in bygone times, like a Guru, and if you have been unable to find a teacher in the human form, enter your inner temple and consult this Great Guru who accompanies you everywhere, and ask Him to show you the way. He knows best what is best, for you. Unlike mortal beings, He is beyond the past and the future, will either send one of His agents to guide you or lead you to one and put you on the right track. He is always anxious to teach the earnest seekers, and waits for you to offer Him an opportunity to do so. But if you have not done your duty and prepared yourself worthy of entering His door, and try to gain access to His presence, laden with your unclean burden, stinking with Kama, Krodha, Lobha, and Moha, be sure He will keep you off from Him.

The Âsanas are a means of gaining steadiness of position and help to gain success in contemplation, without any distraction of the mind. If the position be not comfortable, the slightest inconvenience will draw the mind away from the lakśya (aim), and so no peace of mind will be possible till the posture has ceased to cause pain by regular exercise.

Of all the various methods for concentrating the mind, repetition of Praṇava or Ajapâ Jâpa and contemplation on its meaning is the best. It is impossible for the mind to sit idle even for a single moment, and, therefore, in order to keep it well occupied and to keep other antagonistic thoughts from entering it, repetition of Praṇava should be practised. It should be repeated till Yoga Nidrâ is induced which, when experienced, should be encouraged by slackening all the muscles of the body. This will fill the mind with sacred and divine thoughts and will bring about its one-pointedness, without much effort.

Anâhata Nâda is awakened by the exercise of Prâṇâyâma. A couple of weeks' practice with 80 prâṇâyâmas in the morning and the same number in the evening will cause distinct sounds to be heard; and, as the practice will go on increasing, varied sounds become audible to the practiser. By hearing these sounds attentively one gets concentration of the mind, and thence Sahaja Samâdhi. When Yoga sleep is experienced, the student should give himself up to it and make no efforts to check it. By and by, these sounds become subtle and they become less and less intense, so the mind loses its waywardness and becomes calm and docile; and, on this practice becoming well-established, Samâdhi becomes a voluntary act. This is, however, the highest stage and is the lot of the favoured and fortunate few only.

During contemplation one sees, not with his eyes, as he does the objects of the world, various colours, which the writers on Yoga call the colours of the five elements. Sometimes, stars are seen glittering, and lightning flashes in the sky. But these are all fleeting in their nature.

At first these colours are seen in greatly agitated waves which show the unsteady condition of the mind; and as the practice increases and the mind becomes calm, these colour-waves become steady and motionless and appear as one deep ocean of light. This is the ocean in which One should dive and forget the world and become one with his Lord—which is the condition of highest bliss.

Faith in the practices of Yoga, and in one's own powers to accomplish what others have done before, is of great importance to insure speedy success. I mean "faith that will move mountains," will accomplish anything, be it howsoever difficult. There is nothing which cannot be accomplished by practice. Says Śiva in Śiva Saṃhitâ.

अभ्यासाज्जायते सिद्धिरभ्यासान्मोक्षमाप्नुयात् ॥
संविदंलभतेऽभ्यासा द्योगोभ्यासात्प्रवर्तते ।
मुद्राणांसिद्धिरभ्यासा दभ्यासाद्वायुसाधनम् ॥
कालवञ्चनमभ्यासात्तथामृत्युञ्जयोभवेत् ।
वाक्सिद्धिः कामचारित्वं भवेदभ्यासयोगतः ॥ अ० ४ श्लोक ९—११

Through practice success is obtained; through practice one gains liberation.

Perfect consciousness is gained through practice; Yoga is attained through practice; success in mudrâs comes by practice. Through practice is gained success in Prâṇâyâma. Death can be evaded of its prey through practice, and man becomes the conqueror of death by practice. And then let us gird up our loins, and with a firm resolution engage in the practice, having faith in कर्मण्येवाधिकारस्ते मा फलेषु कदाचन, and the success must be ours. May the Almighty Father, be pleased to shower His blessings on those who thus engage in the performance of their duties. Om Siam.

PANCHAM SINH.

AJMER:
31st *January*, 1915.

THE HAṬHA YOGA PRADIPIKA.

हठ-योग-परदीपिका

haṭha-yogha-pradīpikā

CHAPTER 1.

On Âsanas.

|| १ || परथमोपदेशः

|| 1 || prathamopadeśaḥ

शरी-आदि-नाथाय नमो|अस्तु तस्मै
येनोपदिष्हटा हठ-योग-विद्या |
विभ्राजते परोन्नत-राज-योगम
आरोढुमिछ्छोरधिरोहिणीव || १ || || १ ||

śrī-ādi-nāthāya namo|astu tasmai
yenopadiṣhṭā haṭha-yogha-vidyā |
vibhrājate pronnata-rāja-yogham
ārodhumichchoradhirohiṇīva || 1 || || 1 ||

Salutation to Âdinâtha (Śiva) who expounded the knowledge of Haṭha Yoga, which like a staircase leads the aspirant to the high pinnacled Râja Yoga. 1.

परणम्य शरी-गुरुं नाथं सवात्मारामेण योगिना |
केवलं राज-योगाय हठ-विद्योपदिश्यते || २ ||

praṇamya śrī-ghuruṃ nāthaṃ svātmārāmeṇa yoghinā |
kevalaṃ rāja-yoghāya haṭha-vidyopadiśyate || 2 ||

Yogin Swâtmârâma, after saluting first his Gurû Srinâtha explains Haṭha Yoga for the attainment of Raja Yoga. 2.

भरान्त्या बहुमत-धवान्ते राज-योगमजानताम |
हठ-परदीपिकां धत्ते सवात्मारामः कृपाकरः || ३ |

bhrāntyā bahumata-dhvānte rāja-yoghamajānatām |
haṭha-pradīpikāṃ dhatte svātmārāmaḥ kṝpākaraḥ || 3 |

Owing to the darkness arising from the multiplicity of opinions people are unable to know the Râja Yoga. Compassionate Swâtmârâma composes the Haṭha Yoga Pradipikâ like a torch to dispel it. 3.

हठ-विद्यां हि मत्स्येन्द्र-गोरक्ष्हाद्या विजानते |
सवात्मारामो|अथवा योगी जानीते तत-परसादतः || ४ ||

haṭha-vidyāṃ hi matsyendra-ghorakṣhādyā vijānate |
svātmārāmo|athavā yoghī jānīte tat-prasādataḥ || 4 ||

Matsyendra, Gorakṣa, etc., knew Haṭha Vidyâ, and by their favour Yogî Swâtmârâma also learnt it from them. 4.

The following Siddhas (masters) are said to have existed in former times:—

शरी-आदिनाथ-मत्स्येन्द्र-शावरानन्द-भैरवाः |
छौरङ्गी-मीन-गोरक्ष्ह-विरूपाक्ष्ह-बिलेशयाः || ५ ||

śrī-ādinātha-matsyendra-śāvarānanda-bhairavāḥ |
chaurangghī-mīna-ghorakṣha-virūpākṣha-bileśayāḥ || 5 ||

Sri Âdinâtha (Śiva), Matsyendra, Nâtha, Sâbar, Anand, Bhairava, Chaurangi, Mîna nâtha, Gorakṣanâtha, Virupâkṣa, Bileśaya. 5.

मन्थानो भैरवो योगी सिद्धिर्बुद्धश्छ कन्थडिः |
कोरंटकः सुरानन्दः सिद्धपादश्छ छर्पटिः || ६ ||

manthāno bhairavo yoghī siddhirbuddhaścha kanthaḍiḥ |
koraṃṭakaḥ surānandaḥ siddhapādaścha charpaṭiḥ || 6 ||

Manthâna, Bhairava, Siddhi Buddha, Kanthadi, Karantaka, Surânanda, Siddhipâda, Charapati. 6.

कानेरी पूज्यपादश्छ नित्य-नाथो निरञ्जनः |
कपाली बिन्दुनाथश्छ काकछण्डीश्वराह्वयः || ७ ||

kānerī pūjyapādaścha nitya-nātho nirañjanaḥ |
kapālī bindunāthaścha kākachaṇḍīśvarāhvayaḥ || 7 ||

Kânerî, Pûjyapâda, Nityanâtha, Nirañjana, Kapâli, Vindunâtha, Kâka Chandîśwara. 7.

अल्लामः परभुदेवश्छ घोडा छोली छ टिंटिणिः |
भानुकी नारदेवश्छ खण्डः कापालिकस्तथा || ८ ||

allāmaḥ prabhudevaścha ghoḍā cholī cha ṭiṃṭiṇiḥ |
bhānukī nāradevaścha khaṇḍaḥ kāpālikastathā || 8 ||

Allâma, Prabhudeva, Ghodâ, Cholî, Tintiṇi, Bhânukî Nârdeva, Khanda Kâpâlika, etc. 8.

इत्यादयो महासिद्धा हठ-योग-परभावतः |
खण्डयित्वा काल-दण्डं बरह्माण्डे विछरन्ति ते || ९ ||

ityādayo mahāsiddhā haṭha-yogha-prabhāvataḥ |
khaṇḍayitvā kāla-daṇḍaṃ brahmāṇḍe vicharanti te || 9 ||

These Mahâsiddhas (great masters), breaking the sceptre of death, are roaming in the universe. 9.

अशेष्ह-ताप-तप्तानां समाश्रय-मठो हठः |
अशेष्ह-योग-युक्तानामाधार-कमठो हठः || १० ||

aśeṣha-tāpa-taptānāṃ samāśraya-maṭho haṭhaḥ |
aśeṣha-yogha-yuktānāmādhāra-kamaṭho haṭhaḥ || 10 ||

Like a house protecting one from the heat of the sun, Haṭha Yoga protects its practiser from the burning heat of the three Tâpas; and, similarly, it is the supporting tortoise, as it were, for those who are constantly devoted to the practice of Yoga. 10.

हठ-विद्या परं गोप्या योगिना सिद्धिमिच्छता |
भवेद्वीर्यवती गुप्ता निर्वीर्या तु परकाशिता || ११ ||

haṭha-vidyā paraṃ ghopyā yoghinā siddhimichchatā |
bhavedvīryavatī ghuptā nirvīryā tu prakāśitā || 11 ||

A Yogî desirous of success should keep the knowledge of Haṭha Yoga secret; for it becomes potent by concealing, and impotent by exposing. 11.

सुराज्ये धार्मिके देशे सुभिक्ष्हे निरुपद्रवे |
धनुः परमाण-पर्यन्तं शिलाग्नि-जल-वर्जिते |
एकान्ते मठिका-मध्ये सथातव्यं हठ-योगिना || १२ ||

surājye dhārmike deśe subhikṣhe nirupadrave |
dhanuḥ pramāṇa-paryantaṃ śilāghni-jala-varjite |
ekānte maṭhikā-madhye sthātavyaṃ haṭha-yoghinā || 12 ||

The Yogî should practise Haṭha Yoga in a small room, situated in a solitary place, being 4 cubits square, and free from stones, fire, water, disturbances of all kinds, and in a country where justice is properly administered, where good people live, and food can be obtained easily and plentifully. 12.

अल्प-दवारमरन्ध्र-गर्त-विवरं नात्युछ्छ-नीछायतं
सम्यग-गोमय-सान्द्र-लिप्तममलं निःशेस-जन्तूज्झितम |
बाह्ये मण्डप-वेदि-कूप-रुछिरं पराकार-संवेष्ह्टितं
परोक्तं योग-मठस्य लक्ष्हणमिदं सिद्धैर्हठाभ्यासिभिः || १३ ||

alpa-dvāramarandhra-gharta-vivaraṃ nātyuchcha-nīchāyataṃ
samyagh-ghomaya-sāndra-liptamamalaṃ niḥśesa-jantūjjhitam |
bāhye maṇḍapa-vedi-kūpa-ruchiraṃ prākāra-saṃveṣhṭitaṃ
proktaṃ yogha-maṭhasya lakṣhaṇamidaṃ siddhairhaṭhābhyāsibhiḥ || 13 ||

The room should have a small door, be free from holes, hollows, neither too high nor too low, well plastered with cow-dung and free from dirt, filth and insects. On its outside there should be bowers, raised platform (chabootrâ), a well, and a compound. These characteristics of a room for Haṭha Yogîs have been described by adepts in the practice of Haṭha. 13.

एवं विधे मठे सथित्वा सर्व-छिन्ता-विवर्जितः |
गुरूपदिष्हट-मार्गेण योगमेव समभ्यसेत || १४ ||

evaṃ vidhe maṭhe sthitvā sarva-chintā-vivarjitaḥ |
ghurūpadiṣhṭa-mārgheṇa yoghameva samabhyaset || 14 ||

Having seated in such a room and free from all anxieties, he should practise Yoga, as instructed by his *guru*. 14.

अत्याहारः परयासश्छ परजल्पो नियमाग्रहः |
जन-सङ्गश्छ लौल्यं छ षहड्भिर्योगो विनश्यति || १५ ||

atyāhāraḥ prayāsaścha prajalpo niyamāghrahaḥ |
jana-sangghaścha laulyaṃ cha ṣhaḍbhiryogho vinaśyati || 15 ||

Yoga is destroyed by the following six causes:—Over-eating, exertion, talkativeness, adhering to rules, *i.e.*, cold bath in the morning, eating at night, or eating fruits only, company of men, and unsteadiness. 15.

उत्साहात्साहसाद्धैर्यात्तत्त्व-जज्ञानाश्छ निश्छयात |
जन-सङ्ग-परित्यागात्ष्हड्भिर्योगः परसिद्ध्यति || १६ ||

utsāhātsāhasāddhairyāttattva-jñānāścha niśchayāt |
jana-sanggha-parityāghātṣhaḍbhiryoghaḥ prasiddhyati || 16 ||

The following six bring speedy success:—Courage, daring, perseverance, discriminative knowledge, faith, aloofness. from company. 16.

अथ यम-नियमाः

अहिंसा सत्यमस्तेयं बरह्मछर्यं कष्हमा धृतिः |
दयार्जवं मिताहारः शौछं छैव यमा दश || १७ ||

atha yama-niyamāḥ
ahiṃsā satyamasteyaṃ brahmacharyaṃ kṣhamā dhṝtiḥ |
dayārjavaṃ mitāhāraḥ śauchaṃ chaiva yamā daśa || 17 ||

The ten rules of conduct are: ahiṃsâ (non-injuring), truth, non-stealing, continence, forgiveness, endurance, compassion, meekness, sparing diet and cleanliness. 17.

तपः सन्तोष्ह आस्तिक्यं दानमीश्वर-पूजनम |
सिद्धान्त-वाक्य-शरवणं हरीमती छ तपो हुतम |
नियमा दश सम्प्रोक्ता योग-शास्त्र-विशारदैः || १८ ||

tapaḥ santoṣha āstikyaṃ dānamīśvara-pūjanam |
siddhānta-vākya-śravaṇaṃ hrīmatī cha tapo hutam |
niyamā daśa samproktā yogha-śāstra-viśāradaiḥ || 18 ||

The ten niyamas mentioned by those proficient in the knowledge of yoga are: Tapa, patience, belief in God, charity, adoration of God, hearing discourses on the principles of religion, shame, intellect, Tapa and Yajña. 18.

Âsanas.

अथ आसनम

हठस्य परथमाङ्गत्वादासनं पूर्वमुछ्यते |
कुर्यात्तदासनं सथैर्यमारोग्यं छाङ्ग-लाघवम || १९ ||

atha āsanam
haṭhasya prathamāngghatvādāsanaṃ pūrvamuchyate |
kuryāttadāsanaṃ sthairyamāroghyaṃ chānggha-lāghavam || 19 ||

Being the first accessory of Haṭha Yoga, âsana is described first. It should be practised for gaining steady posture, health and lightness of body. 19.

वशिष्ठाद्यैश्छ मुनिभिर्मत्स्येन्द्राद्यैश्छ योगिभिः |
अङ्गीकृतान्यासनानि कथ्यन्ते कानिछिन्मया || २० ||

vaśiṣhṭhādyaiścha munibhirmatsyendrādyaiścha yoghibhiḥ |
angghīkṝtānyāsanāni kathyante kānichinmayā || 20 ||

I am going to describe certain âsanas which have been adopted by Munîs like Vasiṣṭha, etc., and Yogîs like Matsyendra, etc. 20.

Swastika-âsana.

जानूर्वोरन्तरे सम्यक्कृत्वा पाद-तले उभे |
ऋजु-कायः समासीनः सवस्तिकं तत्प्रछक्ष्हते || २१ ||

jānūrvorantare samyakkṝtvā pāda-tale ubhe |
ṝju-kāyaḥ samāsīnaḥ svastikaṃ tatprachakṣhate || 21 ||

Having kept both the hands under both the thighs, with the body straight, when one sits calmly in this posture, it is called Swastika. 21.

Gomukha-âsana.

सव्ये दक्ष्हिण-गुल्कं तु पृष्ह्ठ-पार्श्वे नियोजयेत |
दक्ष्हिणे|अपि तथा सव्यं गोमुखं गोमुखाकृतिः || २२ ||

savye dakṣhiṇa-ghulkaṃ tu pṝṣhṭha-pārśve niyojayet |
dakṣhiṇe|api tathā savyaṃ ghomukhaṃ ghomukhākṝtiḥ || 22 ||

Placing the right ankle on the left side and the left ankle on the right side, makes Gomukha-âsana, having the appearance of a cow. 22.

Vîrâsana.

एकं पादं तथैकस्मिन्विन्यसेदुरुणि सथिरम |
इतरस्मिंस्तथा छोरुं वीरासनमितीरितम || २३ ||

ekaṃ pādaṃ tathaikasminvinyaseduruṇi sthiram |
itarasmiṃstathā choruṃ vīrāsanamitīritam || 23 ||

One foot is to be placed on the thigh of the opposite side; and so also the other foot on the opposite thigh. This is called Vîrâsana. 23.

Kurmâsana.

गुदं निरुध्य गुल्फाभ्यां वयुत्क्रमेण समाहितः |
कूर्मासनं भवेदेतदिति योग-विदो विदुः || २४ ||

ghudaṃ nirudhya ghulphābhyāṃ vyutkrameṇa samāhitaḥ |
kūrmāsanaṃ bhavedetaditi yogha-vido viduḥ || 24 ||

Placing the right ankle on the left side of anus, and the left ankle on the right side of it, makes what the Yogîs call Kûrma-âsana. 24.

Kukkuṭa âsana.

पद्मासनं तु संस्थाप्य जानूर्वोरन्तरे करौ |
निवेश्य भूमौ संस्थाप्य वयोमस्थं कुक्कुटासनम || २५ ||

padmāsanaṃ tu saṃsthāpya jānūrvorantare karau |
niveśya bhūmau saṃsthāpya vyomasthaṃ kukkuṭāsanam || 25 ||

Taking the posture of Padma-âsana and carrying the hands under the thighs, when the Yogî raises himself above the ground, with his palms resting on the ground, it becomes Kukkuṭa-âsana. 25.

Uttâna Kûrma-âsana.

कुक्कुटासन-बन्ध-सथो दोर्भ्यां सम्बद्य कन्धराम |
भवेद्कूर्मवदुत्तान एतदुत्तान-कूर्मकम || २६ ||

kukkuṭāsana-bandha-stho dorbhyāṃ sambadya kandharām |
bhavedkūrmavaduttāna etaduttāna-kūrmakam || 26 ||

Having assumed Kukkuṭa-âsana, when one grasps his neck by crossing his hands behind his head, and lies in this posture with his back touching the ground, it becomes Uttâna Kûrma-âsana, from its appearance like that of a tortoise. 26.

Dhanura âsana.

पादाङ्गुष्ह्ठौ तु पाणिभ्यां गृहीत्वा शरवणावधि |
धनुराकर्ष्हणं कुर्याद्धनुर-आसनमुछ्यते || २७ ||

pādāngghuṣhṭhau tu pāṇibhyāṃ ghṝhītvā śravaṇāvadhi |
dhanurākarṣhaṇaṃ kuryāddhanur-āsanamuchyate || 27 ||

Having caught the toes of the feet with both the hands and carried them to the ears by drawing the body like a bow, it becomes Dhanura âsana. 27.

Matsya-âsana.

वामोरु-मूलार्पित-दक्ष्ह-पादं
जानोर्बहिर्वेष्ह्टित-वाम-पादम |
परगृह्य तिष्ह्ठेत्परिवर्तिताङ्गः
शरी-मत्य्सनाथोदितमासनं सयात || २८ ||
मत्स्येन्द्र-पीठं जठर-परदीप्तिं
परछण्ड-रुग्मण्डल-खण्डनास्त्रम |
अभ्यासतः कुण्डलिनी-परबोधं
छन्द्र-सथिरत्वं छ ददाति पुंसाम || २९ ||

vāmoru-mūlārpita-dakṣha-pādaṃ
jānorbahirveṣhṭita-vāma-pādam |
praghṝhya tiṣhṭhetparivartitāngghaḥ
śrī-matysanāthoditamāsanaṃ syāt || 28 ||
matsyendra-pīṭhaṃ jaṭhara-pradīptiṃ
prachaṇḍa-rughmaṇḍala-khaṇḍanāstram |
abhyāsataḥ kuṇḍalinī-prabodhaṃ
chandra-sthiratvaṃ cha dadāti puṃsām || 29 ||

Having placed the right foot at the root of the left thigh, let the toe be grasped with the right hand passing over the back, and having placed the left foot on the right thigh at its root, let it be grasped with the left hand passing behind the back. This is the âsana, as explained by Śri Matsyanâtha. It increases appetite and is an instrument for destroying the group of the most deadly diseases. Its practice awakens the Kundalinî, stops the nectar shedding from the moon in people. 28-29.

Paśchima Tâna.

परसार्य पादौ भुवि दण्ड-रूपौ
दोर्भ्यां पदाग्र-दवितयं गृहीत्वा |
जानूपरिन्यस्त-ललाट-देशो
वसेदिदं पश्छिमतानमाहुः || ३० ||

prasārya pādau bhuvi daṇḍa-rūpau
dorbhyāṃ padāghra-dvitayaṃ ghṝhītvā |
jānūparinyasta-lalāṭa-deśo
vasedidaṃ paśchimatānamāhuḥ || 30 ||

Having stretched the feet on the ground, like a stick, and having grasped the toes of both the feet with both the hands, when one sits with his forehead resting on the thighs, it is called Paśchima Tâna. 30.

इति पश्छिमतानमासनाग्र्यं
पवनं पश्छिम-वाहिनं करोति |
उदयं जठरानलस्य कुर्याद
उदरे कार्श्यमरोगतां छ पुंसाम || ३१ ||

iti paśchimatānamāsanāghryaṃ
pavanaṃ paśchima-vāhinaṃ karoti |
udayaṃ jaṭharānalasya kuryād
udare kārśyamaroghatāṃ cha puṃsām || 31 ||

This Paśchima Tâna carries the air from the front to the back part of the body (*i.e.*, to the suṣumna). It kindles gastric fire, reduces obesity and cures all diseases of men. 31.

Mayûra-âsana.

धरामवष्ह्टभ्य कर-दवयेन
तत-कूर्पर-सथापित-नाभि-पार्श्वः ।
उछ्छासनो दण्डवदुत्थितः खे
मायूरमेतत्प्रवदन्ति पीठम ॥ ३२ ॥

dharāmavaṣhṭabhya kara-dvayena
tat-kūrpara-sthāpita-nābhi-pārśvaḥ |
uchchāsano daṇḍavadutthitaḥ khe
māyūrametatpravadanti pīṭham || 32 ||

Place the palms of both the hands on the ground, and place the navel on both the elbows and balancing thus, the body should be stretched backward like a stick. This is called Mayûra-âsana. 32.

हरति सकल-रोगानाशु गुल्मोदरादीन
अभिभवति छ दोष्हानासनं शरी-मयूरम ।
बहु कदशन-भुक्तं भस्म कुर्यादशेष्हं
जनयति जठराग्निं जारयेत्काल-कूटम ॥ ३३ ॥

harati sakala-roghānāśu ghulmodarādīn
abhibhavati cha doṣhānāsanaṃ śrī-mayūram |
bahu kadaśana-bhuktaṃ bhasma kuryādaśeṣhaṃ
janayati jaṭharāghniṃ jārayetkāla-kūṭam || 33 ||

This Âsana soon destroys all diseases, and removes abdominal disorders, and also those arising from irregularities of phlegm, bile and wind, digests unwholesome food taken in excess, increases appetite and destroys the most deadly poison. 33.

Śava-âsana.

उत्तानं शबवद्भूमौ शयनं तछ्छवासनम ।
शवासनं शरान्ति-हरं छित्त-विश्रान्ति-कारकम ॥ ३४ ॥

uttānaṃ śabavadbhūmau śayanaṃ tachchavāsanam |
śavāsanaṃ śrānti-haraṃ chitta-viśrānti-kārakam || 34 ||

Lying down on the ground, like a corpse, is called Śava-âsana. It removes fatigue and gives rest to the mind. 34.

छतुरशीत्यासनानि शिवेन कथितानि छ |
तेभ्यश्छतुष्हकमादाय सारभूतं बरवीम्यहम || ३५ ||

chaturaśītyāsanāni śivena kathitāni cha |
tebhyaśchatuṣhkamādāya sārabhūtaṃ bravīmyaham || 35 ||

Śiva taught 84 âsanas. Of these the first four being essential ones, I am going to explain them here. 35.

सिद्धं पद्मं तथा सिंहं भद्रं वेति छतुष्हटयम |
शरेष्हठं तत्रापि छ सुखे तिष्हठेत्सिद्धासने सदा || ३६ ||

siddhaṃ padmaṃ tathā siṃhaṃ bhadraṃ veti chatuṣhṭayam |
śreṣhṭhaṃ tatrāpi cha sukhe tiṣhṭhetsiddhāsane sadā || 36 ||

These four are:—The Siddha, Padma, Sinha and Bhadra. Even of these, the Siddha-âsana, being very comfortable, one should always practise it. 36.

The Siddhâsana

अथ सिद्धासनम
योनि-सथानकमङ्घ्रि-मूल-घटितं कृत्वा दृढं विन्यसेत
मेण्ढ्रे पादमथैकमेव हृदये कृत्वा हनुं सुस्थिरम |
सथाणुः संयमितेन्द्रियो|अछल-दृशा पश्येद्भ्रुवोरन्तरं
हयेतन्मोक्ष्ह-कपाट-भेद-जनकं सिद्धासनं परोछ्यते || ३७ ||

atha siddhāsanam
yoni-sthānakamangghri-mūla-ghaṭitaṃ kṝtvā dṝḍhaṃ vinyaset
meṇḍhre pādamathaikameva hṝdaye kṝtvā hanuṃ susthiram |
sthāṇuḥ saṃyamitendriyo|achala-dṝśā paśyedbhruvorantaraṃ
hyetanmokṣha-kapāṭa-bheda-janakaṃ siddhāsanaṃ prochyate || 37 ||

Press firmly the heel of the left foot against the perineum, and the right heel above the male organ. With the chin pressing on the chest, one should sit calmly, having restrained the senses, and gaze steadily the space between the eyebrows. This is called the Siddha Âsana, the opener of the door of salvation. 37.

मेण्ढ्रादुपरि विन्यस्य सव्यं गुल्फं तथोपरि |
गुल्फान्तरं छ निक्षिह्प्य सिद्धासनमिदं भवेत || ३८ ||

meṇḍhrādupari vinyasya savyaṃ ghulphaṃ tathopari |
ghulphāntaraṃ cha nikṣhipya siddhāsanamidaṃ bhavet || 38 ||

This Siddhâsana is performed also by placing the left heel on Meḍhra (above the male organ), and then placing the right one on it. 38.

एतत्सिद्धासनं पराहुरन्ये वज्रासनं विदुः |
मुक्तासनं वदन्त्येके पराहुर्गुप्तासनं परे || ३९ ||

etatsiddhāsanaṃ prāhuranye vajrāsanaṃ viduḥ |
muktāsanaṃ vadantyeke prāhurghuptāsanaṃ pare || 39 ||

Some call this Siddhâsana, some Vajrâsana. Others call it Mukta Âsana or Gupta Âsana. 39.

यमेष्ह्विव मिताहारमहिंसा नियमेष्ह्विव |
मुख्यं सर्वासनेष्ह्वेकं सिद्धाः सिद्धासनं विदुः || ४० ||

yameṣhviva mitāhāramahiṃsā niyameṣhviva |
mukhyaṃ sarvāsaneṣhvekaṃ siddhāḥ siddhāsanaṃ viduḥ || 40 ||

Just as sparing food is among Yamas, and Ahiṃsâ among the Niyamas, so is Siddhâsana called by adepts the chief of all the âsanas. 40.

छतुरशीति-पीठेष्हु सिद्धमेव सदाभ्यसेत |
दवासप्तति-सहस्राणां नाडीनां मल-शोधनम || ४१ ||

chaturaśīti-pīṭheṣhu siddhameva sadābhyaset |
dvāsaptati-sahasrāṇāṃ nāḍīnāṃ mala-śodhanam || 41 ||

Out of the 84 Âsanas Siddhâsana should always be practised, because it cleanses the impurities of 72,000 nâḍîs. 41.

आत्म-धयायी मिताहारी यावद्द्वादश-वत्सरम |
सदा सिद्धासनाभ्यासाद्योगी निष्ह्पत्तिमाप्नुयात || ४२ ||

ātma-dhyāyī mitāhārī yāvaddvādaśa-vatsaram |
sadā siddhāsanābhyāsādyoghī niṣhpattimāpnuyāt || 42 ||

By contemplating on oneself, by eating sparingly, and by practising Siddhâsana for 12 years, the Yogî obtains success. 42.

किमन्यैर्बहुभिः पीठैः सिद्धे सिद्धासने सति |
पराणानिले सावधाने बद्धे केवल-कुम्भके |
उत्पद्यते निरायासात्स्वयमेवोन्मनी कला || ४३ ||

kimanyairbahubhiḥ pīṭhaiḥ siddhe siddhāsane sati |
prāṇānile sāvadhāne baddhe kevala-kumbhake |
utpadyate nirāyāsātsvayamevonmanī kalā || 43 ||

Other postures are of no use, when success has been achieved in Siddhâsana, and Prâṇa Vâyû becomes calm and restrained by Kevala Kumbhaka. 43.

तथैकास्मिन्नेव दृढे सिद्धे सिद्धासने सति |
बन्ध-तरयमनायासात्स्वयमेवोपजायते || ४४ ||

tathaikāsminneva dṛḍhe siddhe siddhāsane sati |
bandha-trayamanāyāsātsvayamevopajāyate || 44 ||

Success in one Siddhâsana alone becoming firmly established, one gets Unmanî at once, and the three bonds (Bandhas) are accomplished of themselves. 44.

नासनं सिद्ध-सदृशं न कुम्भः केवलोपमः |
न खेछरी-समा मुद्रा न नाद-सदृशो लयः || ४५ ||

nāsanaṃ siddha-sadṝśaṃ na kumbhaḥ kevalopamaḥ |
na khecharī-samā mudrā na nāda-sadṝśo layaḥ || 45 ||

There is no Âsana like the Siddhâsana and no Kumbhaka like the Kevala. There is no mudrâ like the Khechari and no *laya* like the Nâda (Anâhata Nâda.) 45.

Padmâsana.

अथ पद्मासनम
वामोरूपरि दक्षिहणं छ छरणं संस्थाप्य वामं तथा
दक्ष्होरूपरि पश्छिमेन विधिना धृत्वा कराभ्यां दृढम |
अङ्गुष्ह्ठौ हृदये निधाय छिबुकं नासाग्रमालोकयेत
एतद्व्याधि-विनाश-कारि यमिनां पद्मासनं परोछ्यते || ४६ ||

atha padmāsanam
vāmorūpari dakṣhiṇaṃ cha charaṇaṃ saṃsthāpya vāmaṃ tathā
dakṣhorūpari paśchimena vidhinā dhṛtvā karābhyāṃ dṛḍham |
angghuṣhṭhau hṛdaye nidhāya chibukaṃ nāsāghramālokayet
etadvyādhi-vināśa-kāri yamināṃ padmāsanaṃ prochyate || 46 ||

Place the right foot on the left thigh and the left foot on the right thigh, and grasp the toes with the hands crossed over the back. Press the chin against the chest and gaze on the tip of the nose. This is called the Padmâsana, the destroyer of the diseases of the Yamîs. 46.

उत्तानौ छरणौ कृत्वा ऊरु-संस्थौ परयत्नतः |
ऊरु-मध्ये तथोत्तानौ पाणी कृत्वा ततो दृशौ || ४७ ||

uttānau charaṇau kṛtvā ūru-saṃsthau prayatnataḥ |
ūru-madhye tathottānau pāṇī kṛtvā tato dṛśau || 47 ||

Place the feet on the thighs, with the soles upwards, and place the hands on the thighs, with the palms upwards. 47.

नासाग्रे विन्यसेद्राजद-अन्त-मूले तु जिह्वया |
उत्तम्भ्य छिबुकं वक्ष्हस्युत्थाप्य पवनं शनैः || ४८ ||

nāsāghre vinyasedrājad-anta-mūle tu jihvayā |
uttambhya chibukaṃ vakṣhasyutthāpy pavanaṃ śanaiḥ || 48 ||

Gaze on the tip of the nose, keeping the tongue pressed against the root of the teeth of the upper jaw, and the chin against the chest, and raise the air up slowly, *i.e.*, pull the apâna-vâyû gently upwards. 48.

इदं पद्मासनं परोक्तं सर्व-वयाधि-विनाशनम |
दुर्लभं येन केनापि धीमता लभ्यते भुवि || ४९ ||

idaṃ padmāsanaṃ proktaṃ sarva-vyādhi-vināśanam |
durlabhaṃ yena kenāpi dhīmatā labhyate bhuvi || 49 ||

This is called the Padmâsana, the destroyer of all diseases. It is difficult of attainment by everybody, but can be learnt by intelligent people in this world. 49.

कृत्वा सम्पुटितौ करौ दृढतरं बद्ध्वा तु पद्ममासनं
गाढं वक्ष्हसि सन्निधाय छिबुकं धयायंश्छ तछ्छेतसि |
वारं वारमपानमूर्ध्वमनिलं परोत्सारयन्पूरितं
नयञ्छन्प्राणमुपैति बोधमतुलं शक्ति-परभावान्नरः || ५० ||

kṛtvā samputitau karau dṛḍhataraṃ baddhvā tu padmamāsanaṃ
ghāḍhaṃ vakṣhasi sannidhāya chibukaṃ dhyāyaṃścha tachchetasi |
vāraṃ vāramapānamūrdhvamanilaṃ protsārayanpūritaṃ
nyañchanprāṇamupaiti bodhamatulaṃ śakti-prabhāvānnaraḥ || 50 ||

Having kept both the hands together in the lap, performing the Padmâsana firmly, keeping the chin Fixed to the chest and contemplating on Him in the mind, by drawing the apâna-vâyû up (performing Mûla Bandha) and pushing down the air after inhaling it, joining thus the prâṇa and apâna in the navel, one gets the highest intelligence by awakening the śakti (kundalinî) thus. 50.

NḄ.—When Apâna Vâyû is drawn gently up and after filling in the lungs with the air from outside, the prâṇa is forced down by and by so as to join both of them in the navel, they both enter then the Kundalinî and, reaching the Brahma randhra (the great hole), they make the mind calm. Then the mind can contemplate on the nature of the âtmana and can enjoy the highest bliss.

पद्मासने सथितो योगी नाडी-दवारेण पूरितम |
मारुतं धारयेद्यस्तु स मुक्तो नात्र संशयः || ५१ ||

padmāsane sthito yoghī nāḍī-dvāreṇa pūritam |
mārutaṃ dhārayedyastu sa mukto nātra saṃśayaḥ || 51 ||

The Yogî who, sitting with Padmâsana, can control breathing, there is no doubt, is free from bondage. 51.

The Siṃhâsana.

अथ सिंहासनम
गुल्फौ छ वृष्हणस्याधः सीवन्त्याः पार्श्वयोः क्ष्हिपेत |
दक्ष्हिणे सव्य-गुल्फं तु दक्ष्ह-गुल्फं तु सव्यके || ५२ ||

atha siṃhāsanam
ghulphau cha vṝshaṇasyādhaḥ sīvantyāḥ pārśvayoḥ kṣhipet |
dakṣhiṇe savya-ghulphaṃ tu dakṣha-ghulphaṃ tu savyake || 52 ||

Press the heels on both sides of the seam of Perineum, in such a way that the left heel touches the right side and the right heel touches the left side of it. 52.

हस्तौ तु जान्वोः संस्थाप्य सवाङ्गुलीः सम्प्रसार्य छ |
वयात्त-वक्तो निरीक्ष्हेत नासाग्रं सुसमाहितः || ५३ ||

hastau tu jānvoḥ saṃsthāpya svāngghulīḥ samprasārya cha |
vyātta-vakto nirīkṣheta nāsāghraṃ susamāhitaḥ || 53 ||

Place the hands on the thighs, with stretched fingers, and keeping the mouth open and the mind collected, gaze on the tip of the nose. 53.

सिंहासनं भवेदेतत्पूजितं योगि-पुणगवैः |
बन्ध-तरितय-सन्धानं कुरुते छासनोत्तमम || ५४ ||

siṃhāsanaṃ bhavedetatpūjitaṃ yoghi-pungghavaiḥ |
bandha-tritaya-sandhānaṃ kurute chāsanottamam || 54 ||

This is Siṃhâsana, held sacred by the best of Yogîs. This excellent Âsana effects the completion of the three Bandhas (The Mûlabandha, Kanṭha or Jâlandhar Bandha and Uḍḍiyâna Bandha). 54.

The Bhadrâsana.

अथ भद्रासनम
गुल्फौ छ वृष्हणस्याधः सीवन्त्याः पार्श्वयोः क्ष्हिप्ते |

सव्य-गुल्फं तथा सव्ये दक्ष्ह-गुल्फं तु दक्ष्हिणे || ५५ ||
पार्श्व-पादौ छ पाणिभ्यां दृढं बद्ध्वा सुनिश्छलम |
भद्रासनं भवेदेतत्सर्व-वयाधि-विनाशनम |
गोरक्ष्हासनमित्याहुरिदं वै सिद्ध-योगिनः || ५६ ||

atha bhadrāsanam
ghulphau cha vṝṣhaṇasyādhaḥ sīvantyāḥ pārśvayoḥ kṣhipte |
savya-ghulphaṃ tathā savye dakṣha-ghulphaṃ tu dakṣhiṇe || 55 ||
pārśva-pādau cha pāṇibhyāṃ dṝḍhaṃ baddhvā suniśchalam |
bhadrāsanaṃ bhavedetatsarva-vyādhi-vināśanam |
ghorakṣhāsanamityāhuridaṃ vai siddha-yoghinaḥ || 56 ||

Place the heels on either side of the seam of the Perineum, keeping the left heel on the left side and the right one on the right side, hold the feet firmly joined to one another with both the hands. This Bhadrâsana is the destroyer of all the diseases. 55 and 56.

एवमासन-बन्धेष्हु योगीन्द्रो विगत-शरमः |
अभ्यसेन्नाडिका-शुद्धिं मुद्रादि-पवनी-करियाम || ५७ ||

evamāsana-bandheṣhu yoghīndro vighata-śramaḥ |
abhyasennāḍikā-śuddhiṃ mudrādi-pavanī-kriyām || 57 ||

The expert Yogîs call this Gorakśa âsana. By sitting with this âsana, the Yogî gets rid of fatigue 57.

आसनं कुम्भकं छित्रं मुद्राख्यं करणं तथा |
अथ नादानुसन्धानमभ्यासानुक्रमो हठे || ५८ ||

āsanaṃ kumbhakaṃ chitraṃ mudrākhyaṃ karaṇaṃ tathā |
atha nādānusandhānamabhyāsānukramo haṭhe || 58 ||

The Nâdis should be cleansed of their impurities by performing the mudrâs, etc., (which are the practices relating to the air) Âsanas, Kumbhakas and various curious mûdrâs. 58.

बरह्मछारी मिताहारी तयागी योग-परायणः |
अब्दादूर्ध्वं भवेद्सिद्धो नात्र कार्या विछारणा || ५९ ||

brahmachārī mitāhārī tyāghī yogha-parāyaṇaḥ |
abdādūrdhvaṃ bhavedsiddho nātra kāryā vichāraṇā || 59 ||

By regular and close attention to Nâda (anâhata nâda) in Haṭha Yoga, a Brahmachari, sparing in diet, unattached to objects of enjoyment, and devoted to Yoga, gains success, no doubt, within a year. 59.

सुस्निग्ध-मधुराहारश्छतुर्थांश-विवर्जितः |
भुज्यते शिव-सम्प्रीत्यै मिताहारः स उछ्यते || ६० ||

susnighdha-madhurāhāraśchaturthāṃśa-vivarjitaḥ |
bhujyate śiva-samprītyai mitāhāraḥ sa uchyate || 60 ||

Abstemious feeding is that in which ¾ of hunger is satisfied with food, well cooked with ghee and sweets, and eaten with the offering of it to Śiva. 60.

Foods injurious to a Yogî.

कट्वाम्ल-तीक्ष्हण-लवणोष्हण-हरीत-शाक-
सौवीर-तैल-तिल-सर्ष्हप-मद्य-मत्स्यान |
आजादि-मांस-दधि-तक्र-कुलत्थकोल-
पिण्याक-हिङ्गु-लशुनाद्यमपथ्यमाहुः || ६१ ||

kaṭvāmla-tīkṣhṇa-lavaṇoṣhṇa-harīta-śāka-
sauvīra-taila-tila-sarṣhapa-madya-matsyān |
ājādi-māṃsa-dadhi-takra-kulatthakola-
piṇyāka-hingghu-laśunādyamapathyamāhuḥ || 61 ||

Bitter, sour, saltish, hot, green vegetables, fermented, oily, mixed with til seed, rape seed, intoxicating liquors, fish, meat, curds, chhaasa pulses, plums, oil-cake, asafœtida (hînga), garlic, onion, etc., should not be eaten. 61.

भोजनमहितं विद्यात्पुनरस्योष्हणी-कृतं रूक्ष्हम |
अतिलवणमम्ल-युक्तं कदशन-शाकोत्कं वर्ज्यम || ६२ ||

bhojanamahitaṃ vidyātpunarasyoṣhṇī-kṛtaṃ rūkṣham |
atilavaṇamamla-yuktaṃ kadaśana-śākotkaṃ varjyam || 62 ||

Food heated again, dry, having too much salt, sour, minor grains, and vegetables that cause burning sensation, should not be eaten, Fire, women, travelling, etc., should be avoided. 62.

वह्नि-सत्री-पथि-सेवानामादौ वर्जनमाछरेत || ६३ ||

vahni-strī-pathi-sevānāmādau varjanamācharet || 63 ||

As said by Gorakṣa, one should keep aloof from the society of the evil-minded, fire, women, travelling, early morning bath, fasting, and all kinds of bodily exertion. 63.

तथा हि गोरक्ष्ह-वछनम
वर्जयेद्दुर्जन-परान्तं वह्नि-सत्री-पथि-सेवनम |
परातः-सनानोपवासादि काय-कलेश-विधिं तथा || ६४ ||

tathā hi ghorakṣha-vachanam
varjayeddurjana-prāntaṃ vahni-strī-pathi-sevanam |
prātaḥ-snānopavāsādi kāya-kleśa-vidhiṃ tathā || 64 ||

Wheat, rice, barley, shâstik (a kind of rice), good corns, milk, ghee, sugar, butter, sugarcandy, honey, dried ginger, Parwal (a vegetable) the five vegetables, moong, pure water, these are very beneficial to those who practise Yoga. 64.

गोधूम-शालि-यव-षहाष्ह्टिक-शोभनान्नं
कष्हीराज्य-खण्ड-नवनीत-सिद्धा-मधूनि |
शुण्ठी-पटोल-कफलादिक-पञ्छ-शाकं
मुद्गादि-दिव्यमुदकं छ यमीन्द्र-पथ्यम || ६५ ||

ghodhūma-śāli-yava-ṣhāṣhṭika-śobhanānnaṃ
kṣhīrājya-khaṇḍa-navanīta-siddhā-madhūni |
śuṇṭhī-paṭola-kaphalādika-pañcha-śākaṃ
mudghādi-divyamudakaṃ cha yamīndra-pathyam || 65 ||

A Yogî should eat tonics (things giving strength), well sweetened, greasy (made with ghee), milk, butter, etc., which may increase humors of the body, according to his desire. 65.

पुष्ह्टं सुमधुरं सनिग्धं गव्यं धातु-परपोष्हणम |
मनोभिलष्हितं योग्यं योगी भोजनमाछरेत || ६६ ||

puṣhṭaṃ sumadhuraṃ snighdhaṃ ghavyaṃ dhātu-praposhaṇam |
manobhilaṣhitaṃ yoghyaṃ yoghī bhojanamācharet || 66 ||

Whether young, old or too old, sick or lean, one who discards laziness, gets success if he practises Yoga. 66.

युवो वृद्धो|अतिवृद्धो वा वयाधितो दुर्बलो|अपि वा |
अभ्यासात्सिद्धिमाप्नोति सर्व-योगेष्ह्वतन्द्रितः || ६७ ||

yuvo vṛddho|ativṛddho vā vyādhito durbalo|api vā |
abhyāsātsiddhimāpnoti sarva-yogheṣhvatandritaḥ || 67 ||

Success comes to him who is engaged in the practice. How can one get success without practice; for by merely reading books on Yoga, one can never get success. 67.

करिया-युक्तस्य सिद्धिः सयादक्रियस्य कथं भवेत |
न शास्त्र-पाठ-मात्रेण योग-सिद्धिः परजायते || ६८ ||

kriyā-yuktasya siddhiḥ syādakriyasya kathaṃ bhavet |
na śāstra-pāṭha-mātreṇa yogha-siddhiḥ prajāyate || 68 ||

Success cannot be attained by adopting a particular dress (Veṣa). It cannot be gained by telling tales. Practice alone is the means to success. This is true, there is no doubt. 68.

न वेष्ह-धारणं सिद्धेः कारणं न छ तत-कथा |
करियैव कारणं सिद्धेः सत्यमेतन्न संशयः || ६९ ||
पीठानि कुम्भकाश्छित्रा दिव्यानि करणानि छ |
सर्वाण्यपि हठाभ्यासे राज-योग-फलावधि || ७० ||

na veṣha-dhāraṇaṃ siddheḥ kāraṇaṃ na cha tat-kathā |
kriyaiva kāraṇaṃ siddheḥ satyametanna saṃśayaḥ || 69 ||
pīṭhāni kumbhakāśchitrā divyāni karaṇāni cha |
sarvāṇyapi haṭhābhyāse rāja-yogha-phalāvadhi || 70 ||

Âsanas (postures), various Kumbhakas, and other divine means, all should be practised in the practice of Haṭha Yoga, till the fruit—Râja Yoga—is obtained. 69.

End of chapter 1st, on the method of forming the Âsanas.

इति हठ-परदीपिकायां परथमोपदेशः |

iti haṭha-pradīpikāyāṃ prathamopadeśaḥ |

CHAPTER II.

On Prâṇâyâma.

|| २ || दवितीयोपदेशः

|| 2 || dvitīyopadeśaḥ

अथासने दृधे योगी वशी हित-मिताशनः |
गुरूपदिष्ह्ट-मार्गेण पराणायामान्समभ्यसेत || १ ||

athāsane dṟdhe yoghī vaśī hita-mitāśanaḥ |
ghurūpadiṣhṭa-mārgheṇa prāṇāyāmānsamabhyaset || 1 ||

Posture becoming established, a Yogî, master of himself, eating salutary and moderate food, should practise Prâṇâyâma, as instructed by his guru. 1.

छले वाते छलं छित्तं निश्छले निश्छलं भवेत||
योगी सथाणुत्वमाप्नोति ततो वायुं निरोधयेत || २ ||

chale vāte chalaṃ chittaṃ niśchale niśchalaṃ bhavet||
yoghī sthāṇutvamāpnoti tato vāyuṃ nirodhayet || 2 ||

Respiration being disturbed, the mind becomes disturbed. By restraining respiration, the Yogî gets steadiness of mind 2.

यावद्वायुः सथितो देहे तावज्जीवनमुछ्यते |
मरणं तस्य निष्ह्क्रान्तिस्ततो वायुं निरोधयेत || ३ ||

yāvadvāyuḥ sthito dehe tāvajjīvanamuchyate |
maraṇaṃ tasya niṣhkrāntistato vāyuṃ nirodhayet || 3 ||

So long as the (breathing) air stays in the body, it is called life. Death consists in the passing out of the (breathing) air. It is, therefore, necessary to restrain the breath. 3.

मलाकलासु नाडीष्हु मारुतो नैव मध्यगः |
कथं सयादुन्मनीभावः कार्य-सिद्धिः कथं भवेत || ४ ||

malākalāsu nāḍīṣhu māruto naiva madhyaghaḥ |
kathaṃ syādunmanībhāvaḥ kārya-siddhiḥ kathaṃ bhavet || 4 ||

The breath does not pass through the middle channel (suṣumnâ), owing to the impurities of the nâdîs. How can then success be attained, and how can there be the unmanî avasthâ. 4.

शुद्धमेति यदा सर्वं नाडी-छक्रं मलाकुलम |
तदैव जायते योगी पराण-संग्रहणे कष्हमः || ५ ||

śuddhameti yadā sarvaṃ nāḍī-chakraṃ malākulam |
tadaiva jāyate yoghī prāṇa-saṃghrahaṇe kṣhamaḥ || 5 ||

When the whole system of nâdîs which is full of impurities, is cleaned, then the Yogî becomes able to control the Prâṇa. 5.

पराणायामं ततः कुर्यान्नित्यं सात्त्विकया धिया |
यथा सुष्हुम्णा-नाडीस्था मलाः शुद्धिं परयान्ति छ || ६ ||

prāṇāyāmaṃ tataḥ kuryānnityaṃ sāttvikayā dhiyā |
yathā suṣhumṇā-nāḍīsthā malāḥ śuddhiṃ prayānti cha || 6 ||

Therefore, Prâṇâyâma should be performed daily with sâtwika buddhi (intellect free from raja and tama or activity and sloth), in order to drive out the impurities of the suṣumnâ. 6.

Method of performing Prâṇâyâma.

बद्ध-पद्मासनो योगी पराणं छन्द्रेण पूरयेत |
धारयित्वा यथा-शक्ति भूयः सूर्येण रेछयेत || ७ ||

पराणं सूर्येण छाकृष्ह्य पूरयेदुदरं शनैः |
विधिवत्कुम्भकं कृत्वा पुनश्छन्द्रेण रेछयेत || ८ ||

baddha-padmāsano yoghī prāṇaṃ chandreṇa pūrayet |
dhārayitvā yathā-śakti bhūyaḥ sūryeṇa rechayet || 7 ||
prāṇaṃ sūryeṇa chākṟṣhya pūrayedudaraṃ śanaiḥ |
vidhivatkumbhakaṃ kṟtvā punaśchandreṇa rechayet || 8 ||

Sitting in the Padmâsana posture the Yogî should fill in the air through the left nostril (closing the right one); and, keeping it confined according to one's ability, it should be expelled slowly through the sûrya (right nostril). Then, drawing in the air through the sûrya (right nostril) slowly, the belly should be filled, and after performing Kumbhaka as before, it should be expelled slowly through the chandra (left nostril). 7 and 8.

येन तयजेत्तेन पीत्वा धारयेदतिरोधतः |
रेछयेच्छ ततो|अन्येन शनैरेव न वेगतः || ९ ||

yena tyajettena pītvā dhārayedatirodhataḥ |
rechayechcha tato|anyena śanaireva na veghataḥ || 9 ||

Inhaling thus through the one, through which it was expelled, and having restrained it there, till possible, it should be exhaled through the other, slowly and not forcibly. 9.

पराणं छेदिडया पिबेन्नियमितं भूयो|अन्यथा रेछयेत
पीत्वा पिङ्गलया समीरणमथो बद्ध्वा तयजेद्वामया |
सूर्य-छन्द्रमसोरनेन विधिनाभ्यासं सदा तन्वतां
शुद्धा नाडि-गणा भवन्ति यमिनां मास-तरयादूर्ध्वतः || १० ||

prāṇaṃ chediḍayā pibenniyamitaṃ bhūyo|anyathā rechayet
pītvā pingghalayā samīraṇamatho baddhvā tyajedvāmayā |
sūrya-chandramasoranena vidhinābhyāsaṃ sadā tanvatāṃ
śuddhā nāḍi-ghaṇā bhavanti yamināṃ māsa-trayādūrdhvataḥ || 10 ||

If the air be inhaled through the left nostril, it should be expelled again through the other, and filling it through the right nostril, confining it there, it should be expelled through the left nostril. By practising in this way, through the right and the left nostrils alternately, the whole of the collection of the nâdîs of the yamîs (practisers) becomes clean, *i.e.*, free from impurities, after 3 months and over. 10.

परातर्मध्यन्दिने सायमर्ध-रात्रे छ कुम्भकान |
शनैरशीति-पर्यन्तं छतुर्वारं समभ्यसेत || ११ ||

prātarmadhyandine sāyamardha-rātre cha kumbhakān |
śanairaśīti-paryantaṃ chaturvāraṃ samabhyaset || 11 ||

Kumbhakas should be performed gradually 4 times during day and night, *i.e.*, (morning, noon, evening and midnight), till the number of Kumbhakas for one time is 80 and for day and night together it is 320. 11.

कनीयसि भवेद्स्वेद कम्पो भवति मध्यमे |
उत्तमे सथानमाप्नोति ततो वायुं निबन्धयेत || १२ ||

kanīyasi bhavedsveda kampo bhavati madhyame |
uttame sthānamāpnoti tato vāyuṃ nibandhayet || 12 ||

In the beginning there is perspiration, in the middle stage there is quivering, and in the last or the 3rd stage one obtains steadiness; and then the breath should be made steady or motionless. 12.

जलेन शरम-जातेन गात्र-मर्दनमाछरेत |
दृढता लघुता छैव तेन गात्रस्य जायते || १३ ||

jalena śrama-jātena ghātra-mardanamācharet |
dṛḍhatā laghutā chaiva tena ghātrasya jāyate || 13 ||

The perspiration exuding from exertion of practice should be rubbed into the body (and not wiped), as by so doing the body becomes strong. 13.

अभ्यास-काले परथमे शस्तं कष्हीराज्य-भोजनम |
ततो|अभ्यासे दृढीभूते न तादृङ-नियम-गरहः || १४ ||

abhyāsa-kāle prathame śastaṃ kṣhīrājya-bhojanam |
tato|abhyāse dṛḍhībhūte na tādṛng-niyama-ghrahaḥ || 14 ||

During the first stage of practice the food consisting of milk and ghee is wholesome. When the practice becomes established, no such restriction is necessary. 14.

यथा सिंहो गजो वयाघ्रो भवेद्वश्यः शनैः शनैः |
तथैव सेवितो वायुरन्यथा हन्ति साधकम || १५ ||

yathā siṃho ghajo vyāghro bhavedvaśyaḥ śanaiḥ śanaiḥ |
tathaiva sevito vāyuranyathā hanti sādhakam || 15 ||

Just as lions, elephants and tigers are controlled by and by, so the breath is controlled by slow degrees, otherwise (*i.e.*, by being hasty or using too much force) it kills the practiser himself. 15.

पराणायामेन युक्तेन सर्व-रोग-कष्हयो भवेत |
अयुक्ताभ्यास-योगेन सर्व-रोग-समुद्गमः || १६ ||

prāṇāyāmena yuktena sarva-rogha-kṣhayo bhavet |
ayuktābhyāsa-yoghena sarva-rogha-samudghamaḥ || 16 ||

When Prâṇayama, etc., are performed properly, they eradicate all diseases; but an improper practice generates diseases. 16.

हिक्का शवासश्छ कासश्छ शिरः-कर्णाक्षिह-वेदनाः |
भवन्ति विविधाः रोगाः पवनस्य परकोपतः || १७ ||

hikkā śvāsaścha kāsaścha śiraḥ-karṇākṣhi-vedanāḥ |
bhavanti vividhāḥ roghāḥ pavanasya prakopataḥ || 17 ||

Hiccough, asthma, cough, pain in the head, the ears, and the eyes; these and other various kinds of diseases are generated by the disturbance of the breath. 17.

युक्तं युक्तं तयजेद्वायुं युक्तं युक्तं छ पूरयेत |
युक्तं युक्तं छ बध्नीयादेवं सिद्धिमवाप्नुयात || १८ ||

yuktaṃ yuktaṃ tyajedvāyuṃ yuktaṃ yuktaṃ cha pūrayet |
yuktaṃ yuktaṃ cha badhnīyādevaṃ siddhimavāpnuyāt || 18 ||

The air should be expelled with proper tact and should be filled in skilfully; and when it has been kept confined properly it brings success. 18.

NḄ.—The above caution is necessary to warn the aspirants against omitting any instruction; and, in their zeal to gain success or siddhis early, to begin the practice, either by using too much force in filling in, confining and expelling the air, or by omitting any instructions, it may cause unnecessary pressure on their ears, eyes, &c,, and cause pain. Every word in the instructions is full of meaning and is necessarily used in the slokas, and should be followed very carefully and with due attention. Thus there will be nothing to fear whatsoever. We are inhaling and exhaling the air throughout our lives without any sort of danger, and Prâṇayama being only a regular form of it, there should be no cause to fear.

यदा तु नाडी-शुद्धिः सयात्तथा छिह्नानि बाह्यतः |
कायस्य कृशता कान्तिस्तदा जायते निश्छितम || १९ ||

yadā tu nāḍī-śuddhiḥ syāttathā chihnāni bāhyataḥ |
kāyasya kṝśatā kāntistadā jāyate niśchitam || 19 ||

When the nâdîs become free from impurities, and there appear the outward signs of success, such as lean body and glowing colour, then one should feel certain of success. 19.

यथेष्टं धारणं वायोरनलस्य परदीपनम |
नादाभिव्यक्तिरारोग्यं जायते नाडि-शोधनात || २० ||

yatheṣhṭaṃ dhāraṇaṃ vāyoranalasya pradīpanam |
nādābhivyaktirāroghyaṃ jāyate nāḍi-śodhanāt || 20 ||

By removing the impurities, the air can be restrained, according to one's wish and the appetite is increased, the divine sound is awakened, and the body becomes healthy. 20.

मेद-शलेष्हमाधिकः पूर्वं षहट-कर्माणि समाछरेत |
अन्यस्तु नाछरेत्तानि दोष्हाणां समभावतः || २१ ||

meda-śleṣhmādhikaḥ pūrvaṃ ṣhaṭ-karmāṇi samācharet |
anyastu nācharettāni doṣhāṇāṃ samabhāvataḥ || 21 ||

If there be excess of fat or phlegm in the body, the six kinds of kriyâs (duties) should be performed first. But others, not suffering from the excess of these, should not perform them. 21.

धौतिर्बस्तिस्तथा नेतिस्त्राटकं नौलिकं तथा |
कपाल-भातिश्छैतानि षहट-कर्माणि परछक्ष्हते || २२ ||

dhautirbastistathā netistrāṭakaṃ naulikaṃ tathā |
kapāla-bhātiśchaitāni ṣhaṭ-karmāṇi prachakṣhate || 22 ||

The six kinds of duties are: Dhauti, Basti, Neti, Trâtaka, Nauti and Kapâla Bhâti. These are called the six actions वटूकमि 22.

कर्म षहट्कमिदं गोप्यं घट-शोधन-कारकम |
विछित्र-गुण-सन्धाय पूज्यते योगि-पुणगवैः || २३ ||

karma ṣhaṭkamidaṃ ghopyaṃ ghaṭa-śodhana-kārakam |
vichitra-ghuṇa-sandhāya pūjyate yoghi-pungghavaiḥ || 23 ||

These six kinds of actions which cleanse the body should be kept secret. They produce extraordinary attributes and are performed with earnestness by the best of Yogîs. 23.

The Dhauti (धौति)

तत्र धौतिः
छतुर-अङ्गुल-विस्तारं हस्त-पञ्छ-दशायतम |
गुरूपदिष्हट-मार्गेण सिक्तं वस्त्रं शनैर्ग्रसेत |
पुनः परत्याहरेछ्छैतदुदितं धौति-कर्म तत || २४ ||

tatra dhautiḥ
chatur-angghula-vistāraṃ hasta-pañcha-daśāyatam |
ghurūpadiṣhṭa-mārgheṇa siktaṃ vastraṃ śanairghraset |
punaḥ pratyāharechchaitaduditaṃ dhauti-karma tat || 24 ||

A strip of cloth, about 3 inches wide and 15 cubits long, is pushed in (swallowed), when moist with warm water, through the passage shown by the guru, and is taken out again. This is called Dhauti Karma. 24.

NB.—The strip should be moistened with a little warm water, and the end should be held with the teeth. It is swallowed slowly, little by little; thus, first day 1 cubit, 2nd day 2 cubits, 3rd day 3 cubits, and so on.

After swallowing it the stomach should be given a good, round motion from left to right, and then it should be taken out slowly and gently.

कास-शवास-पलीह-कुष्ह्ठं कफरोगाश्छ्छ विंशतिः |
धौति-कर्म-परभावेण परयान्त्येव न संशयः || २५ ||

kāsa-śvāsa-plīha-kuṣhṭhaṃ kapharoghāścha viṃśatiḥ |
dhauti-karma-prabhāveṇa prayāntyeva na saṃśayaḥ || 25 ||

There is no doubt, that cough, asthma, enlargement of the spleen, leprosy, and 20 kinds of diseases born of phlegm, disappear by the practice of Dhauti Karma. 25.

The Basti (बस्तिकर्म)

अथ बस्तिः
नाभि-दघ्न-जले पायौ नयस्त-नालोत्कटासनः |
आधाराकुनछ्नं कुर्यात्क्ष्हालनं बस्ति-कर्म तत || २६ ||

atha bastiḥ
nābhi-daghna-jale pāyau nyasta-nālotkaṭāsanaḥ |
ādhārākuñchanaṃ kuryātkṣhālanaṃ basti-karma tat || 26 ||

Squatting in navel-deep water, and introducing a six inches long, smooth piece of ½ an inch diameter pipe, open at both ends, half inside the anus; it (anus) should he drawn up (contracted) and then expelled. This washing is called the Basti Karma. 26.

गुल्म-पलीहोदरं छापि वात-पित्त-कफोद्भवाः |
बस्ति-कर्म-परभावेण कष्हीयन्ते सकलामयाः || २७ ||

ghulma-plīhodaraṃ chāpi vāta-pitta-kaphodbhavāḥ |
basti-karma-prabhāveṇa kṣhīyante sakalāmayāḥ || 27 ||

By practising this Basti Karma, colic, enlarged spleen, and dropsy, arising from the disorders of Vâta (air), pitta (bile) and kapha (phlegm), are all cured. 27.

धान्त्वद्रियान्तः-करण-परसादं
दधाच्छ्छ कान्तिं दहन-परदीप्तम |

अशेष्ह-दोष्होपछयं निहन्याद
अभ्यस्यमानं जल-बस्ति-कर्म || २८ ||

dhāntvadriyāntaḥ-karaṇa-prasādaṃ
dadhāchcha kāntiṃ dahana-pradīptam |
aśeṣha-doṣhopachayaṃ nihanyād
abhyasyamānaṃ jala-basti-karma || 28 ||

By practising Basti with water, the Dhâtâs, the Indriyas and the mind become calm. It gives glow and tone to the body and increases the appetite. All the disorders disappear. 28.

The Neti (नेति).

अथ नेतिः
सूत्रं वितस्ति-सुस्निग्धं नासानाले परवेशयेत |
मुखान्निर्गमयेच्छैष्हा नेतिः सिद्धैर्निगद्यते || २९ ||

atha netiḥ
sūtraṃ vitasti-susnighdhaṃ nāsānāle praveśayet |
mukhānnirghamayechchaiṣhā netiḥ siddhairnighadyate || 29 ||

A cord made of threads and about six inches long, should be passed through the passage of the nose and the end taken out in the mouth. This is called by adepts the Neti Karma. 29.

कपाल-शोधिनी छैव दिव्य-दृष्हिट-परदायिनी |
जत्रूर्ध्व-जात-रोगौघं नेतिराशु निहन्ति छ || ३० ||

kapāla-śodhinī chaiva divya-dṛṣhṭi-pradāyinī |
jatrūrdhva-jāta-roghaughaṃ netirāśu nihanti cha || 30 ||

The Neti is the cleaner of the brain and giver of divine sight. It soon destroys all the diseases of the cervical and scapular regions. 30.

The Trâtaka (तराटक).

अथ तराटकम

निरीक्ष्हेन्निश्छल-दृशा सूक्ष्हम-लक्ष्हयं समाहितः |

अश्रु-सम्पात-पर्यन्तमाछार्यैस्त्राटकं समृतम || ३१ ||

atha trāṭakam
nirīkṣhenniśchala-dṝśā sūkṣhma-lakṣhyaṃ samāhitaḥ |
aśru-sampāta-paryantamāchāryaistrāṭakaṃ smṝtam || 31 ||

Being calm, one should gaze steadily at a small mark, till eyes are filled with tears. This is called Trataka by âchâryas. 31.

मोछ्नं नेत्र-रोगाणां तन्दाद्रीणां कपाटकम |

यत्नतस्त्राटकं गोप्यं यथा हाटक-पेटकम || ३२ ||

mochanaṃ netra-roghāṇāṃ tandādrīṇāṃ kapāṭakam |
yatnatastrāṭakaṃ ghopyaṃ yathā hāṭaka-peṭakam || 32 ||

Trâtaka destroys the eye diseases and removes sloth, etc. It should be kept secret very carefully, like a box of jewellery. 32.

The Nauli (नौलि).

अथ नौलिः

अमन्दावर्त-वेगेन तुन्दं सव्यापसव्यतः |

नतांसो भरामयेदेष्हा नौलिः सिद्धैः परशस्यते || ३३ ||

atha nauliḥ
amandāvarta-veghena tundaṃ savyāpasavyataḥ |
natāṃso bhrāmayedeṣhā nauliḥ siddhaiḥ praśasyate || 33 ||

Sitting on the toes with heels raised above the ground, and the palms resting on the ground, and in this bent posture the belly is moved forcibly from left to right just, as in vomiting. This is called by adepts the Nauli Karma. 33.

मन्दाग्नि-सन्दीपन-पाछ्नादि-

सन्धापिकानन्द-करी सदैव |

अशेष्ह-दोष्ह-मय-शोष्हणी छ

हठ-करिया मौलिरियं छ नौलिः || ३४ ||

mandāghni-sandīpana-pāchanādi-
sandhāpikānanda-karī sadaiva |
aśeṣha-doṣha-maya-śoṣhaṇī cha
haṭha-kriyā mauliriyaṃ cha nauliḥ || 34 ||

It removes dyspepsia, increases appetite and digestion, and is like the goddess of creation, and causes happiness. It dries up all the disorders. This Nauli is an excellent exercise in Haṭha Yoga. 34.

The Kapâla Bhâti कपाल भाति.

अथ कपालभातिः

भस्त्रावल्लोह-कारस्य रेछ-पूरौ ससम्भ्रमौ |

कपालभातिर्विख्याता कफ-दोष्ह-विशोष्हणी || ३५ ||

atha kapālabhātiḥ
bhastrāvalloha-kārasya recha-pūrau sasambhramau |
kapālabhātirvikhyātā kapha-doṣha-viśoṣhaṇī || 35 ||

When inhalation and exhalation are performed very quickly, like a pair of bellows of a blacksmith, it dries up all the disorders from the excess of phlegm, and is known as Kapâla Bhâti. 35.

षहट-कर्म-निर्गत-सथौल्य-कफ-दोष्ह-मलादिकः |

पराणायामं ततः कुर्यादनायासेन सिद्ध्यति || ३६ ||

ṣhaṭ-karma-nirghata-sthaulya-kapha-doṣha-malādikaḥ |
prāṇāyāmaṃ tataḥ kuryādanāyāsena siddhyati || 36 ||

When Prâṇâyâma is performed after getting rid of obesity born of the defects phlegm, by the performance of the six duties, it easily brings success 36.

पराणायामैरेव सर्वे परशुष्ह्यन्ति मला इति |
आछार्याणां तु केष्हांछिदन्यत्कर्म न संमतम || ३७ ||

prāṇāyāmaireva sarve praśuṣhyanti malā iti |
āchāryāṇāṃ tu keṣhāṃchidanyatkarma na saṃmatam || 37 ||

Some âchâryâs (teachers) do not advocate any other practice, being of opinion that all the impurities are dried up by the practice of Prâṇâyâma. 37.

Gaja Karaṇi (गजकरणी)

अथ गज-करणी
उदर-गत-पदार्थमुद्वमन्ति
पवनमपानमुदीर्य कण्ठ-नाले |
करम-परिछय-वश्य-नाडि-छक्रा
गज-करणीति निगद्यते हठज्ञैः || ३८ ||

atha ghaja-karaṇī
udara-ghata-padārthamudvamanti
pavanamapānamudīrya kaṇṭha-nāle |
krama-parichaya-vaśya-nāḍi-chakrā
ghaja-karaṇīti nighadyate haṭhajñaiḥ || 38 ||

By carrying the Apâna Vâyû up to the throat, the food, etc., in the stomach are vomited. By degrees, the system of Nâdîs (Śankhinî) becomes known. This is called in Haṭha as Gaja Karaṇi. 38.

बरह्मादयो|अपि तरिदशाः पवनाभ्यास-तत्पराः |
अभूवन्नन्तक-भयात्तस्मात्पवनमभ्यसेत || ३९ ||

brahmādayo|api tridaśāḥ pavanābhyāsa-tatparāḥ |
abhūvannantaka-bhyāttasmātpavanamabhyaset || 39 ||

Brahmâ, and other Devas were always engaged in the exercise of Prâṇâyâma, and, by means of it, got rid of the fear of death. Therefore, one should practise prâṇâyâma regularly. 39.

यावद्बद्धो मरुद-देशे यावच्छित्तं निराकुलम |
यावद्दृष्ट्टिर्भ्रुवोर्मध्ये तावत्काल-भयं कुतः || ४० ||

yāvadbaddho marud-deśe yāvachchittaṃ nirākulam |
yāvaddṝṣhṭirbhruvormadhye tāvatkāla-bhayaṃ kutaḥ || 40 ||

So long as the breath is restrained in the body, so long as the mind is undisturbed, and so long as the gaze is fixed between the eyebrows, there is no fear from Death. 40.

विधिवत्प्राण-संयामैर्नाडी-छक्रे विशोधिते |
सुष्हुम्णा-वदनं भित्त्वा सुखाद्विशति मारुतः || ४१ ||

vidhivatprāṇa-saṃyāmairnāḍī-chakre viśodhite |
suṣhumṇā-vadanaṃ bhittvā sukhādviśati mārutaḥ || 41 ||

When the system of Nâdis becomes clear of the impurities by properly controlling the prâṇa, then the air, piercing the entrance of the Suśumṇâ, enters it easily. 41.

Manomanî. (मनोन्मनी)

अथ मनोन्मनी
मारुते मध्य-संछारे मनः-सथैर्यं परजायते |
यो मनः-सुस्थिरी-भावः सैवावस्था मनोन्मनी || ४२ ||

atha manonmanī
mārute madhya-saṃchāre manaḥ-sthairyaṃ prajāyate |
yo manaḥ-susthirī-bhāvaḥ saivāvasthā manonmanī || 42 ||

Steadiness of mind comes when the air moves Freely in the middle. That is the manonmanî (मनोन्मनी) condition, which is attained when the mind becomes calm. 42.

तत-सिद्धये विधानज्ञाश्छित्रान्कुर्वन्ति कुम्भकान |
विछित्र कुम्भकाभ्यासाद्विछित्रां सिद्धिमाप्नुयात || ४३ ||

tat-siddhaye vidhānajñāśchitrānkurvanti kumbhakān |
vichitra kumbhakābhyāsādvichitrāṃ siddhimāpnuyāt || 43 ||

To accomplish it, various Kumbhakas are performed by those who are expert in the methods; for, by the practice of different Kumbhakas, wonderful success is attained. 43

Different hinds of Kumbhakas.

अथ कुम्भक-भेदाः
सूर्य-भेदनमुज्जायी सीत्कारी शीतली तथा |
भस्त्रिका भरामरी मूछर्छा पलाविनीत्यष्ह्ट-कुम्भकाः || ४४ ||

atha kumbhaka-bhedāḥ
sūrya-bhedanamujjāyī sītkārī śītalī tathā |
bhastrikā bhrāmarī mūrchchā plāvinītyaṣhṭa-kumbhakāḥ || 44 ||

Kumbhakas are of eight kinds, viz., Sûrya Bhedan, Ujjâyî, Sîtkarî, Sîtalî, Bhastrikâ, Bhrâmarî, Mûrchhâ, and Plâvinî. 44

पूरकान्ते तु कर्तव्यो बन्धो जालन्धराभिधः |
कुम्भकान्ते रेछकादौ कर्तव्यस्तूड्डियानकः || ४५ ||

pūrakānte tu kartavyo bandho jālandharābhidhaḥ |
kumbhakānte rechakādau kartavyastūḍḍiyānakaḥ || 45 ||

At the end of Pûraka, Jâlandhara Bandha should be performed, and at the end of Kumbhaka, and at the beginning of Rechaka, Uddiyâna Bandha should be performed. 45

NB.—Pûraka is filling in of the air from outside.

Kumbhaka is the keeping the air confined inside. Rechaka is expelling the confined air. The instructions for Puraka, Kumbhaka and Rechaka will be found at their proper place and should he carefully followed.

अधस्तात्कुनछनेनाशु कण्ठ-सङ्कोछने कृते |
मध्ये पश्छिम-तानेन सयात्प्राणो बरह्म-नाडिगः || ४६ ||

adhastātkuñchanenāśu kaṇṭha-sangkochane kṛte |
madhye paśchima-tānena syātprāṇo brahma-nāḍighaḥ || 46 ||

By drawing up from below (Mûla Bandha) and contracting the throat (Jâlandhara Bandha) and by pulling back the middle of the front portion of the body (*i.e.*, belly), the Prâṇa goes to the Brahma Nâdî (Suṣumnâ). 46

The middle hole, through the vertebral column, through which the spinal cord passes, is called the Su ṣumnâ Nâdî of the Yogîs. The two other sympathetic cords, one on each aide of the spinal cord, are called the Idâ and the Pingalâ Nâdîs. These will be described later on.

आपानमूर्ध्वमुत्थाप्य पराणं कण्ठादधो नयेत |
योगी जरा-विमुक्तः सन्ष्होडशाब्द-वया भवेत || ४७ ||

āpānamūrdhvamutthāpya prāṇaṃ kaṇṭhādadho nayet |
yoghī jarā-vimuktaḥ sanṣhoḍaśābda-vayā bhavet || 47 ||

By pulling up the Apâna Vâyu and by forcing the Prâṇa Vâyu down the throat, the Yogî, liberated from old age, becomes young, as it were 16 years old. 47

Note.—
हृदि प्राणो गुदेऽपानः समानो नाभिमण्डले ।
उदानः कण्ठदेशस्थो व्यानः सर्वशरीरगः । शिवसंहितायाम् अ० ३ श्लो० ७ ।

The seat of the Prâṇa is the heart; of the Apâna anus; of the Samâna the region about the navel; of the Udâna the throat; while the Vyâna moves throughout the body.

Sûrya Bhedana (सूर्य भेदन).

अथ सूर्य-भेदनम
आसने सुखदे योगी बद्ध्वा छैवासनं ततः |
दक्ष्ह-नाड्या समाकृष्ह्य बहिःस्थं पवनं शनैः || ४८ ||

atha sūrya-bhedanam
āsane sukhade yoghī baddhvā chaivāsanaṃ tataḥ |
dakṣha-nāḍyā samākṛṣhya bahiḥsthaṃ pavanaṃ śanaiḥ || 48 ||

Taking any comfortable posture and performing the âsana, the Yogî should draw in the air slowly, through the right nostril. 48

आकेशादानखाग्राच्छ निरोधावधि कुम्भयेत |
ततः शनैः सव्य-नाड्या रेछयेत्पवनं शनैः || ४९ ||

ākeśādānakhāghrāchcha nirodhāvadhi kumbhayet |
tataḥ śanaiḥ savya-nāḍyā rechayetpavanaṃ śanaiḥ || 49 ||

Then it should be confined within, so that it fills from the nails to the tips of the hair, and then let out through the left nostril slowly. 49

Note.—This is to be done alternately with both the nostrils, drawing in through the one, expelling through the other, and vice versa.

कपाल-शोधनं वात-दोष्ह-घनं कृमि-दोष्ह-हृत |
पुनः पुनरिदं कार्यं सूर्य-भेदनमुत्तमम || ५० ||

kapāla-śodhanaṃ vāta-doṣha-ghnaṃ kṝmi-doṣha-hṝt |
punaḥ punaridaṃ kāryaṃ sūrya-bhedanamuttamam || 50 ||

This excellent Sûrya Bhedana cleanses the forehead (frontal sinuses), destroys the disorders of Vâta, and removes the worms, and, therefore, it should be performed again and again.

Note-

योगाभ्यास क्रमं वक्ष्ये योगिनां योगसिद्धये । उषः काले समुत्थाय प्रातःकालेऽथवा बुधः ॥ १ ॥
गुरुं संस्मृत्य शिरसि हृदये स्वेष्टदेवताम् । शौचं कृत्वा दन्तशुद्धिं विदध्याद् भस्मधारणम् ॥ २ ॥
शुचौ देशे मठे रम्ये प्रतिष्ठाप्यासनं मृदु । तत्रोपविश्य संस्मृत्य मनसा गुरुमीश्वरम् ॥ ३ ॥
देशकालौ च संकीर्त्य संकल्प्य विधिपूर्वकम् । अद्येत्यादि श्रीपरमेश्वरप्रसादपूर्वकं समाधि तत्फल सिद्ध्यर्थमासनपूर्वकान् प्राणायामादीन् करिष्ये । अनंतं प्रणमेद्देवं नागेशं पीठसिद्धये ॥ ४ ॥
मणिभ्रात्फणासहस्रविधृतविश्वंभरामंडलायानंताय नागराजायनमः । ततोऽभ्यसेदासनानि श्रमे जाते शवासनम् । अन्ते समभ्यसे त्तु श्रमाभावे तु नाभ्यसेत् ॥ ५ ॥
करणीं विपरीताख्यां कुंभकात्पूर्वमभ्यसेत् । जालंधर प्रसादार्थं कुम्भकात्पूर्वयोगतः ॥ ६ ॥
विधायाचमनं कृत्वा कर्मांगं प्राणसंयमम् । योगींद्रादीन्नमस्कृत्य कौर्म्मोक्त शिववाक्यतः ॥ ७ ॥

कूर्म्मे पुराणे ।

नमस्कृत्याथ योगींद्रान् सशिष्यांश्च विनायकम् । गुरुं चैवाथमां योगी युंजीत सुसमाहितः ॥ ८ ॥
बद्धाभ्यासे सिद्धपीठं कुम्भकाबंधपूर्वकम् । प्रथमे दशकर्तव्या पंचवृद्ध्या दिने दिने ॥ ९ ॥
कार्या अशीति पर्यंतं कुम्भकाः सुसमाहितैः । योगींद्रः प्रथमं कुर्यादभ्यासे चंद्रसूर्ययोः ॥ १० ॥
अनुलोमविलोमाख्य मेतं प्राहुर्मनीषिणः । सूर्यभेदनमभ्यस्य बंधपूर्वकमेकधीः ॥ ११ ॥
उज्जायिनं ततः कुर्यात्सीत्कारीं शीतलींततः । भस्त्रिकांच समभ्यस्य कुर्यादन्यांश्चवापरान् ॥ १२ ॥
मुद्राः समभ्यसेद्बद्ध गुरु वक्त्राद् यथाक्रमम् । ततः पद्मासनं बद्ध्वा कुर्यन्नादानुचिंतनम् ॥ १३ ॥
अभ्यासे सकलं कुर्यादीश्वरार्पणमादतः । अभ्यासादुत्थितः स्नानं कुर्यादुष्णेन वारिणा ॥ १४ ॥
स्नात्वा समापयेन्नित्यं कर्म संक्षेपतः सुधीः । मध्याह्ने पितथाभ्यस्य किञ्चिद्विश्रम्य भोजनम् ॥ १५ ॥

Translation: I am going to describe the procedure of the practice of Yoga, in order that Yogîs may succeed. A wise man should leave his bed in the Uṣâ Kâla (*i.e.*, at the peep of dawn or 4 o'clock) in the morning. 1.

Remembering his guru over his head, and his desired deity in his heart, after answering the calls of nature, and cleaning his mouth, he should apply Bhaṣma (ashes). 2.

In a clean spot, clean room and charming ground, he should spread a soft âsana (cloth for sitting on). Having seated on it and remembering, in his mind his guru and his God. 3.

Having extolled the place and the time and taking up the vow thus: 'To day by the grace of God, I will perform Prâṇâyâmas with âsanas for gaining samâdhi (trance) and its fruits.' He should salute the infinite Deva, Lord of the Nâgas, to ensure success in the âsanas (postures). 4.

Salutation to the Lord of the Nâgas, who is adorned with thousands of heads, set with brilliant jewels (maṇis), and who has sustained the whole universe, nourishes it, and is infinite. After this he should begin his exercise of âsanas and when fatigued, he should practise Śava âsana. Should there be no fatigue, he should not practise it. 5.

Before Kumbhaka, he should perform Viparîta Karṇî mudrâ, in order that he may be able to perform Jâlandhar bandha comfortably. 6.

Sipping a little water, he should begin the exercise of Prâṇâyâma, after saluting Yogindras, as described in the Karma Parana, in the words of Śiva. 7.

Such as "Saluting Yogindras and their disciples and gurû Vinâyaka, the Yogî should unite with me with composed mind." 8.

While practising, he should sit with Siddhâsana, and having performed *bandha* and Kumbhaka, should begin with 10 Prâṇâyâmas the first day, and go on increasing 5 daily. 9.

With composed mind 80 Kumbhakas should be performed at a time; beginning first with the chandra (the left nostril) and then sûrya (the right nostril). 10.

This has been spoken of by wise men as Aṇuloma and Viloma. Having practised Sûrya Bhedan, with Bandhas, the wise rust) should practise Ujjâyî and then Sîtkârî Śîtalî, and Bhastrikâ, he may practice others or not. 11-12.

He should practise mudrâs properly, as instructed by his guru. Then sitting with Padmâsana, he should hear anâhata nâda attentively. 13.

He should *resign the fruits of all his practice reverently to God*, and, on rising on the completion of the practice, a warm bath should be taken. 14.

The bath should bring all the daily duties briefly to an end. At noon also a little rest should be taken at the end of the exercise, and then food should be taken. 15.

Yogîs should always take wholesome food and never anything unwholesome. After dinner he should eat Ilâchî or lavanga. 16.

Some like camphor, and betel leaf. To the Yogîs, practising Prâṇâyâma, betel leaf without powders, i, e., lime, nuts and kâtha, is beneficial. 17.

After taking food he should read books treating of salvation, or hear Purâṇas and repeat the name of God. 18. In the evening the exercise should be begun after finishing sandyhâ, as before, beginning the practice 3 ghatikâ or one hour before the sun sets. 19.

Evening sandhyâ should always be performed after practice, and Haṭha Yoga should be practised at midnight. 20.

Viparîta Karṇi is to be practised in the evening and at midnight, and not just after eating, as it does no good at this time. 21.

Ujjâyî (उज्जायी)

अथ उज्जायी

मुखं संयम्य नाडीभ्यामाकृष्ह्य पवनं शनैः |
यथा लगति कण्ठात्तु हृदयावधि स-सवनम || ५१ ||

atha ujjāyī
mukhaṃ saṃyamya nāḍībhyāmākṛṣhya pavanaṃ śanaiḥ |
yathā laghati kaṇṭhāttu hṛdayāvadhi sa-svanam || 51 ||

Having closed the opening of the Nâdî (Larynx), the air should be drawn in such a way that it goes touching from the throat to the chest, and making noise while passing. 51.

पूर्ववत्कुम्भयेत्प्राणं रेछयेदिडया तथा |
शलेष्हम-दोष्ह-हरं कण्ठे देहानल-विवर्धनम || ५२ ||

pūrvavatkumbhayetprāṇaṃ rechayediḍayā tathā |
śleṣhma-doṣha-haraṃ kaṇṭhe dehānala-vivardhanam || 52 ||

It should be restrained, as before, and then let out through Idâ (the left nostril). This removes śleṣmâ (phlegm) in the throat and increases the appetite. 52.

नाडी-जलोदराधातु-गत-दोष्ह-विनाशनम |
गछछता तिष्हठता कार्यमुज्जाय्याख्यं तु कुम्भकम || ५३ ||

nāḍī-jalodarādhātu-ghata-doṣha-vināśanam |
ghachchatā tiṣhṭhatā kāryamujjāyyākhyaṃ tu kumbhakam || 53 ||

It destroys the defects of the nâdîs, dropsy and disorders of Dhâtu (humours). Ujjâyî should be performed in all conditions of life, even while walking or sitting. 53.

Sîtkârî (सीत्कारी)

अथ सीत्कारी

सीत्कां कुर्यात्तथा वक्त्रे घराणेनैव विजृम्भिकाम |
एवमभ्यास-योगेन काम-देवो दवितीयकः || ५४ ||

atha sītkārī
sītkāṃ kuryāttathā vaktre ghrāṇenaiva vijṝmbhikām |
evamabhyāsa-yoghena kāma-devo dvitīyakaḥ || 54 ||

Sîtkârî is performed by drawing in the air through the mouth, keeping the tongue between the lips. The air thus drawn in should not be expelled through the mouth. By practising in this way, one becomes next to the God of Love in beauty. 54.

योगिनी छक्र-संमान्यः सृष्ह्टि-संहार-कारकः |
न कष्हुधा न तृष्हा निद्रा नैवालस्यं परजायते || ५५ ||

yoghinī chakra-saṃmānyaḥ sṝṣhṭi-saṃhāra-kārakaḥ |
na kṣhudhā na tṝṣhā nidrā naivālasyaṃ prajāyate || 55 ||

He is regarded adorable by the Yoginîs and becomes the destroyer of the cycle of creation, He is not afflicted with hunger, thirst, sleep or lassitude. 55.

भवेत्सत्त्वं छ देहस्य सर्वोपद्रव-वर्जितः |
अनेन विधिना सत्यं योगीन्द्रो भूमि-मण्डले || ५६ ||

bhavetsattvaṃ cha dehasya sarvopadrava-varjitaḥ |
anena vidhinā satyaṃ yoghīndro bhūmi-maṇḍale || 56 ||

The Satwa of his body becomes free from all the disturbances. In truth, he becomes the lord of the Yogîs in this world. 56.

Śîtalî (शीतली)

अथ शीतली
जिह्वया वायुमाकृष्ह्य पूर्ववत्कुम्भ-साधनम |
शनकैर्घ्राण-रन्ध्राभ्यां रेछयेत्पवनं सुधीः || ५७ ||

atha śītalī
jihvayā vāyumākṝṣhya pūrvavatkumbha-sādhanam |
śanakairghrāṇa-randhrābhyāṃ rechayetpavanaṃ sudhīḥ || 57 ||

As in the above (Sîtkári), the tongue to be protruded a little out of the lips, when the air is drawn in. It is kept confined, as before, and then expelled slowly through the nostrils. 57.

गुल्म-पलीहादिकान्रोगान्ज्वरं पित्तं कष्हुधां तृष्हाम |
विष्हाणि शीतली नाम कुम्भिकेयं निहन्ति हि || ५८ ||

ghulma-plīhādikānroghānjvaraṃ pittaṃ kṣhudhāṃ tṝṣhām |
viṣhāṇi śītalī nāma kumbhikeyaṃ nihanti hi || 58 ||

This Śîtalî Ḳumbhikâ cures colic, (enlarged) spleen, fever, disorders of bile, hunger, thirst, and counteracts poisons. 58.

The Bhastrikâ (भस्त्रिका)

अथ भस्त्रिका
ऊर्वोरुपरि संस्थाप्य शुभे पाद-तले उभे |
पद्मासनं भवेदेतत्सर्व-पाप-परणाशनम || ५९ ||

atha bhastrikā
ūrvorupari saṃsthāpya śubhe pāda-tale ubhe |
padmāsanaṃ bhavedetatsarva-pāpa-praṇāśanam || 59 ||

The Padma Âsana consists in crossing the feet and placing them on both the thighs; it is the destroyer of all sins. 59.

सम्यक्पद्मासनं बद्ध्वा सम-गरीवोदरः सुधीः |
मुखं संयम्य यत्नेन पराणं घराणेन रेछयेत || ६० ||

samyakpadmāsanaṃ baddhvā sama-ghrīvodaraḥ sudhīḥ |
mukhaṃ saṃyamya yatnena prāṇaṃ ghrāṇena rechayet || 60 ||

Binding the Padma-Âsana and keeping the body straight, closing the mouth carefully, let the air be expelled through the nose. 60.

यथा लगति हृत-कण्ठे कपालावधि स-सवनम |
वेगेन पूरयेछ्छापि हृत-पद्मावधि मारुतम || ६१ ||

yathā laghati hṝt-kaṇṭhe kapālāvadhi sa-svanam |
veghena pūrayechchāpi hṝt-padmāvadhi mārutam || 61 ||

It should be filled up to the lotus of the heart, by drawing it in with force, making noise and touching the throat, the chest and the head. 61.

पुनर्विरेछयेत्तद्वत्पूरयेछछ पुनः पुनः |
यथैव लोहकारेण भस्त्रा वेगेन छाल्यते || ६२ ||

punarvirechayettadvatpūrayechcha punaḥ punaḥ |
yathaiva lohakāreṇa bhastrā veghena chālyate || 62 ||

It should he expelled again and filled again and again as before, just as a pair of bellows of the blacksmith is worked. 62.

तथैव सव-शरीर-सथं छालयेत्पवनं धिया |
यदा शरमो भवेद्देहे तदा सूर्येण पूरयेत || ६३ ||

tathaiva sva-śarīra-sthaṃ chālayetpavanaṃ dhiyā |
yadā śramo bhaveddehe tadā sūryeṇa pūrayet || 63 ||

In the same way, the air of the body should be moved intelligently, filling it through Sûrya when fatigue is experienced. 63.

यथोदरं भवेत्पूर्णमनिलेन तथा लघु |
धारयेन्नासिकां मध्या-तर्जनीभ्यां विना दृढम || ६४ ||

yathodaraṃ bhavetpūrṇamanilena tathā laghu |
dhārayennāsikāṃ madhyā-tarjanībhyāṃ vinā dṝḍham || 64 ||

The air should be drawn in through the right nostril by pressing the thumb against the left side of the nose, so as to close the left nostril; and when filled to the full, it should be closed with the fourth finger (the one next to the little finger) and kept confined. 64.

विधिवत्कुम्भकं कृत्वा रेछयेदिडयानिलम |
वात-पित्त-शलेष्हम-हरं शरीराग्नि-विवर्धनम || ६५ ||

vidhivatkumbhakaṃ kṝtvā rechayediḍayānilam |
vāta-pitta-śleṣhma-haraṃ śarīrāghni-vivardhanam || 65 ||

Having confined it properly, it should be expelled through the Idâ (left nostril). This destroys Vâta, pitta (bile) and phlegm and increases the digestive power (the gastric fire). 65.

कुण्डली बोधकं क्ष्हिप्रं पवनं सुखदं हितम |
बरह्म-नाडी-मुखे संस्थ-कफाद्य-अर्गल-नाशनम || ६६ ||

kuṇḍalī bodhakaṃ kṣhipraṃ pavanaṃ sukhadaṃ hitam |
brahma-nāḍī-mukhe saṃstha-kaphādy-arghala-nāśanam || 66 ||

It quickly awakens the Kuṇḍalinî, purifies the system, gives pleasure, and is beneficial. It destroys phlegm and the impurities accumulated at the entrance of the Brahma Nâdî. 66.

सम्यग्गात्र-समुद्भूत-गरन्थि-तरय-विभेदकम |
विशेष्हेणैव कर्तव्यं भस्त्राख्यं कुम्भकं तविदम || ६७ ||

samyaghghātra-samudbhūta-ghranthi-traya-vibhedakam |
viśeṣheṇaiva kartavyaṃ bhastrākhyaṃ kumbhakaṃ tvidam || 67 ||

This Bhastrikâ should be performed plentifully, for it breaks the three knots: Brahma granthi (in the chest), Viṣṇu granthi (in the throat), and Rudra granthi (between the eyebrows) of the body. 67.

The Bhrâmari (भरामरी)

अथ भरामरी
वेगाद्घोष्हं पूरकं भृङ्ग-नादं
भृङ्गी-नादं रेछकं मन्द-मन्दम |
योगीन्द्राणमेवमभ्यास-योगाछ
छित्ते जाता काछिदानन्द-लीला || ६८ ||

atha bhrāmarī
veghādghoṣhaṃ pūrakaṃ bhṝnggha-nādaṃ
bhṝngghī-nādaṃ rechakaṃ manda-mandam |

yoghīndrāṇamevamabhyāsa-yoghāch
chitte jātā kāchidānanda-līlā || 68 ||

By filling the air with force, making noise like Bhringi (wasp), and expelling it slowly, making noise in the same way; this practice causes a sort of ecstacy in the minds of Yogîndras. 68.

The Mûrchhâ (मूर्छा).

अथ मूछर्छा
पूरकान्ते गाढतरं बद्ध्वा जालन्धरं शनैः |
रेछयेन्मूछर्छाख्येयं मनो-मूछर्छा सुख-परदा || ६९ ||

atha mūrchchā
pūrakānte ghāḍhataraṃ baddhvā jālandharaṃ śanaiḥ |
rechayenmūrchchākhyeyaṃ mano-mūrchchā sukha-pradā || 69 ||

Closing the passages with Jâlandhar Bandha firmly at the end of Pûraka, and expelling the air slowly, is called Mûrchhâ, from its causing the mind to swoon and giving comfort. 69.

The Plâvinî (पलाविनी).

अथ पलाविनी
अन्तः परवर्तितोदार-मारुतापूरितोदरः |
पयस्यगाधे|अपि सुखात्प्लवते पद्म-पत्रवत || ७० ||

atha plāvinī
antaḥ pravartitodāra-mārutāpūritodaraḥ |
payasyaghādhe|api sukhātplavate padma-patravat || 70 ||

When the belly is filled with air and the inside of the body is filled to its utmost with air, the body floats on the deepest water, like the leaf of a lotus. 70.

पराणायामस्त्रिधा परोक्तो रेछ-पूरक-कुम्भकैः |
सहितः केवलश्छेति कुम्भको दविविधो मतः || ७१ ||

prāṇāyāmastridhā prokto recha-pūraka-kumbhakaiḥ |
sahitaḥ kevalaścheti kumbhako dvividho mataḥ || 71 ||

Considering Pûraka (Filling), Rechaka (expelling) and Kumbhaka (confining), Prâṇâyâma is of three kinds, but considering it accompanied by Pûraka and Rechaka, and without these, it is of two kinds only, *i.e.*, Sahita (with) and Kevala (alone). 71.

यावत्केवल-सिद्धिः सयात्सहितं तावदभ्यसेत |
रेछकं पूरकं मुक्त्वा सुखं यद्वायु-धारणम || ७२ ||

yāvatkevala-siddhiḥ syātsahitaṃ tāvadabhyaset |
rechakaṃ pūrakaṃ muktvā sukhaṃ yadvāyu-dhāraṇam || 72 ||

Exercise in Sahita should be continued till success in Kevala is gained. This latter is simply confining the air with ease, without Rechaka and Pûraka. 72.

पराणायामो|अयमित्युक्तः स वै केवल-कुम्भकः |
कुम्भके केवले सिद्धे रेछ-पूरक-वर्जिते || ७३ ||

prāṇāyāmo|ayamityuktaḥ sa vai kevala-kumbhakaḥ |
kumbhake kevale siddhe recha-pūraka-varjite || 73 ||

In the practice of Kevala Prâṇâyâma when it can be performed successfully without Rechaka and Pûraka, then it is called Kevala Kumbhaka. 73.

न तस्य दुर्लभं किंछित्त्रिष्हु लोकेष्हु विद्यते |
शक्तः केवल-कुम्भेन यथेष्हटं वायु-धारणात || ७४ ||

na tasya durlabhaṃ kiṃchittriṣhu lokeṣhu vidyate |
śaktaḥ kevala-kumbhena yatheṣhṭaṃ vāyu-dhāraṇāt || 74 ||

There is nothing in the three worlds which may be difficult to obtain for him who is able to keep the air confined according to pleasure, by means of Kevala Kumbhaka. 74.

राज-योग-पदं छापि लभते नात्र संशयः |
कुम्भकात्कुण्डली-बोधः कुण्डली-बोधतो भवेत |
अनर्गला सुष्हुम्णा छ हठ-सिद्धिश्छ जायते || ७५ ||

rāja-yogha-padaṃ chāpi labhate nātra saṃśayaḥ |
kumbhakātkuṇḍalī-bodhaḥ kuṇḍalī-bodhato bhavet |
anarghalā suṣhumṇā cha haṭha-siddhiścha jāyate || 75 ||

He obtains the position of Râja Yoga undoubtedly. Kuṇḍalinî awakens by Kumbhaka, and by its awakening, Suṣumnâ becomes free from impurities. 75.

हठं विना राजयोगो राज-योगं विना हठः |
न सिध्यति ततो युग्ममानिष्पत्तेः समभ्यसेत || ७६ ||

haṭhaṃ vinā rājayogho rāja-yoghaṃ vinā haṭhaḥ |
na sidhyati tato yughmamāniṣhpatteḥ samabhyaset || 76 ||

No success in Râja Yoga without Haṭha Yoga, and no success in Haṭha Yoga without Râja Yoga. One should, therefore, practise both of these well, till complete success is gained. 76.

कुम्भक-पराण-रोधान्ते कुर्याच्छित्तं निराश्रयम |
एवमभ्यास-योगेन राज-योग-पदं वरजेत || ७७ ||

kumbhaka-prāṇa-rodhānte kuryāchchittaṃ nirāśrayam |
evamabhyāsa-yoghena rāja-yogha-padaṃ vrajet || 77 ||

On the completion of Kumbhaka, the mind should be given rest. By practising in this way one is raised to the position of (succeeds in getting) Râja Yoga. 77.

Indications of success in the practice of Haṭha Yoga.

वपुः कृशत्वं वदने परसन्नता
नाद-सफुटत्वं नयने सुनिर्मले |
अरोगता बिन्दु-जयो|अग्नि-दीपनं
नाडी-विशुद्धिर्हठ-सिद्धि-लक्ष्हणम || ७८ ||

vapuḥ kṛśatvaṃ vadane prasannatā
nāda-sphuṭatvaṃ nayane sunirmale |
aroghatā bindu-jayo|aghni-dīpanaṃ
nāḍī-viśuddhirhaṭha-siddhi-lakṣhaṇam || 78 ||

When the body becomes lean, the face glows with delight, Anâhatanâda manifests, and eyes are clear, body is healthy, *bindu* under control, and appetite increases, then one should know that the Nâdîs are purified and success in Haṭha Yoga is approaching. 78.

End of Chapter II.

इति हठ-परदीपिकायां दवितीयोपदेशः |

iti haṭha-pradīpikāyāṃ dvitīyopadeśaḥ |

CHAPTER III.

On Mudrâs.

|| ३ || तृतीयोपदेशः

|| 3 || tṛtīyopadeśaḥ

स-शैल-वन-धात्रीणां यथाधारो|अहि-नायकः |
सर्वेष्हां योग-तन्त्राणां तथाधारो हि कुण्डली || १ ||

sa-śaila-vana-dhātrīṇāṃ yathādhāro|ahi-nāyakaḥ |
sarveṣhāṃ yogha-tantrāṇāṃ tathādhāro hi kuṇḍalī || 1 ||

As the chief of the snakes is the support of the earth with all the mountains and forests on it, so all the Tantras (Yoga practices) rest on the Kuṇḍalinî. (The Vertebral column.) 1.

सुप्ता गुरु-परसादेन यदा जागर्ति कुण्डली |
तदा सर्वाणि पद्मानि भिद्यन्ते गरन्थयो|अपि छ || २ ||

suptā ghuru-prasādena yadā jāgharti kuṇḍalī |
tadā sarvāṇi padmāni bhidyante ghranthayo|api cha || 2 ||

When the sleeping Kuṇḍalinî awakens by favour of a guru, then all the lotuses (in the six chakras or centres) and all the knots are pierced through. 2.

पराणस्य शून्य-पदवी तदा राजपथायते |
तदा छित्तं निरालम्बं तदा कालस्य वञ्छनम || ३ ||

prāṇasya śūnya-padavī tadā rājapathāyate |
tadā chittaṃ nirālambaṃ tadā kālasya vañchanam || 3 ||

Suṣumnâ (Sûnya Padavî) becomes a main road for the passage of Prâṇa, and the mind then becomes free from all connections (with its objects of enjoyments) and Death is then evaded. 3.

सुष्हुम्णा शून्य-पदवी बरह्म-रन्ध्रः महापथः |
शमशानं शाम्भवी मध्य-मार्गश्छेत्येक-वाछकाः || ४ ||

suṣhumṇā śūnya-padavī brahma-randhraḥ mahāpathaḥ |
śmaśānaṃ śāmbhavī madhya-mārghaśchetyeka-vāchakāḥ || 4 ||

Suṣumnâ, Sunya Padavî, Brahma Randhra, Mahâ Patha, Śmaśâna, Śambhavî, Madhya Mârga, are names of one and the same thing. 4.

तस्मात्सर्व-परयत्नेन परबोधयितुमीश्वरीम |
बरह्म-दवार-मुखे सुप्तां मुद्राभ्यासं समाछरेत || ५ ||

tasmātsarva-prayatnena prabodhayitumīśvarīm |
brahma-dvāra-mukhe suptāṃ mudrābhyāsaṃ samācharet || 5 ||

In order, therefore, to awaken this goddess, who is sleeping at the entrance of Brahma Dwâra (the great door), mudrâs should be practised well. 5.

The mudrâs.

महामुद्रा महाबन्धो महावेधश्छ खेछरी |
उड्डीयानं मूलबन्धश्छ बन्धो जालन्धराभिधः || ६ ||

mahāmudrā mahābandho mahāvedhaścha khecharī |
uḍḍīyānaṃ mūlabandhaścha bandho jālandharābhidhaḥ || 6 ||

Mahâ Mudrâ, Mahâ Bandha, Mahâ Vedha, Khecharî, Uḍḍiyâna Bandha, Mûla Bandha, Jâlandhara Bandha. 6.

करणी विपरीताख्या वज्रोली शक्ति-छालनम |
इदं हि मुद्रा-दशकं जरा-मरण-नाशनम || ७ ||

karaṇī viparītākhyā vajrolī śakti-chālanam |
idaṃ hi mudrā-daśakaṃ jarā-maraṇa-nāśanam || 7 ||

Viparîta Karaṇî, Vajroli, and Śakti Châlana. These are the ten Mudrâs which annihilate old age and death. 7.

आदिनाथोदितं दिव्यमष्ह्टैश्वर्य-परदायकम |
वल्लभं सर्व-सिद्धानां दुर्लभं मरुतामपि || ८ ||

ādināthoditaṃ divyamaṣhṭaiśvarya-pradāyakam |
vallabhaṃ sarva-siddhānāṃ durlabhaṃ marutāmapi || 8 ||

They have been explained by Âdi Nâtha (Śiva) and give eight kinds of divine wealth. They are loved by all the Siddhas and are hard to attain even by the Marutas. 8.

Note.—The eight *Aiśwaryas* are: Aṇimâ (becoming small, like an atom), Mahimâ (becoming great, like âkâs, by drawing in atoms of Prakṛiti), Garimâ (light things, like cotton becoming very heavy like mountains.)

Prâpti (coming within easy reach of everything; as touching the moon with the little finger, while standing on the earth.)

Prâkâmya (non-resistance to the desires, as entering the earth like water.)

Îsatâ (mastery over matter and objects made of it.)

Vaśitwa (controlling the animate and inanimate objects.)

गोपनीयं परयत्नेन यथा रत्न-करण्डकम |
कस्यछिन्नैव वक्तव्यं कुल-सत्री-सुरतं यथा || ९ ||

ghopanīyaṃ prayatnena yathā ratna-karaṇḍakam |
kasyachinnaiva vaktavyaṃ kula-strī-surataṃ yathā || 9 ||

These Mudrâs should be kept secret by every means, as one keeps one's box of jewellery, and should, on no account be told to any one, just as husband and wife keep their dealings secret. 9.

The mahâ mudrâ.

अथ महा-मुद्रा
पाद-मूलेन वामेन योनिं सम्पीड्य दक्ष्हिणाम |
परसारितं पदं कृत्वा कराभ्यां धारयेद्दृढम || १० ||

atha mahā-mudrā
pāda-mūlena vāmena yoniṃ sampīḍya dakṣhiṇām |
prasāritaṃ padaṃ kṛtvā karābhyāṃ dhārayeddṛḍham || 10 ||

Pressing the Yoni (perineum) with the heel of the left foot, and stretching forth the right foot, its toe should be grasped by the thumb and first finger. 10.

कण्ठे बन्धं समारोप्य धारयेद्वायुमूर्ध्वतः |
यथा दण्ड-हतः सर्पो दण्डाकारः परजायते || ११ ||
ऋज्वीभूता तथा शक्तिः कुण्डली सहसा भवेत |
तदा सा मरणावस्था जायते दविपुटाश्रया || १२ ||

kaṇṭhe bandhaṃ samāropya dhārayedvāyumūrdhvataḥ |
yathā daṇḍa-hataḥ sarpo daṇḍākāraḥ prajāyate || 11 ||
ṛjvībhūtā tathā śaktiḥ kuṇḍalī sahasā bhavet |
tadā sā maraṇāvasthā jāyate dvipuṭāśrayā || 12 ||

By stopping the throat (by Jâlandhara Bandha) the air is drawn in from the outside and carried down. Just as a snake struck with a stick becomes straight like a stick, in the same way, *śakti* (suṣumnâ) becomes straight at once. Then the Kuṇḍalinî, becoming as it were dead, and, leaving both the Idâ and the Pingalâ, enters the suṣumnâ (the middle passage). 11-12.

ततः शनैः शनैरेव रेछयेन्नैव वेगतः |
महा-मुद्रां छ तेनैव वदन्ति विबुधोत्तमाः || १३ ||

tataḥ śanaiḥ śanaireva rechayennaiva veghataḥ |
mahā-mudrāṃ cha tenaiva vadanti vibudhottamāḥ || 13 ||

It should be expelled then, slowly only and not violently. For this very reason, the best of the wise men call it the Mahâ Mudrâ. This Mahâ Mudrâ has been propounded by great masters. 13.

इयं खलु महामुद्रा महा-सिद्धैः परदर्शिता |
महा-कलेशादयो दोष्हाः कष्हीयन्ते मरणादयः |
महा-मुद्रां छ तेनैव वदन्ति विबुधोत्तमाः || १४ ||

iyaṃ khalu mahāmudrā mahā-siddhaiḥ pradarśitā |
mahā-kleśādayo doṣhāḥ kṣhīyante maraṇādayaḥ |
mahā-mudrāṃ cha tenaiva vadanti vibudhottamāḥ || 14 ||

Great evils and pains, like death, are destroyed by it, and for this reason wise men call it the Mahâ Mudrâ. 14.

छन्द्राङ्गे तु समभ्यस्य सूर्याङ्गे पुनरभ्यसेत |
यावत-तुल्या भवेत्सङ्ख्या ततो मुद्रां विसर्जयेत || १५ ||

chandrāngghe tu samabhyasya sūryāngghe punarabhyaset |
yāvat-tulyā bhavetsangkhyā tato mudrāṃ visarjayet || 15 ||

Having practised with the left nostril, it should be practised with the right one; and, when the number on both sides becomes equal, then the mudrâ should be discontinued. 15.

न हि पथ्यमपथ्यं वा रसाः सर्वे|अपि नीरसाः |
अपि भुक्तं विष्हं घोरं पीयूष्हमपि जीर्यति || १६ ||

na hi pathyamapathyaṃ vā rasāḥ sarve|api nīrasāḥ |
api bhuktaṃ viṣhaṃ ghoraṃ pīyūṣhamapi jīryati || 16 ||

There is nothing wholesome or injurious; for the practice of this mudrâ destroys the injurious effects of all the rasas (chemicals). Even the deadliest of poisons, if taken, acts like nectar. 16.

कष्हय-कुष्हठ-गुदावर्त-गुल्माजीर्ण-पुरोगमाः |
तस्य दोष्हाः कष्हयं यान्ति महामुद्रां तु यो|अभ्यसेत || १७ ||

kṣhaya-kuṣhṭha-ghudāvarta-ghulmājīrṇa-puroghamāḥ |
tasya doṣhāḥ kṣhayaṃ yānti mahāmudrāṃ tu yo|abhyaset || 17 ||

Consumption, leprosy, prolapsus anii, colic, and the diseases due to indigestion,—all these irregularities are removed by the practice of this Mahâ Mudrâ. 17.

कथितेयं महामुद्रा महा-सिद्धि-करा नृणाम |
गोपनीया परयत्नेन न देया यस्य कस्यछित || १८ ||

kathiteyaṃ mahāmudrā mahā-siddhi-karā nṝṇām |
ghopanīyā prayatnena na deyā yasya kasyachit || 18 ||

This Mahâ Mudrâ has been described as the giver of great success (Siddhi) to men. It should be kept secret by every effort, and not revealed to any and everyone. 18.

The Mahâ Bandha.

अथ महा-बन्धः
पार्ष्णिं वामस्य पादस्य योनि-सथाने नियोजयेत |
वामोरूपरि संस्थाप्य दक्ष्हिणं छरणं तथा || १९ ||

atha mahā-bandhaḥ
pārṣhṇiṃ vāmasya pādasya yoni-sthāne niyojayet |
vāmorūpari saṃsthāpya dakṣhiṇaṃ charaṇaṃ tathā || 19 ||

Press the left heel to the perineum and place the right foot on the left thigh. 19.

पूरयित्वा ततो वायुं हृदये छुबुकं दृढम |
निष्हपीड्यं वायुमाकुनछ्य मनो-मध्ये नियोजयेत || २० ||

pūrayitvā tato vāyuṃ hṝdaye chubukaṃ dṝḍham |
niṣhpīḍyaṃ vāyumākuñchya mano-madhye niyojayet || 20 ||

Fill in the air, keeping the chin firm against the chest, and, having pressed the air, the mind should he fixed on the middle of the eyebrows or in the suṣumnâ (the spine). 20.

धारयित्वा यथा-शक्ति रेछयेदनिलं शनैः |
सव्याङ्गे तु समभ्यस्य दक्षहाङ्गे पुनरभ्यसेत || २१ ||

dhārayitvā yathā-śakti rechayedanilaṃ śanaiḥ |
savyāngghe tu samabhyasya dakṣhāngghe punarabhyaset || 21 ||

Having kept it confined so long as possible, it should be expelled slowly. Having practised on the left side, it should be practised on the right side. 21.

मतमत्र तु केष्हांछित्कण्ठ-बन्धं विवर्जयेत |
राज-दन्त-सथ-जिह्वाया बन्धः शस्तो भवेदिति || २२ ||

matamatra tu keṣhāṃchitkaṇṭha-bandhaṃ vivarjayet |
rāja-danta-stha-jihvāyā bandhaḥ śasto bhavediti || 22 ||

Some are of opinion that the closing of throat is not necessary here, for keeping the tongue pressed against the roots of the upper teeth makes a good bandha (stop). 22.

अयं तु सर्व-नाडीनामूर्ध्वं गति-निरोधकः |
अयं खलु महा-बन्धो महा-सिद्धि-परदायकः || २३ ||

ayaṃ tu sarva-nāḍīnāmūrdhvaṃ ghati-nirodhakaḥ |
ayaṃ khalu mahā-bandho mahā-siddhi-pradāyakaḥ || 23 ||

This stops the upward motion of all the Nâdîs. Verily this Mahâ Bandha is the giver of great Siddhis. 23.

काल-पाश-महा-बन्ध-विमोछन-विछक्ष्हणः |
तरिवेणी-सङ्गमं धत्ते केदारं परापयेन्मनः || २४ ||

kāla-pāśa-mahā-bandha-vimochana-vichakṣhaṇaḥ |
triveṇī-sangghamaṃ dhatte kedāraṃ prāpayenmanaḥ || 24 ||

This Mahâ Bandha is the most skilful means for cutting away the snares of death. It brings about the conjunction of the Trivenî (Idâ, Pingalâ and Suṣumnâ) and carries the mind to Kedâr (the space between the eyebrows, which is the seat of Śiva). 24.

रूप-लावण्य-सम्पन्ना यथा सत्री पुरुष्हं विना |
महा-मुद्रा-महा-बन्धौ निष्हफलौ वेध-वर्जितौ || २५ ||

rūpa-lāvaṇya-sampannā yathā strī puruṣhaṃ vinā |
mahā-mudrā-mahā-bandhau niṣhphalau vedha-varjitau || 25 ||

As beauty and loveliness, do not avail a woman without husband, so the Mahâ Mudrâ and the Mahâ-Bandha are useless without the Mahâ Vedha. 25.

The Mahâ Vedha.

अथ महा-वेधः
महा-बन्ध-सथितो योगी कृत्वा पूरकमेक-धीः |
वायूनां गतिमावृत्य निभृतं कण्ठ-मुद्रया || २६ ||

atha mahā-vedhaḥ
mahā-bandha-sthito yoghī kṛtvā pūrakameka-dhīḥ |
vāyūnāṃ ghatimāvṛtya nibhṛtaṃ kaṇṭha-mudrayā || 26 ||

Sitting with Mahâ Bandha, the Yogî should fill in the air and keep his mind collected. The movements of the Vâyus (Prâṇa and Apâna) should be stopped by closing the throat.) 26.

सम-हस्त-युगो भूमौ सफिछौ सनाडयेछछनैः |
पुट-दवयमतिक्रम्य वायुः सफुरति मध्यगः || २७ ||

sama-hasta-yugho bhūmau sphichau sanāḍayechchanaiḥ |
puṭa-dvayamatikramya vāyuḥ sphurati madhyaghaḥ || 27 ||

Resting both the hands equally on the ground, he should raise himself a little and strike his buttocks against the ground gently. The air, leaving both the passages (Idâ and Pingalâ), starts into the middle one. 27.

सोम-सूर्याग्नि-सम्बन्धो जायते छामृताय वै |
मृतावस्था समुत्पन्ना ततो वायुं विरेछयेत || २८ ||

soma-sūryāghni-sambandho jāyate chāmṝtāya vai |
mṝtāvasthā samutpannā tato vāyuṃ virechayet || 28 ||

The union of the Idâ and the Pingalâ is effected, in order to bring about immortality. When the air becomes as it were dead (by leaving its course through the Idâ and the Pingalâ) (*i.e.*, when it has been kept confined), then it should be expelled. 28.

महा-वेधो|अयमभ्यासान्महा-सिद्धि-परदायकः |
वली-पलित-वेप-घनः सेव्यते साधकोत्तमैः || २९ ||

mahā-vedho|ayamabhyāsānmahā-siddhi-pradāyakaḥ |
valī-palita-vepa-ghnaḥ sevyate sādhakottamaiḥ || 29 ||

The practice of this Mahâ Vedha, the giver of great Siddhis, destroys old age, grey hair, and shaking of the body, and therefore it is practised by the best masters. 29.

एतत्त्रयं महा-गुह्यं जरा-मृत्यु-विनाशनम |
वह्नि-वृद्धि-करं छैव हयणिमादि-गुण-परदम || ३० ||

etattrayaṃ mahā-ghuhyaṃ jarā-mṝtyu-vināśanam |
vahni-vṝddhi-karaṃ chaiva hyaṇimādi-ghuṇa-pradam || 30 ||

These THREE are the great secrets. They are the destroyers of old age and death, increase the appetite, confer the accomplishments of Anima, etc. 30.

अष्ह्टधा करियते छैव यामे यामे दिने दिने |
पुण्य-संभार-सन्धाय पापौघ-भिदुरं सदा |
सम्यक-शिक्ष्हावतामेवं सवल्पं परथम-साधनम || ३१ ||

aṣhṭadhā kriyate chaiva yāme yāme dine dine |
puṇya-saṃbhāra-sandhāya pāpaugha-bhiduraṃ sadā |
samyak-śikṣhāvatāmevaṃ svalpaṃ prathama-sādhanam || 31 ||

They should, be practised in 8 ways, daily and hourly. They increase collection of good actions and lessen the evil ones. People, instructed well, should begin their practice, little by little, first. 31.

The Khechari.

अथ खेछरी
कपाल-कुहरे जिह्वा परविष्हटा विपरीतगा |
भरुवोरन्तर्गता दृष्हिटर्मुद्रा भवति खेछरी || ३२ ||

atha khecharī
kapāla-kuhare jihvā praviṣhṭā viparītaghā |
bhruvorantarghatā dṝṣhṭirmudrā bhavati khecharī || 32 ||

The Khechari Mudrâ is accomplished by thrusting the tongue into the gullet, by turning it over itself, and keeping the eyesight in the middle of the eyebrows. 32.

छेदन-छालन-दोहैः कलां करमेणाथ वर्धयेत्तावत |
सा यावद्भ्रू-मध्यं सपृशति तदा खेछरी-सिद्धिः || ३३ ||

chedana-chālana-dohaiḥ kalāṃ krameṇātha vardhayettāvat |
sā yāvadbhrū-madhyaṃ spṝśati tadā khecharī-siddhiḥ || 33 ||

To accomplish this, the tongue is lengthened by cutting the frænum linguæ, moving, and pulling it. When it can touch the space between the eyebrows, then Khechari can be accomplished. 33.

सनुही-पत्र-निभं शस्त्रं सुतीक्ष्हणं सनिग्ध-निर्मलम |
समादाय ततस्तेन रोम-मात्रं समुछिछनेत || ३४ ||

snuhī-patra-nibhaṃ śastraṃ sutīkṣhṇaṃ snighdha-nirmalam |
samādāya tatastena roma-mātraṃ samuchchinet || 34 ||

Taking a sharp, smooth, and clean instrument, of the shape of a cactus leaf, the frænum of the tongue should be cut a little (as much as a hair's thickness), at a time. 34.

ततः सैन्धव-पथ्याभ्यां छूर्णिताभ्यां परघर्ष्हयेत |
पुनः सप्त-दिने पराप्ते रोम-मात्रं समुछिछनेत || ३५ ||

tataḥ saindhava-pathyābhyāṃ chūrṇitābhyāṃ pragharṣhayet |
punaḥ sapta-dine prāpte roma-mātraṃ samuchchinet || 35 ||

Then rock salt and yellow myrobalan (both powdered) should be rubbed in. On the 7th day, it should again be cut a hair's breadth. 35.

एवं करमेण षहण-मासं नित्यं युक्तः समाछरेत |
षहण्मासाद्रसना-मूल-शिरा-बन्धः परणश्यति || ३६ ||

evaṃ krameṇa ṣhaṇ-māsaṃ nityaṃ yuktaḥ samācharet |
ṣhaṇmāsādrasanā-mūla-śirā-bandhaḥ praṇaśyati || 36 ||

One should go on doing thus, regularly for six months. At the end of six months, the frænum of the tongue will be completely cut. 36.

कलां पराङ्मुखीं कृत्वा तरिपथे परियोजयेत |
सा भवेत्खेछरी मुद्रा वयोम-छक्रं तदुछ्यते || ३७ ||

kalāṃ parāngmukhīṃ kṝtvā tripathe pariyojayet |
sā bhavetkhecharī mudrā vyoma-chakraṃ taduchyate || 37 ||

Turning the tongue upwards, it is fixed on the three ways (œsophagus, windpipe and palate.) Thus it makes the Khechari Mudrâ, and is called the Vyoma Chakra. 37.

रसनामूर्ध्वगां कृत्वा कष्हणार्धमपि तिष्हठति |
विष्हैर्विमुछ्यते योगी वयाधि-मृत्यु-जरादिभिः || ३८ ||

rasanāmūrdhvaghāṃ kṝtvā kṣhaṇārdhamapi tiṣhṭhati |
viṣhairvimuchyate yoghī vyādhi-mṝtyu-jarādibhiḥ || 38 ||

The Yogî who sits for a minute turning his tongue upwards, is saved from poisons, diseases, death, old age, etc. 38.

न रोगो मरणं तन्द्रा न निद्रा न क्ष्हुधा तृष्हा |
न छ मूछ्र्छा भवेत्तस्य यो मुद्रां वेत्ति खेछरीम || ३९ ||

na rogho maraṇaṃ tandrā na nidrā na kṣhudhā tṛṣhā |
na cha mūrchchā bhavettasya yo mudrāṃ vetti khecharīm || 39 ||

He who knows the Khechari Mudrâ is not afflicted with disease, death, sloth, sleep, hunger, thirst, and swooning. 39.

पीड्यते न स रोगेण लिप्यते न छ कर्मणा |
बाध्यते न स कालेन यो मुद्रां वेत्ति खेछरीम || ४० ||

pīḍyate na sa rogheṇa lipyate na cha karmaṇā |
bādhyate na sa kālena yo mudrāṃ vetti khecharīm || 40 ||

He who knows the Khechari Mudrâ, is not troubled by diseases, is not stained with karmas, and is not snared by time. 40.

छित्तं छरति खे यस्माज्जिह्वा छरति खे गता |
तेनैष्हा खेछरी नाम मुद्रा सिद्धैर्निरूपिता || ४१ ||

chittaṃ charati khe yasmājjihvā charati khe ghatā |
tenaiṣhā khecharī nāma mudrā siddhairnirūpitā || 41 ||

खेछर्या मुद्रितं येन विवरं लम्बिकोर्ध्वतः |
न तस्य क्ष्हरते बिन्दुः कामिन्याः शलेष्हितस्य छ || ४२ ||

khecharyā mudritaṃ yena vivaraṃ lambikordhvataḥ |
na tasya kṣharate binduḥ kāminyāḥ śleṣhitasya cha || 42 ||

The Siddhas have devised this Khechari Mudrâ from the fact that the mind and the tongue reach âkâśa by its practice. 41.

छलितो|अपि यदा बिन्दुः सम्प्राप्तो योनि-मण्डलम |
वरजत्यूर्ध्वं हृतः शक्त्या निबद्धो योनि-मुद्रया || ४३ ||

chalito|api yadā binduḥ samprāpto yoni-maṇḍalam |
vrajatyūrdhvaṃ hṝtaḥ śaktyā nibaddho yoni-mudrayā || 43 ||

If the hole behind the palate be stopped with Khechari by turning the tongue upwards, then bindu cannot leave its place even if a woman were embraced. 42.

ऊर्ध्व-जिह्वः सथिरो भूत्वा सोमपानं करोति यः |
मासार्धेन न सन्देहो मृत्युं जयति योगवित || ४४ ||

ūrdhva-jihvaḥ sthiro bhūtvā somapānaṃ karoti yaḥ |
māsārdhena na sandeho mṝtyuṃ jayati yoghavit || 44 ||

If the Yogî drinks Somarasa (juice) by sitting with the tongue turned backwards and mind concentrated, there is no doubt he conquers death within 15 days. 43.

नित्यं सोम-कला-पूर्णं शरीरं यस्य योगिनः |
तक्ष्हकेणापि दष्ह्टस्य विष्हं तस्य न सर्पति || ४५ ||

nityaṃ soma-kalā-pūrṇaṃ śarīraṃ yasya yoghinaḥ |
takṣhakeṇāpi daṣhṭasya viṣhaṃ tasya na sarpati || 45 ||

If the Yogî, whose body is full of Somarasa (juice), were bitten by Takshaka (snake), its poison cannot permeate his body. 44.

As fire is inseparably connected with the wood and light is connected with the wick and oil, so does the soul not leave the body full of nectar exuding from the Soma. 45.

Note.—Soma (Chandra) is described later on located in the thousand-petalled lotus in the human brain, and is the same as is seen on Śivas' head in pictures, and from which a sort of juice exudes. It is the retaining of this exudation which makes one immortal.

इन्धनानि यथा वह्निस्तैल-वर्ति छ दीपकः |
तथा सोम-कला-पूर्णं देही देहं न मुनछति || ४६ ||

indhanāni yathā vahnistaila-varti cha dīpakaḥ |
tathā soma-kalā-pūrṇaṃ dehī dehaṃ na muñchati || 46 ||

Those who eat the flesh of the cow and drink the immortal liquor daily, are regarded by me men of noble family. Others are but a disgrace to their families.

कृतार्थौ पितरौ तेन धन्यो देशः कुलं च तत् ।
जायते योगवान्यत्र दत्तमक्षय्यतां व्रजेत् ॥
दृष्टः संभाषितः स्पृष्टः पुंप्रकृत्या विवेकवान् ।
भवकोटि शतापातं पुनाति वृजिनं नृणाम् ॥
ब्रह्मवैवर्त्ते

Translation: Fortunate are the parents and blessed is the country and the family where a Yogî is born. Anything given to such a Yogî, becomes immortal. One, who discriminates between Puruṣa and Prakṛiti, purges the sins of a million incarnations, by seeing, speaking, and touching such men (*i.e.*, Yogî.)

[illegible]

A Yogî far exceeds a thousand householders, a hundred vânaprasthas, and a thousand Brahmacharîs.

राजयोगस्य महात्म्यं कोविजानातितत्वतः । तञ्ज्ञानीवसतैयत्र सदेशोपुण्यभाजनम् ॥
दर्शनादर्चनादस्य त्रिसप्तकुल संयुताः । अज्ञामुक्तिपदंयान्ति किं पुनस्तत्परायणाः ॥
अंतर्योगं बहिर्योगं यो जानातिविशेषतः त्वया मयाप्यसौवंद्यः शेषैर्वंद्यस्तु कापुनः ॥
राजयोग, कूर्म्मपुराणे
एक कालं द्विकालं वा त्रिकालं नित्यमेववा । ये युञ्जतेमहायोगं विज्ञे यास्ते महेश्वराः ॥

Who can know the reality of the Raja Yoga? That country is very sacred where resides a man who knows it. By seeing and honouring him, generations of ignorant men get mokṣa, what to speak of those who are actually engaged in it. He who knows internal and external yoga, deserves adoration from you and me, what if he is adored by the rest of mankind!

Those who engage in the great yoga, once, twice or thrice daily, are to be known as masters of great wealth (maheshwaras) or Lords.

गोमांसं भक्ष्हयेन्नित्यं पिबेदमर-वारुणीम |
कुलीनं तमहं मन्ये छेतरे कुल-घातकाः || ४७ ||

ghomāṃsaṃ bhakṣhayennityaṃ pibedamara-vāruṇīm |
kulīnaṃ tamahaṃ manye chetare kula-ghātakāḥ || 47 ||

गो-शब्देनोदिता जिह्वा तत्प्रवेशो हि तालुनि |
गो-मांस-भक्ष्हणं तत्तु महा-पातक-नाशनम || ४८ ||

gho-śabdenoditā jihvā tatpraveśo hi tāluni |
gho-māṃsa-bhakṣhaṇaṃ tattu mahā-pātaka-nāśanam || 48 ||

The word गी means tongue; eating it is thrusting it in the gullet which destroys great sins..

जिह्वा-परवेश-सम्भूत-वह्निनोत्पादितः खलु |
छन्द्रात्स्रवति यः सारः सा सयादमर-वारुणी || ४९ ||

jihvā-praveśa-sambhūta-vahninotpāditaḥ khalu |
chandrātsravati yaḥ sāraḥ sā syādamara-vāruṇī || 49 ||

Immortal liquor is the nectar exuding from the moon (Chandra situated on the left side of the space between the eyebrows). It is produced by the fire which is generated by thrusting the tongue. 48.

छुम्बन्ती यदि लम्बिकाग्रमनिशं जिह्वा-रस-सयन्दिनी
स-कष्हारा कटुकाम्ल-दुग्ध-सदृशी मध्वाज्य-तुल्या तथा |
वयाधीनां हरणं जरान्त-करणं शस्त्रागमोदीरणं
तस्य सयादमरत्वमष्ह्ट-गुणितं सिद्धाङ्गनाकर्ष्हणम || ५० ||

chumbantī yadi lambikāghramaniśaṃ jihvā-rasa-syandinī
sa-kṣhārā kaṭukāmla-dughdha-sadṝśī madhvājya-tulyā tathā |
vyādhīnāṃ haraṇaṃ jarānta-karaṇaṃ śastrāghamodīraṇaṃ
tasya syādamaratvamaṣhṭa-ghuṇitaṃ siddhāngghanākarṣhaṇam || 50 ||

If the tongue can touch with its end the hole from which falls the rasa (juice) which is saltish, bitter, sour, milky and similar to ghee and honey, one can drive away disease, destroy old age, can evade an attack of arms, become immortal in eight ways and can attract fairies. 49.

ऊर्द्व्हास्यो रसनां नियम्य विवरे शक्तिं परां छिन्तयन |
उत्कल्लोल-कला-जलं छ विमलं धारामयं यः पिबेन
निर्व्याधिः स मृणाल-कोमल-वपुर्योगी छिरं जीवति || ५१ ||

ūrdvhāsyo rasanāṃ niyamya vivare śaktiṃ parāṃ chintayan |
utkallola-kalā-jalaṃ cha vimalaṃ dhārāmayaṃ yaḥ piben
nirvyādhiḥ sa mṝṇāla-komala-vapuryoghī chiraṃ jīvati || 51 ||

He who drinks the clear stream of liquor of the moon (soma) falling from the brain to the sixteen-petalled lotus (in the heart), obtained by means of Prâṇa, by applying the tongue to the hole of the pendant in the palate, and by meditating on the great power (Kuṇḍalinî), becomes free from disease and tender in body, like the stalk of a lotus, and the Yogî lives a very long life. 50.

यत्प्रालेयं परहित-सुष्हिरं मेरु-मूर्धान्तर-सथं
तस्मिंस्तत्त्वं परवदति सुधीस्तन-मुखं निम्नगानाम |
छन्द्रात्सारः सरवति वपुष्हस्तेन मृत्युर्नराणां
तद्बध्नीयात्सुकरणमधो नान्यथा काय-सिद्धिः || ५२ ||

yatprāleyaṃ prahita-suṣhiraṃ meru-mūrdhāntara-sthaṃ
tasmiṃstattvaṃ pravadati sudhīstan-mukhaṃ nimnaghānām |
chandrātsāraḥ sravati vapuṣhastena mṝtyurnarāṇāṃ
tadbadhnīyātsukaraṇamadho nānyathā kāya-siddhiḥ || 52 ||

On the top of the Merû (vertebral column), concealed in a hole, is the Somarasa (nectar of Chandra); the wise, whose intellect is not overpowered by Raja and Tama guṇas, but in whom Satwa guṇa is predominant, say there is the (universal spirit) âtma in it. It is the source of the down-going Idâ, Pingalâ and Suṣumnâ Nâdis, which are the Ganges, the Yamuna and the Sarasvati. From that Chandra is shed the essence of the body which causes death of men. It should, therefore, be stopped from shedding. This (Khechari Mudrâ) is a very good instrument for this purpose. There is no other means of achieving this end. 51.

सुष्हिरं जञान-जनकं पञ्छ-सरोतः-समन्वितम |
तिष्हठते खेछरी मुद्रा तस्मिन्शून्ये निरञ्जने || ५३ ||

suṣhiraṃ jñāna-janakaṃ pañcha-srotaḥ-samanvitam |
tiṣhṭhate khecharī mudrā tasminśūnye nirañjane || 53 ||

This hole is the generator of knowledge and is the source of the five streams (Idâ, Pingalâ, &c.). In that colorless vacuum, Khecharî Mudrâ should be established. 52.

एकं सृष्ह्टिमयं बीजमेका मुद्रा छ खेछरी |
एको देवो निरालम्ब एकावस्था मनोन्मनी || ५४ ||

ekaṃ sṝshṭimayaṃ bījamekā mudrā cha khecharī |
eko devo nirālamba ekāvasthā manonmanī || 54 ||

There is only one seed germinating the whole universe from it; and there is only one Mudrâ, called Khecharî. There is only one deva (god) without any one's support, and there is one condition called Manonmaṇi. 53.

The Uḍḍiyâna Bandha.

Uḍḍiyâna is so called by the Yogîs, because by its practice the Prâṇa (Vâyu,) flies (flows) in the Suṣumnâ. 54.

अथ उड्डीयान-बन्धः
बद्धो येन सुष्हुम्णायां पराणस्तूड्डीयते यतः |
तस्मादुड्डीयनाख्यो|अयं योगिभिः समुदाहृतः || ५५ ||

atha uḍḍīyāna-bandhaḥ
baddho yena suṣhumṇāyāṃ prāṇastūḍḍīyate yataḥ |
tasmāduḍḍīyanākhyo|ayaṃ yoghibhiḥ samudāhṝtaḥ || 55 ||

Uḍḍiyâna is so called, because the great bird, Prâṇa, tied to it, flies without being fatigued. It is explained below. 55.

उड्डीनं कुरुते यस्मादविश्रान्तं महा-खगः |
उड्डीयानं तदेव सयात्तव बन्धो|अभिधीयते || ५६ ||

uḍḍīnaṃ kurute yasmādaviśrāntaṃ mahā-khaghaḥ |
uḍḍīyānaṃ tadeva syāttava bandho|abhidhīyate || 56 ||

उदरे पश्छिमं तानं नाभेरूर्ध्वं छ कारयेत |
उड्डीयानो हयसौ बन्धो मृत्यु-मातङ्ग-केसरी || ५७ ||

udare paśchimaṃ tānaṃ nābherūrdhvaṃ cha kārayet |
uḍḍīyāno hyasau bandho mṝtyu-mātanggha-kesarī || 57 ||

The belly above the navel is pressed backwards towards the spine. This Uḍḍiyâna Bandha is like a lion for the elephant of death. 56.

उड्डीयानं तु सहजं गुरुणा कथितं सदा |
अभ्यसेत्सततं यस्तु वृद्धो|अपि तरुणायते || ५८ ||

uḍḍīyānaṃ tu sahajaṃ ghuruṇā kathitaṃ sadā |
abhyasetsatataṃ yastu vṝddho|api taruṇāyate || 58 ||

Uḍḍiyâna is always very easy, when learnt from a guru. The practiser of this, if old, becomes young again. 57.

The portions above and below the navel, should be drawn backwards towards the spine. By practising this for six months one can undoubtedly conquer death. 58.

नाभेरूर्ध्वमधश्छापि तानं कुर्यात्प्रयत्नतः |
षहण्मासमभ्यसेन्मृत्युं जयत्येव न संशयः || ५९ ||

nābherūrdhvamadhaśchāpi tānaṃ kuryātprayatnataḥ |
ṣhaṇmāsamabhyasenmṝtyuṃ jayatyeva na saṃśayaḥ || 59 ||

सर्वेष्हामेव बन्धानां उत्तमो हयुड्डीयानकः |
उड्डियाने दृढे बन्धे मुक्तिः सवाभाविकी भवेत || ६० ||

sarveṣhāmeva bandhānāṃ uttamo hyuḍḍīyānakaḥ |
uḍḍiyāne dṝḍhe bandhe muktiḥ svābhāvikī bhavet || 60 ||

Of all the Bandhas, Uḍḍiyâna is the best; for by binding it firmly liberation comes spontaneously. 59.

The Mûla Bandha.

Pressing Yoni (perineum) with the heel, contract up the anus. By drawing the Apâna thus, Mûla Bandha is made. 60.

अथ मूल-बन्धः
पार्ष्णि-भागेन सम्पीड्य योनिमाकुनछयेद्गुदम |
अपानमूर्ध्वमाकृष्हय मूल-बन्धो|अभिधीयते || ६१ ||

atha mūla-bandhaḥ
pārṣhṇi-bhāghena sampīḍya yonimākuñchayedghudam |
apānamūrdhvamākṝṣhya mūla-bandho|abhidhīyate || 61 ||

The Apâna, naturally inclining downward, is made to go up by force. This Mûla Bandha is spoken of by Yogîs as done by contracting the anus. 61.

अधो-गतिमपानं वा ऊर्ध्वगं कुरुते बलात |
आकुनछनेन तं पराहुर्मूल-बन्धं हि योगिनः || ६२ ||

adho-ghatimapānaṃ vā ūrdhvaghaṃ kurute balāt |
ākuñchanena taṃ prāhurmūla-bandhaṃ hi yoghinaḥ || 62 ||

Pressing the heel well against the anus, draw up the air by force, again and again till it (air) goes up. 62.

गुदं पार्ष्ण्या तु सम्पीड्य वायुमाकुनछयेद्बलात |
वारं वारं यथा छोर्ध्वं समायाति समीरणः || ६३ ||

ghudaṃ pārṣhṇyā tu sampīḍya vāyumākuñchayedbalāt |
vāraṃ vāraṃ yathā chordhvaṃ samāyāti samīraṇaḥ || 63 ||

Prâṇa, Apâna, Nâda and Bindu uniting into one in this way, give success in Yoga, undoubtedly. 63.

पराणापानौ नाद-बिन्दू मूल-बन्धेन छैकताम |
गत्वा योगस्य संसिद्धिं यछछतो नात्र संशयः || ६४ ||

prāṇāpānau nāda-bindū mūla-bandhena chaikatām |
ghatvā yoghasya saṃsiddhiṃ yachchato nātra saṃśayaḥ || 64 ||

By the purification of Prâṇa, and Apâna, urine and excrements decrease. Even an old man becomes young by constantly practising Mûla Bandha. 64.

अपान-पराणयोरैक्यं कष्हयो मूत्र-पुरीष्हयोः |
युवा भवति वृद्धो|अपि सततं मूल-बन्धनात || ६५ ||

apāna-prāṇayoraikyaṃ kṣhayo mūtra-purīṣhayoḥ |
yuvā bhavati vṛddho|api satataṃ mūla-bandhanāt || 65 ||

Going up, the Apâna enters the zone of fire, *i.e.*, the stomach. The flame of fire struck by the air is thereby lengthened. 65.

Note.—

In the centre of the body is the seat of fire, like heated gold.

In men it is triangular, in quadrupeds square, in birds circular. There is a long thin flame in this fire.

It is gastric fire.

अपान ऊर्ध्वगे जाते परयाते वह्नि-मण्डलम |
तदानल-शिखा दीर्घा जायते वायुनाहता || ६६ ||

apāna ūrdhvaghe jāte prayāte vahni-maṇḍalam |
tadānala-śikhā dīrghā jāyate vāyunāhatā || 66 ||

These, fire and Apâna, go to the naturally hot Prâṇa, which, becoming inflamed thereby, causes burning sensation in the body. 66.

ततो यातो वह्न्य-अपानौ पराणमुष्ह्ण-सवरूपकम |
तेनात्यन्त-परदीप्तस्तु जवलनो देहजस्तथा || ६७ ||

tato yāto vahny-apānau prāṇamuṣhṇa-svarūpakam |
tenātyanta-pradīptastu jvalano dehajastathā || 67 ||

The Kuṇḍalinî, which has been sleeping all this time, becomes well heated by this means and awakens well. It becomes straight like a serpent, struck dead with a stick. 67.

तेन कुण्डलिनी सुप्ता सन्तप्ता सम्प्रबुध्यते |
दण्डाहता भुजङ्गीव निश्वस्य ऋजुतां वरजेत || ६८ ||

tena kuṇḍalinī suptā santaptā samprabudhyate |
daṇḍāhatā bhujangghīva niśvasya ṝjutāṃ vrajet || 68 ||

It enters the Brahma Nâdî, just as a serpent enters its hole. Therefore, the Yogî should always practise this Mûla Bandha. 68.

बिलं परविष्हटेव ततो बरह्म-नाड्यं तरं वरजेत |
तस्मान्नित्यं मूल-बन्धः कर्तव्यो योगिभिः सदा || ६९ ||

bilaṃ praviṣhṭeva tato brahma-nāḍyaṃ taraṃ vrajet |
tasmānnityaṃ mūla-bandhaḥ kartavyo yoghibhiḥ sadā || 69 ||

The Jâlandhara Bandha.

अथ जलन्धर-बन्धः
कण्ठमाकुनछ्य हृदये सथापयेच्छिबुकं दृढम |
बन्धो जालन्धराख्यो|अयं जरा-मृत्यु-विनाशकः || ७० ||

atha jalandhara-bandhaḥ
kaṇṭhamākuñchya hṝdaye sthāpayechchibukaṃ dṝḍham |
bandho jālandharākhyo|ayaṃ jarā-mṝtyu-vināśakaḥ || 70 ||

Contract the throat and press the chin firmly against the chest. This is called Jâlandhara Bandha, which destroys old age and death. 69.

बध्नाति हि सिराजालमधो-गामि नभो-जलम |
ततो जालन्धरो बन्धः कण्ठ-दुःखौघ-नाशनः || ७१ ||

badhnāti hi sirājālamadho-ghāmi nabho-jalam |
tato jālandharo bandhaḥ kaṇṭha-duḥkhaugha-nāśanaḥ || 71 ||

It stops the opening (hole) of the group of the Nâdîs, through which the juice from the sky (from the Soma or Chandra in the brain) falls down. It is, therefore, called the Jâlandhara Bandha —the destroyer of a host of diseases of the throat. 70.

जालन्धरे कृते बन्धे कण्ठ-संकोछ-लक्ष्हणे |
न पीयूष्हं पतत्यग्नौ न छ वायुः परकुप्यति || ७२ ||

jālandhare kṛte bandhe kaṇṭha-saṃkocha-lakṣhaṇe |
na pīyūṣhaṃ patatyaghnau na cha vāyuḥ prakupyati || 72 ||

In Jâlandhara Bandha, the indications of a perfect contraction of throat are, that the nectar does not fall into the fire (the Sûrya situated in the navel), and the air is not disturbed. 71.

कण्ठ-संकोछनेनैव दवे नाड्यौ सतम्भयेद्दृढम |
मध्य-छक्रमिदं जञेयं षहोडशाधार-बन्धनम || ७३ ||

kaṇṭha-saṃkochanenaiva dve nāḍyau stambhayeddṛḍham |
madhya-chakramidaṃ jñeyaṃ ṣhoḍaśādhāra-bandhanam || 73 ||

The two Nâdîs should be stopped firmly by contracting the throat. This is called the middle circuit or centre (Madhya Chakra), and it stops the 16 âdhâras (*i.e.*, vital parts). 72.

Note.

The sixteen vital parts mentioned by renowned Yogîs are the (1) thumbs, (2) ankles, (3) knees, (4) thighs, (5) the prepuce, (6) organs of generation, (17) the navel, (8) the heart, (9) the neck, (10) the throat, (11) the palate, (12) the nose, (13) the middle of the eyebrows, (14) the forehead, (15) the head and (16) the Brahma randhra.

मूल-सथानं समाकुनछ्य उड्डियानं तु कारयेत |
इडां छ पिङ्गलां बद्ध्वा वाहयेत्पश्छिमे पथि || ७४ ||

mūla-sthānaṃ samākuñchya uḍḍiyānaṃ tu kārayet |
iḍāṃ cha pingghalāṃ baddhvā vāhayetpaśchime pathi || 74 ||

By drawing up the mûlasthâna (anus,) Uḍḍiyâna Bandha should be performed. The flow of the air should be directed to the Suṣumnâ, by closing the Idâ, and the Pingalâ. 73.

अनेनैव विधानेन परयाति पवनो लयम |
ततो न जायते मृत्युर्जरा-रोगादिकं तथा || ७५ ||

anenaiva vidhānena prayāti pavano layam |
tato na jāyate mṛtyurjarā-roghādikaṃ tathā || 75 ||

The Prâna becomes calm and latent by this means, and thus there is no death, old age, disease, etc. 74.

बन्ध-तरयमिदं शरेष्हठं महा-सिद्धैश्छ सेवितम |
सर्वेष्हां हठ-तन्त्राणां साधनं योगिनो विदुः || ७६ ||

bandha-trayamidaṃ śreshṭhaṃ mahā-siddhaiścha sevitam |
sarveṣhāṃ haṭha-tantrāṇāṃ sādhanaṃ yoghino viduḥ || 76 ||

These three Bandhas are the best of all and have been practised by the masters. Of all the means of success in the Haṭha Yoga, they are known to the Yogîs as the chief ones. 75.

यत्किंछित्स्रवते छन्द्रादमृतं दिव्य-रूपिणः |
तत्सर्वं गरसते सूर्यस्तेन पिण्डो जरायुतः || ७७ ||

yatkiṃchitsravate chandrādamṝtaṃ divya-rūpiṇaḥ |
tatsarvaṃ ghrasate sūryastena piṇḍo jarāyutaḥ || 77 ||

The whole of the nectar, possessing divine qualities, which exudes from the Soma (Chandra) is devoured by the Sûrya; and, owing to this, the body becomes old. 76.

To remedy this, the opening of the Sûrya is avoided by excellent means. It is to be learnt best by instructions from a guru; but not by even a million discussions. 77.

The Viparîta Karaṇî.

अथ विपरीत-करणी मुद्रा
तत्रास्ति करणं दिव्यं सूर्यस्य मुख-वञ्छनम |
गुरूपदेशतो जञेयं न तु शास्त्रार्थ-कोटिभिः || ७८ ||

atha viparīta-karaṇī mudrā
tatrāsti karaṇaṃ divyaṃ sūryasya mukha-vañchanam |
ghurūpadeśato jñeyaṃ na tu śāstrārtha-koṭibhiḥ || 78 ||

Above the navel and below the palate respectively, are the Sûrya and the Chandra. The exercise, called the Viparîta Karaṇî, is learnt from the guru's instructions. 78.

ऊर्ध्व-नाभेरधस्तालोरूर्ध्वं भानुरधः शशी |
करणी विपरीताखा गुरु-वाक्येन लभ्यते || ७९ ||

ūrdhva-nābheradhastālorūrdhvaṃ bhānuradhaḥ śaśī |
karaṇī viparītākhā ghuru-vākyena labhyate || 79 ||

This exercise increases the appetite; and, therefore, one who practises it, should obtain a good supply of food. If the food be scanty, it will burn him at once. 79.

नित्यमभ्यास-युक्तस्य जठराग्नि-विवर्धनी |
आहारो बहुलस्तस्य सम्पाद्यः साधकस्य छ || ८० ||

nityamabhyāsa-yuktasya jaṭharāghni-vivardhanī |
āhāro bahulastasya sampādyaḥ sādhakasya cha || 80 ||

Place the head on the ground and the feet up into the sky, for a second only the first day, and increase this time daily. 80.

अल्पाहारो यदि भवेदग्निर्दहति तत-कष्हणात |
अधः-शिराश्छोर्ध्व-पादः कष्हणं सयात्प्रथमे दिने || ८१ ||

alpāhāro yadi bhavedaghnirdahati tat-kṣhaṇāt |
adhaḥ-śirāśchordhva-pādaḥ kṣhaṇaṃ syātprathame dine || 81 ||

कष्हणाछ्छ किंछिदधिकमभ्यसेछ्छ दिने दिने |
वलितं पलितं छैव षहण्मासोर्ध्वं न दृश्यते |
याम-मात्रं तु यो नित्यमभ्यसेत्स तु कालजित || ८२ ||

kṣhaṇāchcha kiṃchidadhikamabhyasechcha dine dine |
valitaṃ palitaṃ chaiva ṣhaṇmāsordhvaṃ na dṛśyate |
yāma-mātraṃ tu yo nityamabhyasetsa tu kālajit || 82 ||

After six months, the wrinkles and grey hair are not seen. He who practises it daily, even for two hours, conquers death. 81.

The Vajrolî.

अथ वज्रोली

सवेच्छया वर्तमानो|अपि योगोक्तैर्नियमैर्विना |
वज्रोलीं यो विजानाति स योगी सिद्धि-भाजनम || ८३ ||

atha vajrolī
svechchayā vartamāno|api yoghoktairniyamairvinā |
vajrolīṃ yo vijānāti sa yoghī siddhi-bhājanam || 83 ||

Even if one who lives a wayward life, without observing any rules of Yoga, but performs Vajrolî, deserves success and is a Yogî. 82.

तत्र वस्तु-दवयं वक्ष्ह्ये दुर्लभं यस्य कस्यछित |
कष्हीरं छैकं दवितीयं तु नारी छ वश-वर्तिनी || ८४ ||

tatra vastu-dvayaṃ vakṣhye durlabhaṃ yasya kasyachit |
kṣhīraṃ chaikaṃ dvitīyaṃ tu nārī cha vaśa-vartinī || 84 ||

Two things are necessary for this, and these are difficult to get for the ordinary people—(1) milk and (2) a woman behaving, as desired. 83.

मेहनेन शनैः सम्यगूर्ध्वाकुनछनमभ्यसेत |
पुरुष्हो|अप्यथवा नारी वज्रोली-सिद्धिमाप्नुयात || ८५ ||

mehanena śanaiḥ samyaghūrdhvākuñchanamabhyaset |
puruṣho|apyathavā nārī vajrolī-siddhimāpnuyāt || 85 ||

By practising to draw in the *bindu*, discharged during cohabitation, whether one be a man or a woman, one obtains success in the practice of Vajrolî. 84.

यत्नतः शस्त-नालेन फूत्कारं वज्र-कन्दरे |
शनैः शनैः परकुर्वीत वायु-संछार-कारणात || ८६ ||

yatnataḥ śasta-nālena phūtkāraṃ vajra-kandare |
śanaiḥ śanaiḥ prakurvīta vāyu-saṃchāra-kāraṇāt || 86 ||

By means of a pipe, one should blow air slowly into the passage in the male organ. 85.

नारी-भगे पदद-बिन्दुमभ्यासेनोर्ध्वमाहरेत |
छलितं छ निजं बिन्दुमूर्ध्वमाकृष्ह्य रक्ष्हयेत || ८७ ||

nārī-bhaghe padad-bindumabhyāsenordhvamāharet |
chalitaṃ cha nijaṃ bindumūrdhvamākṝṣhya rakṣhayet || 87 ||

By practice, the discharged *bindu* is drawn out. One can draw back and preserve one's own discharged bindu. 86.

एवं संरक्ष्हयेद्बिन्दुं जयति योगवित |
मरणं बिन्दु-पातेन जीवनं बिन्दु-धारणात || ८८ ||

evaṃ saṃrakṣhayedbinduṃ jayati yoghavit |
maraṇaṃ bindu-pātena jīvanaṃ bindu-dhāraṇāt || 88 ||

The Yogî who can protect his *bindu* thus, overcomes death; because death comes by discharging *bindu*, and life is prolonged by its preservation. 87.

सुगन्धो योगिनो देहे जायते बिन्दु-धारणात |
यावद्बिन्दुः सथिरो देहे तावत्काल-भयं कुतः || ८९ ||

sughandho yoghino dehe jāyate bindu-dhāraṇāt |
yāvadbinduḥ sthiro dehe tāvatkāla-bhayaṃ kutaḥ || 89 ||

By preserving *bindu*, the body of the Yogî emits a pleasing smell. There is no fear of death, so long as the *bindu* is well-established in the body. 88.

छित्तायत्तं नृणां शुक्रं शुक्रायत्तं छ जीवितम |
तस्माछ्छुक्रं मनश्छैव रक्ष्हणीयं परयत्नतः || ९० ||

chittāyattaṃ nṝṇāṃ śukraṃ śukrāyattaṃ cha jīvitam |
tasmāchchukraṃ manaśchaiva rakṣhaṇīyaṃ prayatnataḥ || 90 ||

ऋतुमत्या रजो|अप्येवं निजं बिन्दुं छ रक्ष्हयेत |
मेढ्रेणाकर्ष्हयेदूर्ध्वं सम्यगभ्यास-योग-वित || ९१ ||

ṝtumatyā rajo|apyevaṃ nijaṃ binduṃ cha rakṣhayet |
meḍhreṇākarṣhayedūrdhvaṃ samyaghabhyāsa-yogha-vit || 91 ||

The *bindu* of men is under the control of the mind, and life is dependent on the *bindu*. Hence, mind and *bindu* should be protected by all means. 89.

The Sahajolî.

अथ सहजोलिः
सहजोलिश्छामरोलिर्वज्रोल्या भेद एकतः |
जले सुभस्म निक्ष्हिप्य दग्ध-गोमय-सम्भवम || ९२ ||

atha sahajoliḥ
sahajoliśchāmarolirvajrolyā bheda ekataḥ |
jale subhasma nikṣhipya daghdha-ghomaya-sambhavam || 92 ||

Sahajolî and Amarolî are only the different kinds of Vajrolî. Ashes from burnt up cowdung should be mixed with water. 90.

वज्रोली-मैथुनादूर्ध्वं सत्री-पुंसोः सवाङ्ग-लेपनम |
आसीनयोः सुखेनैव मुक्त-वयापारयोः कष्हणात || ९३ ||

vajrolī-maithunādūrdhvaṃ strī-puṃsoḥ svānggha-lepanam |
āsīnayoḥ sukhenaiva mukta-vyāpārayoḥ kṣhaṇāt || 93 ||

Being free from the exercise of Vajrolî, man and woman should both rub it on their bodies. 91.

सहजोलिरियं परोक्ता शरद्धेया योगिभिः सदा |
अयं शुभकरो योगो भोग-युक्तो|अपि मुक्तिदः || ९४ ||

sahajoliriyaṃ proktā śraddheyā yoghibhiḥ sadā |
ayaṃ śubhakaro yogho bhogha-yukto|api muktidaḥ || 94 ||

This is called Sahajolî, and should be relied on by Yogîs. It does good and gives mokṣa. 92.

अयं योगः पुण्यवतां धीराणां तत्त्व-दर्शिनाम |
निर्मत्सराणां वै सिध्येन्न तु मत्सर-शालिनाम || ९५ ||

ayaṃ yoghaḥ puṇyavatāṃ dhīrāṇāṃ tattva-darśinām |
nirmatsarāṇāṃ vai sidhyenna tu matsara-śālinām || 95 ||

This Yoga is achieved by courageous wise men, who are free from sloth, and cannot he accomplished by the slothful. 93.

The Amarolî.

अथ अमरोली
पित्तोल्बणत्वात्प्रथमाम्बु-धारां
विहाय निःसारतयान्त्यधाराम |
निष्हेव्यते शीतल-मध्य-धारा
कापालिके खण्डमते|अमरोली || ९६ ||

atha amarolī
pittolbaṇatvātprathamāmbu-dhārāṃ
vihāya niḥsāratayāntyadhārām |
niṣhevyate śītala-madhya-dhārā
kāpālike khaṇḍamate|amarolī || 96 ||

In the doctrine of the sect of the Kapâlikas, the Amarolî is the drinking of the mid stream; leaving the 1st, as it is a mixture of too much bile and the last, which is useless. 94.

अमरीं यः पिबेन्नित्यं नस्यं कुर्वन्दिने दिने |
वज्रोलीमभ्यसेत्सम्यक्सामरोलीति कथ्यते || ९७ ||

amarīṃ yaḥ pibennityaṃ nasyaṃ kurvandine dine |
vajrolīmabhyasetsamyaksāmarolīti kathyate || 97 ||

He who drinks Amarî, snuffs it daily, and practices Vajrolî, is called practising Amarolî. 95.

अभ्यासान्निःसृतां छान्द्रीं विभूत्या सह मिश्रयेत |
धारयेदुत्तमाङ्गेष्हु दिव्य-दृष्हिटः परजायते || ९८ ||

abhyāsānniḥsṛtāṃ chāndrīṃ vibhūtyā saha miśrayet |
dhārayeduttamānggheṣhu divya-dṛṣhṭiḥ prajāyate || 98 ||

पुंसो बिन्दुं समाकुनछ्य सम्यगभ्यास-पाटवात |
यदि नारी रजो रक्ष्हेद्वज्रोल्या सापि योगिनी || ९९ ||

puṃso binduṃ samākuñchya samyaghabhyāsa-pāṭavāt |
yadi nārī rajo rakṣhedvajrolyā sāpi yoghinī || 99 ||

The *bindu* discharged in the practice of Vajrolî should be mixed with ashes, and the rubbing it on the best parts of the body gives divine sight. 96.

तस्याः किंछिद्रजो नाशं न गछ्छति न संशयः |
तस्याः शरीरे नादश्छ बिन्दुतामेव गछ्छति || १०० ||

tasyāḥ kiṃchidrajo nāśaṃ na ghachchati na saṃśayaḥ |
tasyāḥ śarīre nādaścha bindutāmeva ghachchati || 100 ||

स बिन्दुस्तद्रजश्छैव एकीभूय सवदेहगौ |
वज्रोल्य-अभ्यास-योगेन सर्व-सिद्धिं परयछ्छतः || १०१ ||

sa bindustadrajaśchaiva ekībhūya svadehaghau |
vajroly-abhyāsa-yoghena sarva-siddhiṃ prayachchataḥ || 101 ||

रक्ष्हेदाकुनछनादूर्ध्वं या रजः सा हि योगिनी |
अतीतानागतं वेत्ति खेछरी छ भवेद्ध्रुवम || १०२ ||

rakṣhedākuñchanādūrdhvaṃ yā rajaḥ sā hi yoghinī |
atītānāghataṃ vetti khecharī cha bhaveddhruvam || 102 ||

देह-सिद्धिं छ लभते वज्रोल्य-अभ्यास-योगतः |
अयं पुण्य-करो योगो भोगे भुक्ते|अपि मुक्तिदः || १०३ ||

deha-siddhiṃ cha labhate vajroly-abhyāsa-yoghataḥ |
ayaṃ puṇya-karo yogho bhoghe bhukte|api muktidaḥ || 103 ||

The Śakti châlana.

अथ शक्ति-छालनम
कुटिलाङ्गी कुण्डलिनी भुजङ्गी शक्तिरीश्वरी |
कुण्डल्यरुन्धती छैते शब्दाः पर्याय-वाछकाः || १०४ ||

atha śakti-chālanam
kuṭilāngghī kuṇḍalinī bhujangghī śaktirīśvarī |
kuṇḍalyarundhatī chaite śabdāḥ paryāya-vāchakāḥ || 104 ||

Kutilângî (crooked-bodied), Kuṇḍalinî, Bhujangî (a she-serpent) Śakti, Iśhwarî, Kundalî, Arundhatî,—all these words are synonymous. 97.

उद्घाटयेत्कपाटं तु यथा कुंछिकया हठात |
कुण्डलिन्या तथा योगी मोक्ष्हद्वारं विभेदयेत || १०५ ||

udghāṭayetkapāṭaṃ tu yathā kuṃchikayā haṭhāt |
kuṇḍalinyā tathā yoghī mokṣhadvāraṃ vibhedayet || 105 ||

As a door is opened with a key, so the Yogî opens the door of mukti by opening Kuṇḍalinî by means of Haṭha Yoga. 98.

येन मार्गेण गन्तव्यं बरह्म-सथानं निरामयम |
मुखेनाछछाद्य तद्वारं परसुप्ता परमेश्वरी || १०६ ||

yena mārgheṇa ghantavyaṃ brahma-sthānaṃ nirāmayam |
mukhenāchchādya tadvāraṃ prasuptā parameśvarī || 106 ||

The Parameśwarî (Kuṇḍalinî) sleeps, covering the hole of the passage by which one can go to the seat of Brahma which is free from pains. 99.

Keeping the feet in Vajra-âsana (Padma-âsana), hold them firmly with the hands. The position of the bulb then will be near the ankle joint, where it should be pressed. 107.

कन्दोर्ध्वे कुण्डली शक्तिः सुप्ता मोक्ष्हाय योगिनाम |
बन्धनाय छ मूढानां यस्तां वेत्ति स योगवित || १०७ ||

kandordhve kuṇḍalī śaktiḥ suptā mokṣhāya yoghinām |
bandhanāya cha mūḍhānāṃ yastāṃ vetti sa yoghavit || 107 ||

Kuṇḍalî Sakti sleeps on the bulb, for the purpose of giving moksa to Yogîs and bondage to the ignorant. He who knows it, knows Yoga. 100.

कुण्डली कुटिलाकारा सर्पवत्परिकीर्तिता |
सा शक्तिश्छालिता येन स मुक्तो नात्र संशयः || १०८ ||

kuṇḍalī kuṭilākārā sarpavatparikīrtitā |
sā śaktiśchālitā yena sa mukto nātra saṃśayaḥ || 108 ||

Kuṇḍalî is of a bent shape, and has been described to be like a serpent. He who has moved that Śakti is no doubt Mukta (released from bondage). 101.

गङ्गा-यमुनयोर्मध्ये बाल-रण्डां तपस्विनीम |
बलात्कारेण गृह्णीयात्तद्विष्ह्णोः परमं पदम || १०९ ||

ghanggha-yamunayormadhye bāla-raṇḍāṃ tapasvinīm |
balātkāreṇa ghṝhṇīyāttadviṣhṇoḥ paramaṃ padam || 109 ||

Youngster Tapaswini (a she-ascetic), lying between the Ganges and the Yamunâ, (Idâ and Pingalâ) should be caught hold of by force, to get the highest position. 102.

इडा भगवती गङ्गा पिङ्गला यमुना नदी |
इडा-पिङ्गलयोर्मध्ये बालरण्डा छ कुण्डली || ११० ||

iḍā bhaghavatī ghanggha pinggalā yamunā nadī |
iḍā-pingghalayormadhye bālaraṇḍā cha kuṇḍalī || 110 ||

Idâ is called goddess Ganges, Pingalâ goddess Yamunâ. In the middle of the Idâ and the Pingalâ is the infant widow, Kuṇḍalî. 103.

पुच्छे परगृहय भुजङ्गीं सुप्तामुद्बोधयेच्छ ताम |
निद्रां विहाय सा शक्तिरूर्ध्वमुत्तिष्हठते हठात || १११ ||

puchche praghṝhya bhujangghīṃ suptāmudbodhayechcha tām |
nidrāṃ vihāya sā śaktirūrdhvamuttiṣhṭhate haṭhāt || 111 ||

This sleeping she-serpent should be awakened by catching hold of her tail. By the force of Haṭha, the Śakti leaves her sleep, and starts upwards. 104.

अवस्थिता छैव फणावती सा
परातश्छ सायं परहरार्ध-मात्रम |
परपूर्य सूर्यात्परिधान-युक्त्या
परगृहय नित्यं परिछालनीया || ११२ ||

avasthitā chaiva phaṇāvatī sā
prātaścha sāyaṃ praharārdha-mātram |
prapūrya sūryātparidhāna-yuktyā
praghṝhya nityaṃ parichālanīyā || 112 ||

This she-serpent is situated in Mûlâdhâr. She should be caught and moved daily, morning and evening, for ½ a prahar (1½ hours), by filling with air through Pingalâ by the Paridhana method. 105.

ऊर्ध्वं वितस्ति-मात्रं तु विस्तारं छतुरङ्गुलम |
मृदुलं धवलं परोक्तं वेष्ह्टिताम्बर-लक्ष्हणम || ११३ ||

ūrdhvaṃ vitasti-mātraṃ tu vistāraṃ chaturangghulam |
mṝdulaṃ dhavalaṃ proktaṃ veṣhṭitāmbara-lakṣhaṇam || 113 ||

The bulb is above the anus, a vitasti (12 angulas) long, and measures 4 angulas (3 inches) in extent and is soft and white, and appears as if a folded cloth. 106.

सति वज्रासने पादौ कराभ्यां धारयेद्दृढम |
गुल्फ-देश-समीपे छ कन्दं तत्र परपीडयेत || ११४ ||

sati vajrāsane pādau karābhyāṃ dhārayeddṛḍham |
ghulpha-deśa-samīpe cha kandaṃ tatra prapīḍayet || 114 ||

Keeping the feet in Vajra-âsana (Padma-âsana), hold them firmly with the hands. The position of the bulb then will be near the ankle joint, where it should be pressed. 107.

वज्रासने सथितो योगी छालयित्वा छ कुण्डलीम |
कुर्यादनन्तरं भस्त्रां कुण्डलीमाशु बोधयेत || ११५ ||

vajrāsane sthito yoghī chālayitvā cha kuṇḍalīm |
kuryādanantaraṃ bhastrāṃ kuṇḍalīmāśu bodhayet || 115 ||

The Yogî, sitting with Vajra-âsana and having moved Kuṇḍalî, should perform Bhastrikâ to awaken the Kuṇḍalî soon. 108.

भानोराकुनछनं कुर्यात्कुण्डलीं छालयेत्ततः |
मृत्यु-वक्त्र-गतस्यापि तस्य मृत्यु-भयं कुतः || ११६ ||

bhānorākuñchanaṃ kuryātkuṇḍalīṃ chālayettataḥ |
mṛtyu-vaktra-ghatasyāpi tasya mṛtyu-bhayaṃ kutaḥ || 116 ||

Bhânu (Sûrya, near the navel) should be contracted (by contracting the navel) which will move the Kuṇḍalî. There is no fear for him who does so, even if he has entered the mouth of death. 109.

मुहूर्त-दवय-पर्यन्तं निर्भयं छालनादसौ |
ऊर्ध्वमाकृष्ह्यते किंछित्सुष्हुम्णायां समुद्गता || ११७ ||

muhūrta-dvaya-paryantaṃ nirbhayaṃ chālanādasau |
ūrdhvamākṛṣhyate kiṃchitsuṣhumṇāyāṃ samudghatā || 117 ||

By moving this, for two muhûrtas, it is drawn up a little by entering the Suṣumnâ (spinal column). 110.

तेन कुण्डलिनी तस्याः सुष्हुम्णाया मुखं धरुवम |
जहाति तस्मात्प्राणो|अयं सुष्हुम्णां वरजति सवतः || ११८ ||

tena kuṇḍalinī tasyāḥ suṣhumṇāyā mukhaṃ dhruvam |
jahāti tasmātprāṇo|ayaṃ suṣhumṇāṃ vrajati svataḥ || 118 ||

By this Kuṇḍalinî leaves the entrance of the Suṣumnâ at once, and the Prâṇa enters it of itself. 111.

तस्मात्संछालयेन्नित्यं सुख-सुप्तामरुन्धतीम |
तस्याः संछालनेनैव योगी रोगैः परमुछ्यते || ११९ ||

tasmātsaṃchālayennityaṃ sukha-suptāmarundhatīm |
tasyāḥ saṃchālanenaiva yoghī roghaiḥ pramuchyate || 119 ||

Therefore, this comfortably sleeping Arundhatî should always be moved; for by so doing the Yogî gets rid of diseases. 112.

येन संछालिता शक्तिः स योगी सिद्धि-भाजनम |
किमत्र बहुनोक्तेन कालं जयति लीलया || १२० ||

yena saṃchālitā śaktiḥ sa yoghī siddhi-bhājanam |
kimatra bahunoktena kālaṃ jayati līlayā || 120 ||

The Yogî, who has been able to move the Śakti deserves success. It is useless to say more, suffice it to say that he conquers death playfully. 113.

बरह्मछर्य-रतस्यैव नित्यं हित-मिताशिनः |
मण्डलाद्दृश्यते सिद्धिः कुण्डल्य-अभ्यास-योगिनः || १२१ ||

brahmacharya-ratasyaiva nityaṃ hita-mitāśinaḥ |
maṇḍalāddṛśyate siddhiḥ kuṇḍaly-abhyāsa-yoghinaḥ || 121 ||

The Yogî observing Brahmacharya (continence and always eating sparingly, gets success within 40 days by practice with the Kuṇḍalinî. 114.

कुण्डलीं छालयित्वा तु भस्त्रां कुर्याद्विशेष्हतः |
एवमभ्यस्यतो नित्यं यमिनो यम-भीः कुतः || १२२ ||

kuṇḍalīṃ chālayitvā tu bhastrāṃ kuryādviśeṣhataḥ |
evamabhyasyato nityaṃ yamino yama-bhīḥ kutaḥ || 122 ||

After moving the Kuṇḍalî, plenty of Bhastrâ should be performed. By such practice, he has no fear from the god of death. 115.

दवा-सप्तति-सहस्राणां नाडीनां मल-शोधने |
कुतः परक्ष्हालनोपायः कुण्डल्य-अभ्यसनादृते || १२३ ||

dvā-saptati-sahasrāṇāṃ nāḍīnāṃ mala-śodhane |
kutaḥ prakṣhālanopāyaḥ kuṇḍaly-abhyasanādṝte || 123 ||

There is no other way, but the practice of the Kuṇḍalî, for washing away the impurities of 72,000 Nâdîs. 116.

इयं तु मध्यमा नाडी दृढाभ्यासेन योगिनाम |
आसन-पराण-संयाम-मुद्राभिः सरला भवेत || १२४ ||

iyaṃ tu madhyamā nāḍī dṝḍhābhyāsena yoghinām |
āsana-prāṇa-saṃyāma-mudrābhiḥ saralā bhavet || 124 ||

This middle Nâdî becomes straight by steady practice of postures; Prâṇâyâma and Mudrâs of Yogîs. 117.

अभ्यासे तु विनिद्राणां मनो धृत्वा समाधिना |
रुद्राणी वा परा मुद्रा भद्रां सिद्धिं परयछ्छति || १२५ ||

abhyāse tu vinidrāṇāṃ mano dhṝtvā samādhinā |
rudrāṇī vā parā mudrā bhadrāṃ siddhiṃ prayachchati || 125 ||

Those whose sleep has decreased by practice and mind has become calm by samâdhi, get beneficial accomplishments by Sâmbhavî and other Mudrâs. 118.

राज-योगं विना पृथ्वी राज-योगं विना निशा |
राज-योगं विना मुद्रा विछित्रापि न शोभते || १२६ ||

rāja-yogham vinā pṛthvī rāja-yogham vinā niśā |
rāja-yogham vinā mudrā vichitrāpi na śobhate || 126 ||

Without Raja Yoga, this earth, the night, and the Mudrâs, be they howsoever wonderful, do not appear beautiful. 119.

Note.—Raja Yoga = âsana. Earth = steadiness, calmness. Night = Kumbhaka; cessations of the activity of the Prâṇa, just as King's officials cease moving at night. Hence night means absence of motion, *i.e.*, Kumbhaka.

मारुतस्य विधिं सर्वं मनो-युक्तं समभ्यसेत |
इतरत्र न कर्तव्या मनो-वृत्तिर्मनीष्हिणा || १२७ ||

mārutasya vidhiṃ sarvaṃ mano-yuktaṃ samabhyaset |
itaratra na kartavyā mano-vṛttirmanīṣhiṇā || 127 ||

All the practices relating to the air should be performed with concentrated mind. A wise man should not allow his mind to wander away. 120.

इति मुद्रा दश परोक्ता आदिनाथेन शम्भुना |
एकैका तासु यमिनां महा-सिद्धि-परदायिनी || १२८ ||

iti mudrā daśa proktā ādināthena śambhunā |
ekaikā tāsu yamināṃ mahā-siddhi-pradāyinī || 128 ||

These are the Mudrâs, as explained by Âdinâtha (Śiva). Every one of them is the giver of great accomplishments to the practiser. 121.

उपदेशं हि मुद्राणां यो दत्ते साम्प्रदायिकम |
स एव शरी-गुरुः सवामी साक्ष्हादीश्वर एव सः || १२९ ||

upadeśaṃ hi mudrāṇāṃ yo datte sāmpradāyikam |
sa eva śrī-ghuruḥ svāmī sākṣhādīśvara eva saḥ || 129 ||

He is really the *guru* and to be considered as Îśvara in human form who teaches the Mudrâs as handed down from guru to guru. 122.

तस्य वाक्य-परो भूत्वा मुद्राभ्यासे समाहितः |
अणिमादि-गुणैः सार्धं लभते काल-वञ्छनम || १३० ||

tasya vākya-paro bhūtvā mudrābhyāse samāhitaḥ |
aṇimādi-ghuṇaiḥ sārdhaṃ labhate kāla-vañchanam || 130 ||

Engaging in practice, by putting faith in his words, one gets the Siddhis of Anima, etc., as also evades death. 123.

End of chapter III, on the Exposition of the Mudrâs.

इति हठ-परदीपिकायां तृतीयोपदेशः |

iti haṭha-pradīpikāyāṃ tṛtīyopadeśaḥ |

CHAPTER IV.

On Samâdhi.

|| ४ || छतुर्थोपदेशः

|| 4 || chaturthopadeśaḥ

नमः शिवाय गुरवे नाद-बिन्दु-कलात्मने |
निरञ्जन-पदं याति नित्यं तत्र परायणः || १ ||

namaḥ śivāya ghurave nāda-bindu-kalātmane |
nirañjana-padaṃ yāti nityaṃ tatra parāyaṇaḥ || 1 ||

Salutation to the Gurû, the dispenser of happiness to all, appearing as Nâda, Vindû and Kalâ. One who is devoted to Him, obtains the highest bliss. 1.

अथेदानीं परवक्ष्ह्यामि समाधिक्रममुत्तमम |
मृत्युघ्नं छ सुखोपायं बरह्मानन्द-करं परम || २ ||

athedānīṃ pravakṣhyāmi samādhikramamuttamam |
mṛtyughnaṃ cha sukhopāyaṃ brahmānanda-karaṃ param || 2 ||

Now I will describe a regular method of attaining to Samâdhi, which destroys death, is the means for obtaining happiness, and gives the Brahmânanda. 2.

राज-योगः समाधिश्छ उन्मनी छ मनोन्मनी |
अमरत्वं लयस्तत्त्वं शून्याशून्यं परं पदम || ३ ||
अमनस्कं तथाद्वैतं निरालम्बं निरञ्जनम |
जीवन्मुक्तिश्छ सहजा तुर्या छेत्येक-वाछकाः || ४ ||

rāja-yoghaḥ samādhiścha unmanī cha manonmanī |
amaratvaṃ layastattvaṃ śūnyāśūnyaṃ paraṃ padam || 3 ||
amanaskaṃ tathādvaitaṃ nirālambaṃ nirañjanam |
jīvanmuktiścha sahajā turyā chetyeka-vāchakāḥ || 4 ||

Raja Yogî, Samâdhi, Unmani, Mauonmanî, Amarativa, Laya, Tatwa, Sûnya, Aśûnya, Parama Pada, Amanaska, Adwaitama, Nirālamba, Nirañjana, Jîwana Mukti, Sahajâ, Turyâ, are all synonymous. 3-4.

सलिले सैन्धवं यद्वत्साम्यं भजति योगतः |
तथात्म-मनसोरैक्यं समाधिरभिधीयते || ५ ||

salile saindhavaṃ yadvatsāmyaṃ bhajati yoghataḥ |
tathātma-manasoraikyaṃ samādhirabhidhīyate || 5 ||

As salt being dissolved in water becomes one with it, so when Âtmâ and mind become one, it is called Samâdhi. 5.

यदा संक्षीयते पराणो मानसं छ परलीयते |
तदा समरसत्वं छ समाधिरभिधीयते || ६ ||

yadā saṃkṣhīyate prāṇo mānasaṃ cha pralīyate |
tadā samarasatvaṃ cha samādhirabhidhīyate || 6 ||

When the Prâṇa becomes lean (vigourless) and the mind becomes absorbed, then their becoming equal is called Samâdhi. 6.

तत-समं छ दवयोरैक्यं जीवात्म-परमात्मनोः |
परनष्ह्टट-सर्व-सङ्कल्पः समाधिः सो|अभिधीयते || ७ ||

tat-samaṃ cha dvayoraikyaṃ jīvātma-paramātmanoḥ |
pranaṣhṭa-sarva-sangkalpaḥ samādhiḥ so|abhidhīyate || 7 ||

This equality and oneness of the self and the ultra self, when all Saṃkalpas cease to exist, is called Samâdhi. 7.

राज-योगस्य माहात्म्यं को वा जानाति तत्त्वतः |
जञानं मुक्तिः सथितिः सिद्धिर्गुरु-वाक्येन लभ्यते || ८ ||

rāja-yoghasya māhātmyaṃ ko vā jānāti tattvataḥ |
jñānaṃ muktiḥ sthitiḥ siddhirghuru-vākyena labhyate || 8 ||

Or, who can know the true greatness of the Raja Yoga. Knowledge, mukti, condition, and Siddhîs can be learnt by instructions from a *gurû* alone. 8.

दुर्लभो विष्हय-तयागो दुर्लभं तत्त्व-दर्शनम |
दुर्लभा सहजावस्था सद-गुरोः करुणां विना || ९ ||

durlabho viṣhaya-tyāgho durlabhaṃ tattva-darśanam |
durlabhā sahajāvasthā sad-ghuroḥ karuṇāṃ vinā || 9 ||

Indifference to worldly enjoyments is very difficult to obtain, and equally difficult is the knowledge of the Realities to obtain. It is very difficult to get the condition of Samâdhi, without the favour of a true *guru*. 9.

विविधैरासनैः कुभैर्विछित्रैः करणैरपि |
परबुद्धायां महा-शक्तौ पराणः शून्ये परलीयते || १० ||

vividhairāsanaiḥ kubhairvichitraiḥ karaṇairapi |
prabuddhāyāṃ mahā-śaktau prāṇaḥ śūnye pralīyate || 10 ||

By means of various postures and different Kumbhakas, when the great power (Kuṇḍalî) awakens, then the Prâṇa becomes absorbed in Sûnya (Samâdhi). 10.

उत्पन्न-शक्ति-बोधस्य तयक्त-निःशेष्ह-कर्मणः |
योगिनः सहजावस्था सवयमेव परजायते || ११ ||

utpanna-śakti-bodhasya tyakta-niḥśeṣha-karmaṇaḥ |
yoghinaḥ sahajāvasthā svayameva prajāyate || 11 ||

The Yogî whose śakti has awakened, and who has renounced all actions, attains to the condition of Samâdhi, without any effort. 11.

सुष्हुम्णा-वाहिनि पराणे शून्ये विशति मानसे |
तदा सर्वाणि कर्माणि निर्मूलयति योगवित || १२ ||

suṣhumṇā-vāhini prāṇe śūnye viśati mānase |
tadā sarvāṇi karmāṇi nirmūlayati yoghavit || 12 ||

When the Prâṇa flows in the Suṣumnâ, and the mind has entered śûnya, then the Yogî is free from the effects of Karmas. 12.

अमराय नमस्तुभ्यं सो|अपि कालस्त्वया जितः |
पतितं वदने यस्य जगदेतच्छराछरम || १३ ||

amarāya namastubhyaṃ so|api kālastvayā jitaḥ |
patitaṃ vadane yasya jaghadetachcharācharam || 13 ||

O Immortal one (that is, the yogi who has attained to the condition of Samâdhi), I salute thee! Even death itself, into whose mouth the whole of this movable and immovable world has fallen, has been conquered by thee. 13.

छित्ते समत्वमापन्ने वायौ वरजति मध्यमे |
तदामरोली वज्रोली सहजोली परजायते || १४ ||

chitte samatvamāpanne vāyau vrajati madhyame |
tadāmarolī vajrolī sahajolī prajāyate || 14 ||

Amarolî, Vajrolî and Sahajolî are accomplished when the mind becomes calm and Prâṇa has entered the middle channel. 14.

जञानं कुतो मनसि सम्भवतीह तावत
पराणो|अपि जीवति मनो मरियते न यावत |
पराणो मनो दवयमिदं विलयं नयेद्यो
मोक्ष्हं स गच्छति नरो न कथंछिदन्यः || १५ ||

jñānaṃ kuto manasi sambhavatīha tāvat
prāṇo|api jīvati mano mriyate na yāvat |
prāṇo mano dvayamidaṃ vilayaṃ nayedyo
mokṣhaṃ sa ghachchati naro na kathaṃchidanyaḥ || 15 ||

How can it he possible to get knowledge, so long as the Prâṇa is living and the mind has not died? No one else can get mokṣa, except one who can make one's Prâṇa and mind latent. 15.

जञात्वा सुष्हुम्णासद-भेदं कृत्वा वायुं छ मध्यगम |
सथित्वा सदैव सुस्थाने बरह्म-रन्ध्रे निरोधयेत || १६ ||

jñātvā suṣhumṇāsad-bhedaṃ kṛtvā vāyuṃ cha madhyagham |
sthitvā sadaiva susthāne brahma-randhre nirodhayet || 16 ||

Always living in a good locality and having known the secret of the Suṣumnâ, which has a middle course, and making the Vâyu move in it., (the Yogî) should restrain the Vâyu in the Brahma randhra. 16.

सूर्य-छन्द्रमसौ धत्तः कालं रात्रिन्दिवात्मकम |
भोक्त्री सुष्हुम्ना कालस्य गुह्यमेतदुदाहृतम || १७ ||

sūrya-chandramasau dhattaḥ kālaṃ rātrindivātmakam |
bhoktrī suṣhumnā kālasya ghuhyametadudāhṛtam || 17 ||

Time, in the form of night and day, is made by the sun and the moon. That, the Suṣumnâ devours this time (death) even, is a great secret. 17.

दवा-सप्तति-सहस्राणि नाडी-दवाराणि पञ्जरे |
सुष्हुम्णा शाम्भवी शक्तिः शेष्हास्त्वेव निरर्थकाः || १८ ||

dvā-saptati-sahasrāṇi nāḍī-dvārāṇi pañjare |
suṣhumṇā śāmbhavī śaktiḥ śeṣhāstveva nirarthakāḥ || 18 ||

In this body there are 72,000 openings of Nâdis; of these, the Suṣumnâ, which has the Śâmhhavî Sakti in it, is the only important one, the rest are useless. 18.

वायुः परिछितो यस्मादग्निना सह कुण्डलीम |
बोधयित्वा सुष्हुम्णायां परविशेदनिरोधतः || १९ ||

vāyuḥ parichito yasmādaghninā saha kuṇḍalīm |
bodhayitvā suṣhumṇāyāṃ praviśedanirodhataḥ || 19 ||

The Vâyu should be made to enter the Suṣumnâ without restraint by him who has practised the control of breathing and has awakened the Kuṇḍali by the (gastric) fire. `19

सुष्हुम्णा-वाहिनि पराणे सिद्ध्यत्येव मनोन्मनी |
अन्यथा तवितराभ्यासाः परयासायैव योगिनाम || २० ||

suṣhumṇā-vāhini prāṇe siddhyatyeva manonmanī |
anyathā tvitarābhyāsāḥ prayāsāyaiva yoghinām || 20 ||

The Prâṇa, flowing through the Suṣumnâ, brings about the condition of manonmaṇî; other practices are simply futile for the Yogî. 20.

पवनो बध्यते येन मनस्तेनैव बध्यते |
मनश्छ बध्यते येन पवनस्तेन बध्यते || २१ ||

pavano badhyate yena manastenaiva badhyate |
manaścha badhyate yena pavanastena badhyate || 21 ||

By whom the breathing has been controlled, by him the activities of the mind also have been controlled; and, conversely, by whom the activities of the mind have been controlled, by him the breathing also has been controlled. 21.

हेतु-दवयं तु छित्तस्य वासना छ समीरणः |
तयोर्विनष्ह्ट एकस्मिन्तौ दवावपि विनश्यतः || २२ ||

hetu-dvayaṃ tu chittasya vāsanā cha samīraṇaḥ |
tayorvinaṣhṭa ekasmintau dvāvapi vinaśyataḥ || 22 ||

There are two causes of the activities of the mind: (1) Vâsanâ (desires) and (2) the respiration (the Prâṇa). Of these, the destruction of the one is the destruction of both. 22.

मनो यत्र विलीयेत पवनस्तत्र लीयते |
पवनो लीयते यत्र मनस्तत्र विलीयते || २३ ||

mano yatra vilīyeta pavanastatra līyate |
pavano līyate yatra manastatra vilīyate || 23 ||

Breathing is lessened when the mind becomes absorbed, and the mind becomes absorbed when the Prâṇa is restrained. 23.

दुग्धाम्बुवत्संमिलितावुभौ तौ
तुल्य-करियौ मानस-मारुतौ हि |
यतो मरुत्तत्र मनः-परवृत्तिर
यतो मनस्तत्र मरुत-परवृत्तिः || २४ ||

dughdhāmbuvatsaṃmilitāvubhau tau
tulya-kriyau mānasa-mārutau hi |
yato maruttatra manaḥ-pravṝttir
yato manastatra marut-pravṝttiḥ || 24 ||

Both the mind and the breath are united together, like milk and water; and both of them are equal in their activities. Mind begins its activities where there is the breath, and the Parana begins its activities where there is the mind. 24.

तत्रैक-नाशादपरस्य नाश
एक-परवृत्तेरपर-परवृत्तिः |
अध्वस्तयोश्छेन्द्रिय-वर्ग-वृत्तिः
परध्वस्तयोर्मोक्श्ह-पदस्य सिद्धिः || २५ ||

tatraika-nāśādaparasya nāśa
eka-pravṝtterapara-pravṝttiḥ |

adhvastayośchendriya-vargha-vṝttiḥ
pradhvastayormokṣha-padasya siddhiḥ || 25 ||

By the suspension of the one, therefore, comes the suspension of the other, and by the operations of the one are brought about the operations of the other. When they are present, the Indriyas (the senses) remain engaged in their proper functions, and when they become latent then there is moksa. 25.

रसस्य मनसश्छैव छञ्छलत्वं सवभावतः |
रसो बद्धो मनो बद्धं किं न सिद्ध्यति भूतले || २६ ||

rasasya manasaśchaiva chañchalatvaṃ svabhāvataḥ |
raso baddho mano baddhaṃ kiṃ na siddhyati bhūtale || 26 ||

By nature, Mercury and mind are unsteady: there is nothing in the world which cannot be accomplished when these are made steady. 26.

मूर्छ्छितो हरते वयाधीन्मृतो जीवयति सवयम |
बद्धः खेछरतां धत्ते रसो वायुश्छ पार्वति || २७ ||

mūrchchito harate vyādhīnmṝto jīvayati svayam |
baddhaḥ khecharatāṃ dhatte raso vāyuścha pārvati || 27 ||

O Pârvati! Mercury and breathing, when made steady, destroy diseases and the dead himself comes to life (by their means). By their (proper) control, moving in the air is attained. 27.

मनः सथैर्यं सथिरो वायुस्ततो बिन्दुः सथिरो भवेत |
बिन्दु-सथैर्यात्सदा सत्त्वं पिण्ड-सथैर्यं परजायते || २८ ||

manaḥ sthairyaṃ sthiro vāyustato binduḥ sthiro bhavet |
bindu-sthairyātsadā sattvaṃ piṇḍa-sthairyaṃ prajāyate || 28 ||

The breathing is calmed when the mind becomes steady and calm; and hence the preservation of *bindu*. The preservation of this latter makes the satwa established in the body. 28.

इन्द्रियाणां मनो नाथो मनोनाथस्तु मारुतः |
मारुतस्य लयो नाथः स लयो नादमाश्रितः || २९ ||

indriyāṇāṃ mano nātho manonāthastu mārutaḥ |
mārutasya layo nāthaḥ sa layo nādamāśritaḥ || 29 ||

Mind is the master of the senses, and the breath is the master of the mind. The breath in its turn is subordinate to the laya (absorption), and that laya depends on the nâda. 29.

सो|अयमेवास्तु मोक्ष्हाख्यो मास्तु वापि मतान्तरे |
मनः-पराण-लये कश्छिदानन्दः सम्प्रवर्तते || ३० ||

so|ayamevāstu mokṣhākhyo māstu vāpi matāntare |
manaḥ-prāṇa-laye kaśchidānandaḥ sampravartate || 30 ||

This very laya is what is called mokṣa, or, being a sectarian, you may not call it mokṣa; but when the mind becomes absorbed, a sort of ecstacy is experienced. 30.

परनष्ह्ट-शवास-निश्वासः परध्वस्त-विष्हय-गरहः |
निश्छेष्ह्टो निर्विकारश्छ लयो जयति योगिनाम || ३१ ||

pranaṣhṭa-śvāsa-niśvāsaḥ pradhvasta-viṣhaya-ghrahaḥ |
niścheṣhṭo nirvikāraścha layo jayati yoghinām || 31 ||

By the suspension of respiration and the annihilation of the enjoyments of the senses, when the mind becomes devoid of all the activities and remains changeless, then the Yogî attains to the Laya Stage. 31.

उछ्छिन्न-सर्व-सङ्कल्पो निःशेष्हाशेष्ह-छेष्ह्टितः |
सवावगम्यो लयः को|अपि जायते वाग-अगोछरः || ३२ ||

uchchinna-sarva-sangkalpo niḥśeṣhāśeṣha-cheṣhṭitaḥ |
svāvaghamyo layaḥ ko|api jāyate vāgh-aghocharaḥ || 32 ||

When all the thoughts and activities are destroyed, then the Laya Stage is produced, to describe which is beyond the power of speech, being known by self-experience alone. 32.

यत्र दृष्हिटर्लयस्तत्र भूतेन्द्रिय-सनातनी |
सा शक्तिर्जीव-भूतानां दवे अलक्ष्हये लयं गते || ३३ ||

yatra dṝshṭirlayastatra bhūtendriya-sanātanī |
sā śaktirjīva-bhūtānāṃ dve alakṣhye layaṃ ghate || 33 ||

They often speak of Laya, Laya; but what is meant by it?

लयो लय इति पराहुः कीदृशं लय-लक्ष्हणम |
अपुनर-वासनोत्थानाल्लयो विष्हय-विस्मृतिः || ३४ ||

layo laya iti prāhuḥ kīdṝśaṃ laya-lakṣhaṇam |
apunar-vāsanotthānāllayo viṣhaya-vismṝtiḥ || 34 ||

Laya is simply then forgetting of the objects of senses when the Vâsanâs (desires) do not rise into existence again. 33.

The Sâmbhavî Mudrâ.

वेद-शास्त्र-पुराणानि सामान्य-गणिका इव |
एकैव शाम्भवी मुद्रा गुप्ता कुल-वधूरिव || ३५ ||

veda-śāstra-purāṇāni sāmānya-ghaṇikā iva |
ekaiva śāmbhavī mudrā ghuptā kula-vadhūriva || 35 ||

The Vedas and the Śâstras are like ordinary public women. Śâmhhavî Mudrâ is the one, which is secluded like a respectable lady. 34.

अथ शाम्भवी
अन्तर्लक्ष्हयं बहिर्दृष्हिटर्निमेष्होन्मेष्ह-वर्जिता |
एष्हा सा शाम्भवी मुद्रा वेद-शास्त्रेष्हु गोपिता || ३६ ||

atha śāmbhavī
antarlakṣhyaṃ bahirdṝshṭirnimeṣhonmeṣha-varjitā |
eṣhā sā śāmbhavī mudrā veda-śāstreṣhu ghopitā || 36 ||

Aiming at Brahman inwardly, while keeping the sight directed to the external objects, without blinking the eyes, is called the Sâmbhavî Mudrâ, hidden in the Vedas and the Sâstras. 35.

अन्तर्लक्ष्ह्य-विलीन-छित्त-पवनो योगी यदा वर्तते
दृष्ह्ट्या निश्छल-तारया बहिरधः पश्यन्नपश्यन्नपि |
मुद्रेयं खलु शाम्भवी भवति सा लब्धा परसादाद्गुरोः
शून्याशून्य-विलक्ष्हणं सफुरति तत्तत्त्वं पदं शाम्भवम || ३७ ||

antarlakṣhya-vilīna-chitta-pavano yoghī yadā vartate
dṛṣhṭyā niśchala-tārayā bahiradhaḥ paśyannapaśyannapi |
mudreyaṃ khalu śāmbhavī bhavati sā labdhā prasādādghuroḥ
śūnyāśūnya-vilakṣhaṇaṃ sphurati tattattvaṃ padaṃ śāmbhavam || 37 ||

When the Yogî remains inwardly attentive to the Brahman, keeping the mind and the Prâṇa absorbed, and the sight steady, as if seeing everything while in reality seeing nothing outside, below, or above, verily then it is called the Sâmbhavî Mudrâ, which is learnt by the favour of a *guru*. Whatever, wonderful, Sûnya or Asûnya is perceived, is to be regarded as the manifestation of that great Śambhû (Śiva.) 36.

शरी-शाम्भव्याश्छ खेछर्या अवस्था-धाम-भेदतः |
भवेछ्छित्त-लयानन्दः शून्ये छित-सुख-रूपिणि || ३८ ||

śrī-śāmbhavyāścha khecharyā avasthā-dhāma-bhedataḥ |
bhavechchitta-layānandaḥ śūnye chit-sukha-rūpiṇi || 38 ||

The two states, the Sâmbhavî and the Khecharî, are different because of their seats (being the heart and the space between the eyebrows respectively); but both cause happiness, for the mind becomes absorbed in the Chita-sukha-Rupa-âtmana which is void. 37.

The Unmanî.

तारे जयोतिष्हि संयोज्य किंछिदुन्नमयेद्भ्रुवौ |
पूर्व-योगं मनो युनजन्नुन्मनी-कारकः कष्हणात || ३९ ||

tāre jyotiṣhi saṃyojya kiṃchidunnamayedbhruvau |
pūrva-yoghaṃ mano yuñjannunmanī-kārakaḥ kṣhaṇāt || 39 ||

Fix the gaze on the light (seen on the tip of the nose) and raise the eyebrows a little, with the mind contemplating as before (in the Śambhavî Mudrâ, that is, inwardly thinking of Brahma, but apparently looking outside.) This will create the Unmanî avasthâ at once. 38.

The Târaka.

केछिदागम-जालेन केछिन्निगम-सङ्कुलैः |
केछित्तर्केण मुह्यन्ति नैव जानन्ति तारकम || ४० ||

kechidāghama-jālena kechinnighama-sangkulaiḥ |
kechittarkeṇa muhyanti naiva jānanti tārakam || 40 ||

Some are devoted to the Vedas, some to Nigama, while others are enwrapt in Logic, but none knows the value of this mudrâ, which enables one to cross the ocean of existence 39.

अर्धोन्मीलित-लोछनः सथिर-मना नासाग्र-दत्तेक्ष्हणश
छन्द्रार्कावपि लीनतामुपनयन्निस्पन्द-भावेन यः |
जयोती-रूपमशेष्ह-बीजमखिलं देदीप्यमानं परं
तत्त्वं तत-पदमेति वस्तु परमं वाछ्यं किमत्राधिकम || ४१ ||

ardhonmīlita-lochanaḥ sthira-manā nāsāghra-dattekṣhaṇaś
chandrārkāvapi līnatāmupanayannispanda-bhāvena yaḥ |
jyotī-rūpamaśeṣha-bījamakhilaṃ dedīpyamānaṃ paraṃ
tattvaṃ tat-padameti vastu paramaṃ vāchyaṃ kimatrādhikam || 41 ||

With steady calm mind and half closed eyes, fixed on the tip of the nose, stopping the Idâ and the Pingalâ without blinking, he who can see the light which is the all, the seed, the entire brilliant, great Tatwama, approaches Him, who is the great object. What is the use of more talk? 40.

दिवा न पूजयेल्लिङ्गं रात्रौ छैव न पूजयेत |
सर्वदा पूजयेल्लिङ्गं दिवारात्रि-निरोधतः || ४२ ||

divā na pūjayellinggham rātrau chaiva na pūjayet |
sarvadā pūjayellinggham divārātri-nirodhataḥ || 42 ||

One should not meditate on the Linga (*i.e.*, Âtman) in the day (*i.e.*, while Sûrya or Pingalâ is working) or at night (when Idâ is working), but should always contemplate after restraining both. 41.

The Khecharî.

अथ खेछरी
सव्य-दक्ष्हिण-नाडी-सथो मध्ये छरति मारुतः |
तिष्हठते खेछरी मुद्रा तस्मिन्स्थाने न संशयः || ४३ ||

atha khecharī
savya-dakṣhiṇa-nāḍī-stho madhye charati mārutaḥ |
tiṣhṭhate khecharī mudrā tasminsthāne na saṃśayaḥ || 43 ||

When the air has ceased to move in the right and the left nostrils, and has begun to flow in the middle path, then the Khecharî Mudrâ, can be accomplished there. There is no doubt of this. 42.

इडा-पिङ्गलयोर्मध्ये शून्यं छैवानिलं गरसेत |
तिष्हठते खेछरी मुद्रा तत्र सत्यं पुनः पुनः || ४४ ||

iḍā-pingghalayormadhye śūnyaṃ chaivānilaṃ ghraset |
tiṣhṭhate khecharī mudrā tatra satyaṃ punaḥ punaḥ || 44 ||

If the Prâṇa can he drawn into the Sûnya (Suṣumnâ), which is between the Idâ and the Pingalâ, and male motionless there, then the Khecharî Mudrâ can truly become steady there. 43.

सूछर्याछन्द्रमसोर्मध्ये निरालम्बान्तरे पुनः |
संस्थिता वयोम-छक्रे या सा मुद्रा नाम खेछरी || ४५ ||

sūrchyāchandramasormadhye nirālambāntare punaḥ |
saṃsthitā vyoma-chakre yā sā mudrā nāma khecharī || 45 ||

That Mudrâ is called Khecharî which is performed in the supportless space between the Sûrya and the Chandra (the Idâ and the Pingalâ) and called the Vyoma Chakra. 44.

सोमाद्यत्रोदिता धारा साक्ष्हात्सा शिव-वल्लभा |
पूरयेदतुलां दिव्यां सुष्हुम्णां पश्छिमे मुखे || ४६ ||

somādyatroditā dhārā sākṣhātsā śiva-vallabhā |
pūrayedatulāṃ divyāṃ suṣhumṇāṃ paśchime mukhe || 46 ||

The Khecharî which causes the stream to flow from the Chandra (Śoma) is beloved of Śiva. The incomparable divine Suṣumnâ should be closed by the tongue drawn back. 45.

पुरस्ताछ्छैव पूर्येत निश्छिता खेछरी भवेत |
अभ्यस्ता खेछरी मुद्राप्युन्मनी सम्प्रजायते || ४७ ||

purastāchchaiva pūryeta niśchitā khecharī bhavet |
abhyastā khecharī mudrāpyunmanī samprajāyate || 47 ||

It can be closed from the front also (by stopping the movements of the Prâṇa), and then surely it becomes the Khecharî. By practice, this Khecharî leads to Unmanî. 46.

भरुवोर्मध्ये शिव-सथानं मनस्तत्र विलीयते |
जञातव्यं तत-पदं तुर्यं तत्र कालो न विद्यते || ४८ ||

bhruvormadhye śiva-sthānaṃ manastatra vilīyate |
jñātavyaṃ tat-padaṃ turyaṃ tatra kālo na vidyate || 48 ||

The seat of Śiva is between the eyebrows, and the mind becomes absorbed there. This condition (in which the mind is thus absorbed) is known as Tûrya, and death has no access there. 47.

अभ्यसेत्खेछरीं तावद्यावत्स्याद्योग-निद्रितः |
सम्प्राप्त-योग-निद्रस्य कालो नास्ति कदाछन || ४९ ||

abhyasetkhecharīṃ tāvadyāvatsyādyogha-nidritaḥ |
samprāpta-yogha-nidrasya kālo nāsti kadāchana || 49 ||

The Khecharî should be practised till there is Yoga-nidrâ (Samâdhi). One who has induced Yoga-nidrâ, cannot fall a victim to death. 48.

निरालम्बं मनः कृत्वा न किंछिदपि छिन्तयेत |
स-बाह्याभ्यन्तरं वयोम्नि घटवत्तिष्ठति धरुवम || ५० ||

nirālambaṃ manaḥ kṝtvā na kiṃchidapi chintayet |
sa-bāhyābhyantaraṃ vyomni ghaṭavattiṣhṭhati dhruvam || 50 ||

Freeing the mind from all thoughts and thinking of nothing, one should sit firmly like a pot in the space (surrounded and filled with the ether). 49.

बाह्य-वायुर्यथा लीनस्तथा मध्यो न संशयः |
सव-सथाने सथिरतामेति पवनो मनसा सह || ५१ ||

bāhya-vāyuryathā līnastathā madhyo na saṃśayaḥ |
sva-sthāne sthiratāmeti pavano manasā saha || 51 ||

As the air, in and out of the body, remains unmoved, so the breath with mind becomes steady in its place (*i.e.*, in Brahma randhra). 50.

एवमभ्यस्यतस्तस्य वायु-मार्गे दिवानिशम |
अभ्यासाज्जीर्यते वायुर्मनस्तत्रैव लीयते || ५२ ||

evamabhyasyatastasya vāyu-mārghe divāniśam |
abhyāsājjīryate vāyurmanastatraiva līyate || 52 ||

By thus practising, night and day, the breathing is brought under control, and, as the practice increases, the mind becomes calm and steady. 51.

अमृतैः पलावयेद्देहमापाद-तल-मस्तकम |
सिद्ध्यत्येव महा-कायो महा-बल-पराक्रमः || ५३ ||

amṝtaiḥ plāvayeddehamāpāda-tala-mastakam |
siddhyatyeva mahā-kāyo mahā-bala-parākramaḥ || 53 ||

By rubbing the body over with Amrita (exuding from the moon), from head to foot, one gets Mahâkâyâ, *i.e.*, great strength and energy. 52.

End of the Khecharî.

शक्ति-मध्ये मनः कृत्वा शक्तिं मानस-मध्यगाम |
मनसा मन आलोक्य धारयेत्परमं पदम || ५४ ||

śakti-madhye manaḥ kṛtvā śaktiṃ mānasa-madhyaghām |
manasā mana ālokya dhārayetparamaṃ padam || 54 ||

Placing the mind into the Kuṇḍalini, and getting the latter into the mind, by looking upon the Buddhi (intellect) with mind (reflexively), the Param Pada (Brahma) should be obtained. 53.

ख-मध्ये कुरु छात्मानमात्म-मध्ये छ खं कुरु |
सर्वं छ ख-मयं कृत्वा न किंछिदपि छिन्तयेत || ५५ ||

kha-madhye kuru chātmānamātma-madhye cha khaṃ kuru |
sarvaṃ cha kha-mayaṃ kṛtvā na kiṃchidapi chintayet || 55 ||

Keep the âtmâ inside the Kha (Brahma) and place Brahma inside your âtmâ. Having made everything pervaded with Kha (Brahma), think of nothing else. 54.

अन्तः शून्यो बहिः शून्यः शून्यः कुम्भ इवाम्बरे |
अन्तः पूर्णो बहिः पूर्णः पूर्णः कुम्भ इवार्णवे || ५६ ||

antaḥ śūnyo bahiḥ śūnyaḥ śūnyaḥ kumbha ivāmbare |
antaḥ pūrṇo bahiḥ pūrṇaḥ pūrṇaḥ kumbha ivārṇave || 56 ||

One should become void in and void out, and voice like a pot in the space. Full in and full outside, like a jar in the ocean. 55.

बाह्य-छिन्ता न कर्तव्या तथैवान्तर-छिन्तनम |
सर्व-छिन्तां परित्यज्य न किंछिदपि छिन्तयेत || ५७ ||

bāhya-chintā na kartavyā tathaivāntara-chintanam |
sarva-chintāṃ parityajya na kiṃchidapi chintayet || 57 ||

He should be neither of his inside nor of outside world; and, leaving all thoughts, he should think of nothing. 56.

सङ्कल्प-मात्र-कलनैव जगत्समग्रं
सङ्कल्प-मात्र-कलनैव मनो-विलासः |
सङ्कल्प-मात्र-मतिमुत्सृज निर्विकल्पम
आश्रित्य निश्छयमवाप्नुहि राम शान्तिम || ५८ ||

sangkalpa-mātra-kalanaiva jaghatsamaghraṃ
sangkalpa-mātra-kalanaiva mano-vilāsaḥ |
sangkalpa-mātra-matimutsṛja nirvikalpam
āśritya niśchayamavāpnuhi rāma śāntim || 58 ||

The whole of this world and all the schemes of the mind are but the creations of thought. Discarding these thoughts and taking leave of all conjectures, O Râma! obtain peace. 57.

कर्पूरमनले यद्वत्सैन्धवं सलिले यथा |
तथा सन्धीयमानं छ मनस्तत्त्वे विलीयते || ५९ ||

karpūramanale yadvatsaindhavaṃ salile yathā |
tathā sandhīyamānaṃ cha manastattve vilīyate || 59 ||

As camphor disappears in fire, and rock salt in water, so the mind united with the âtmâ loses its identity. 58.

जज्ञेयं सर्वं परतीतं छ जज्ञानं छ मन उछ्यते |
जज्ञानं जज्ञेयं समं नष्हटं नान्यः पन्था दवितीयकः || ६० ||

jñeyaṃ sarvaṃ pratītaṃ cha jñānaṃ cha mana uchyate |
jñānaṃ jñeyaṃ samaṃ nashṭaṃ nānyaḥ panthā dvitīyakaḥ || 60 ||

When the knowable, and the knowledge, are both destroyed equally, then there is no second way (*i.e.*, Duality is destroyed). 59.

मनो-दृश्यमिदं सर्वं यत्किंछित्स-छराछरम |
मनसो हयुन्मनी-भावाद्द्वैतं नैवोलभ्यते || ६१ ||

mano-dṛśyamidaṃ sarvaṃ yatkiṃchitsa-charācharam |
manaso hyunmanī-bhāvāddvaitaṃ naivolabhyate || 61 ||

All this movable and immovable world is mind. When the mind has attained to the unmanî avasthâ, there is no dwaita (from the absence of the working of the mind.) 60

जञेय-वस्तु-परित्यागाद्विलयं याति मानसम |
मनसो विलये जाते कैवल्यमवशिष्हयते || ६२ ||

jñeya-vastu-parityāghādvilayaṃ yāti mānasam |
manaso vilaye jāte kaivalyamavaśiṣhyate || 62 ||

Mind disappears by removing the knowable, and, on its disappearance, âtmâ only remains behind. 61.

एवं नाना-विधोपायाः सम्यक्स्वानुभवान्विताः |
समाधि-मार्गाः कथिताः पूर्वाछार्यैर्महात्मभिः || ६३ ||

evaṃ nānā-vidhopāyāḥ samyaksvānubhavānvitāḥ |
samādhi-mārghāḥ kathitāḥ pūrvāchāryairmahātmabhiḥ || 63 ||

The high-souled Âchâryas (Teachers) of yore gained experience in the various methods of Samâdhi themselves, and then they preached them to others. 62.

सुष्हुम्णायै कुण्डलिन्यै सुधायै छन्द्र-जन्मने |
मनोन्मन्यै नमस्तुभ्यं महा-शक्त्यै छिद-आत्मने || ६४ ||

suṣhumṇāyai kuṇḍalinyai sudhāyai chandra-janmane |
manonmanyai namastubhyaṃ mahā-śaktyai chid-ātmane || 64 ||

Salutations to Thee, O Suṣumnâ, to Thee O Kuṇḍalinî, to Thee O Sudhâ, born of Chandra, to Thee O Manomnanî! to Thee O great power, energy and the intelligent spirit. 63.

अशक्य-तत्त्व-बोधानां मूढानामपि संमतम |
परोक्तं गोरक्ष्ह-नाथेन नादोपासनमुछ्यते || ६५ ||

aśakya-tattva-bodhānāṃ mūḍhānāmapi saṃmatam |
proktaṃ ghorakṣha-nāthena nādopāsanamuchyate || 65 ||

I will describe now the practice of anâhata nâda, as propounded by Gorakṣa Nâtha, for the benefit of those who are unable to understand the principles of knowledge—a method, which is liked by the ignorant also. 64.

शरी-आदिनाथेन स-पाद-कोटि-
लय-परकाराः कथिता जयन्ति |
नादानुसन्धानकमेकमेव
मन्यामहे मुख्यतमं लयानाम || ६६ ||

śrī-ādināthena sa-pāda-koṭi-
laya-prakārāḥ kathitā jayanti |
nādānusandhānakamekameva
manyāmahe mukhyatamaṃ layānām || 66 ||

Âdinâtha propounded 1¼ crore methods of trance, and they are all extant. Of these, the hearing of the anâhata nâda is the Only one, the chief, in my opinion. 65.

मुक्तासने सथितो योगी मुद्रां सन्धाय शाम्भवीम |
शृणुयाद्दक्षिहणे कर्णे नादमन्तास्थमेकधीः || ६७ ||

muktāsane sthito yoghī mudrāṃ sandhāya śāmbhavīm |
śṝṇuyāddakṣhiṇe karṇe nādamantāsthamekadhīḥ || 67 ||

Sitting with Mukta Âsana and with the Sâmbhavî Madill, the Yogî should hear the sound inside his right ear, with collected mind. 66.

शरवण-पुट-नयन-युगल
घराण-मुखानां निरोधनं कार्यम |
शुद्ध-सुष्हुम्णा-सरणौ
सफुटममलः शरूयते नादः || ६८ ||

śravaṇa-puṭa-nayana-yughala
ghrāṇa-mukhānāṃ nirodhanaṃ kāryam |
śuddha-suṣhumṇā-saraṇau
sphuṭamamalaḥ śrūyate nādaḥ || 68 ||

The ears, the eyes, the nose, and the mouth should be closed and then the clear sound is heard in the passage of the Suṣumnâ which has been cleansed of all its impurities. 67.

आरम्भश्छ घटश्छैव तथा परिछयो|अपि छ |
निष्हपत्तिः सर्व-योगेष्हु सयादवस्था-छतुष्हटयम || ६९ ||

ārambhaścha ghaṭaśchaiva tathā parichayo|api cha |
niṣhpattiḥ sarva-yogheṣhu syādavasthā-chatuṣhṭayam || 69 ||

In all the Yogas, there are four states: (1) ârambha or the preliminary, (2) Ghata, or the state of a jar, (3) Parichaya (known), (4) niṣpatti (consumate.) 68.

Ârambha Avasthâ.

अथ आरम्भावस्था
बरह्म-गरन्थेर्भवेद्भेदो हयानन्दः शून्य-सम्भवः |
विछित्रः क्वणको देहे|अनाहतः शरूयते धवनिः || ७० ||

atha ārambhāvasthā
brahma-ghrantherbhavedbhedo hyānandaḥ śūnya-sambhavaḥ |
vichitraḥ kvaṇako dehe|anāhataḥ śrūyate dhvaniḥ || 70 ||

When the Brahma granthi (in the heart) is pierced through by Prâṇâyâma, then a sort of happiness is experienced in the vacuum of the heart, and the anâhat sounds, like various tinkling sounds of ornaments, are heard in the body. 69.

दिव्य-देहश्छ तेजस्वी दिव्य-गन्धस्त्वरोगवान |
सम्पूर्ण-हृदयः शून्य आरम्भे योगवान्भवेत || ७१ ||

divya-dehaścha tejasvī divya-ghandhastvaroghavān |
sampūrṇa-hṛdayaḥ śūnya ārambhe yoghavānbhavet || 71 ||

In the ârambha, a Yogî's body becomes divine, glowing, healthy, and emits a divine swell. The whole of his heart becomes void. 70.

The Ghata Avasthâ.

अथ घटावस्था
दवितीयायां घटीकृत्य वायुर्भवति मध्यगः |
दृढासनो भवेद्योगी जज्ञानी देव-समस्तदा || ७२ ||

atha ghaṭāvasthā
dvitīyāyāṃ ghaṭīkṝtya vāyurbhavati madhyaghaḥ |
dṝḍhāsano bhavedyoghī jñānī deva-samastadā || 72 ||

In the second stage, the airs are united into one and begin moving in the middle channel. The Yogî's posture becomes firm, and he becomes wise like a god. 71.

विष्ह्णु-गरन्थेस्ततो भेदात्परमानन्द-सूछकः |
अतिशून्ये विमर्दश्छ भेरी-शब्दस्तदा भवेत || ७३ ||

viṣhṇu-ghranthestato bhedātparamānanda-sūchakaḥ |
atiśūnye vimardaścha bherī-śabdastadā bhavet || 73 ||

By this means the Viṣṇu knot (in the throat) is pierced which is indicated by highest pleasure experienced, And then the Bherî sound (like the beating of a kettle drain) is evolved in the vacuum in the throat. 72.

The Parichaya Avasthâ.

अथ परिछयावस्था
तृतीयायां तु विज्ञेयो विहायो मर्दल-धवनिः |
महा-शून्यं तदा याति सर्व-सिद्धि-समाश्रयम || ७४ ||

atha parichayāvasthā
tṝtīyāyāṃ tu vijñeyo vihāyo mardala-dhvaniḥ |
mahā-śūnyaṃ tadā yāti sarva-siddhi-samāśrayam || 74 ||

In the third stage, the sound of a drum is known to arise in tie Sûnya between the eyebrows, and then the Vâyu goes to the Mahâsûnya, which is the home of all the siddhîs. 73.

छित्तानन्दं तदा जित्वा सहजानन्द-सम्भवः |
दोष्ह-दुःख-जरा-वयाधि-कष्हुधा-निद्रा-विवर्जितः || ७५ ||

chittānandaṃ tadā jitvā sahajānanda-sambhavaḥ |
doṣha-duḥkha-jarā-vyādhi-kṣhudhā-nidrā-vivarjitaḥ || 75 ||

Conquering, then, the pleasures of the mind, ecstacy is spontaneously produced which is devoid of evils, pains, old age, disease, hunger and sleep. 74.

अथ निष्हपत्त्य-अवस्था
रुद्र-गरन्थिं यदा भित्त्वा शर्व-पीठ-गतो|अनिलः |
निष्हपत्तौ वैणवः शब्दः कवणद-वीणा-कवणो भवेत || ७६ ||

atha niṣhpatty-avasthā
rudra-ghranthiṃ yadā bhittvā śarva-pīṭha-ghato|anilaḥ |
niṣhpattau vaiṇavaḥ śabdaḥ kvaṇad-vīṇā-kvaṇo bhavet || 76 ||

When the Rudra granthi is pierced and the air enters the seat of the Lord (the space between the eyebrows), then the perfect sound like that of a flute is produced. 75.

एकीभूतं तदा छित्तं राज-योगाभिधानकम |
सृष्हिट-संहार-कर्तासौ योगीश्वर-समो भवेत || ७७ ||

ekībhūtaṃ tadā chittaṃ rāja-yoghābhidhānakam |
sṛṣhṭi-saṃhāra-kartāsau yoghīśvara-samo bhavet || 77 ||

The union of the mind and the sound is called the Râja-Yoga. The (real) Yogî becomes the creator and destroyer of the universe, like God. 76.

अस्तु वा मास्तु वा मुक्तिरत्रैवाखण्डितं सुखम |
लयोद्भवमिदं सौख्यं राज-योगादवाप्यते || ७८ ||

astu vā māstu vā muktiratraivākhaṇḍitaṃ sukham |
layodbhavamidaṃ saukhyaṃ rāja-yoghādavāpyate || 78 ||

Perpetual Happiness is achieved by this; I do not care if the mukti be not attained. This happiness, resulting from absorption [in Brahma], is obtained by means of Raja-Yoga. 77.

राज-योगमजानन्तः केवलं हठ-कर्मिणः |
एतानभ्यासिनो मन्ये परयास-फल-वर्जितान || ७९ ||

rāja-yoghamajānantaḥ kevalaṃ haṭha-karmiṇaḥ |
etānabhyāsino manye prayāsa-phala-varjitān || 79 ||

Those who are ignorant of the Râja-Yoga and practise only the Haṭha-Yoga, will, in my opinion, waste their energy fruitlessly. 78.

उन्मन्य-अवाप्तये शीघ्रं भरू-धयानं मम संमतम |
राज-योग-पदं पराप्तुं सुखोपायो|अल्प-छेतसाम |
सद्यः परत्यय-सन्धायी जायते नादजो लयः || ८० ||

unmany-avāptaye śīghraṃ bhrū-dhyānaṃ mama saṃmatam |
rāja-yogha-padaṃ prāptuṃ sukhopāyo|alpa-chetasām |
sadyaḥ pratyaya-sandhāyī jāyate nādajo layaḥ || 80 ||

Contemplation on the space between the eyebrows is, in my opinion, best for accomplishing soon the *Unmanî* state. For people of small intellect, it is a very easy method for obtaining perfection in the Raja-Yoga. The Laya produced by nâda, at once gives experience (of spiritual powers). 79.

नादानुसन्धान-समाधि-भाजां
योगीश्वराणां हृदि वर्धमानम |
आनन्दमेकं वछसामगम्यं
जानाति तं शरी-गुरुनाथ एकः || ८१ ||

nādānusandhāna-samādhi-bhājāṃ
yoghīśvarāṇāṃ hṛdi vardhamānam |
ānandamekaṃ vachasāmaghamyaṃ
jānāti taṃ śrī-ghurunātha ekaḥ || 81 ||

The happiness which increases in the hearts of Yogiśwaras, who have gained success in Samâdhi by means of attention to the nâda, is beyond description, and is known to *Śri Gurû Nâtha* alone. 80.

कर्णौ पिधाय हस्ताभ्यां यः शृणोति ध्वनिं मुनिः |
तत्र छित्तं सथिरीकुर्याद्यावत्स्थिर-पदं वरजेत || ८२ ||

karṇau pidhāya hastābhyāṃ yaḥ śṝṇoti dhvaniṃ muniḥ |
tatra chittaṃ sthirīkuryādyāvatsthira-padaṃ vrajet || 82 ||

The sound which a muni hears by closing his ears with his fingers, should be heard attentively, till the mind becomes steady in it. 81.

अभ्यस्यमानो नादो|अयं बाह्यमावृणुते ध्वनिम |
पक्ष्हाद्विक्ष्हेपमखिलं जित्वा योगी सुखी भवेत || ८३ ||

abhyasyamāno nādo|ayaṃ bāhyamāvṝṇute dhvanim |
pakṣhādvikṣhepamakhilaṃ jitvā yoghī sukhī bhavet || 83 ||

By practising with this nâda, all other external sounds are stopped. The Yogî becomes happy by overcoming all distractions within 15 days. 82.

शरूयते परथमाभ्यासे नादो नाना-विधो महान |
ततो|अभ्यासे वर्धमाने शरूयते सूक्ष्हम-सूक्ष्हमकः || ८४ ||

śrūyate prathamābhyāse nādo nānā-vidho mahān |
tato|abhyāse vardhamāne śrūyate sūkṣhma-sūkṣhmakaḥ || 84 ||

In the beginning, the sounds heard are of great variety and very loud; but, as the practice increases, they become more and more subtle. 83.

आदौ जलधि-जीमूत-भेरी-झर्झर-सम्भवाः |
मध्ये मर्दल-शङ्खोत्था घण्टा-काहलजास्तथा || ८५ ||

ādau jaladhi-jīmūta-bherī-jharjhara-sambhavāḥ |
madhye mardala-śangkhotthā ghaṇṭā-kāhalajāstathā || 85 ||

In the first stage, the sounds are surging, thundering like the beating of kettle drums and jingling ones. In the intermediate stage, they are like those produced by conch, *Mridanga*, bells, &c. 84.

अन्ते तु किङ्किणी-वंश-वीणा-भरमर-निःस्वनाः |
इति नानाविधा नादाः शरूयन्ते देह-मध्यगाः || ८६ ||

ante tu kingkiṇī-vaṃśa-vīṇā-bhramara-niḥsvanāḥ |
iti nānāvidhā nādāḥ śrūyante deha-madhyaghāḥ || 86 ||

In the last stage, the sounds resemble those from tinklets, flute, Vîṇâ, bee, &c. These various kinds of sounds are heard as being produced in the body. 85.

महति शरूयमाणे|अपि मेघ-भेर्य-आदिके धवनौ |
तत्र सूक्ष्हमात्सूक्ष्हमतरं नादमेव परामृशेत || ८७ ||

mahati śrūyamāṇe|api megha-bhery-ādike dhvanau |
tatra sūkṣhmātsūkṣhmataraṃ nādameva parāmṝśet || 87 ||

Though hearing loud sounds like those of thunder, kettle drums, etc., one should practise with the subtle sounds also. 86.

घनमुत्सृज्य वा सूक्ष्हमे सूक्ष्हममुत्सृज्य वा घने |
रममाणमपि कष्हिप्तं मनो नान्यत्र छालयेत || ८८ ||

ghanamutsṝjya vā sūkṣhme sūkṣhmamutsṝjya vā ghane |
ramamāṇamapi kṣhiptaṃ mano nānyatra chālayet || 88 ||

Leaving the loudest, taking up the subtle one, and leaving the subtle one, taking up the loudest, thus practising, the distracted mind does not wander elsewhere. 87.

यत्र कुत्रापि वा नादे लगति परथमं मनः |
तत्रैव सुस्थिरीभूय तेन सार्धं विलीयते || ८९ ||

yatra kutrāpi vā nāde laghati prathamaṃ manaḥ |
tatraiva susthirībhūya tena sārdhaṃ vilīyate || 89 ||

Wherever the mind attaches itself first, it becomes steady there; and then it becomes absorbed in it. 88.

मकरन्दं पिबन्भृङ्गी गन्धं नापेक्ष्हते यथा |
नादासक्तं तथा छित्तं विष्हयान्नहि काङ्क्ष्हते || ९० ||

makarandaṃ pibanbhṝngghī ghandhaṃ nāpekṣhate yathā |
nādāsaktaṃ tathā chittaṃ viṣhayānnahi kāngkṣhate || 90 ||

Just as a bee, drinking sweet juice, does not care for the smell of the flower; so the mind, absorbed in the nâda, does not desire the objects of enjoyment. 89.

मनो-मत्त-गजेन्द्रस्य विष्हयोद्यान-छारिणः |
समर्थो|अयं नियमने निनाद-निशिताङ्कुशः || ९१ ||

mano-matta-ghajendrasya viṣhayodyāna-chāriṇaḥ |
samartho|ayaṃ niyamane nināda-niśitāngkuśaḥ || 91 ||

The mind, like an elephant habituated to wander in the garden of enjoyments, is capable of being controlled by the sharp goad of anâhata nâda. 90.

बद्धं तु नाद-बन्धेन मनः सन्त्यक्त-छापलम |
परयाति सुतरां सथैर्यं छिन्न-पक्ष्हः खगो यथा || ९२ ||

baddhaṃ tu nāda-bandhena manaḥ santyakta-chāpalam |
prayāti sutarāṃ sthairyaṃ chinna-pakṣhaḥ khagho yathā || 92 ||

The mind, captivated in the snare of nâda, gives up all its activity; and, like a bird with clipped wings, becomes calm at once. 91.

सर्व-छिन्तां परित्यज्य सावधानेन छेतसा |
नाद एवानुसन्धेयो योग-साम्राज्यमिछ्छता || ९३ ||

sarva-chintāṃ parityajya sāvadhānena chetasā |
nāda evānusandheyo yogha-sāmrājyamichchatā || 93 ||

Those desirous of the kingdom of Yoga, should take up the practice of hearing the anâhata nâda, with mind collected and free from all cares. 92.

नादो|अन्तरङ्ग-सारङ्ग-बन्धने वागुरायते |
अन्तरङ्ग-कुरङ्गस्य वधे वयाधायते|अपि छ || ९४ ||

nādo|antaranggha-sāranggha-bandhane vāghurāyate |
antaranggha-kurangghasya vadhe vyādhāyate|api cha || 94 ||

Nada is the snare for catching the mind; and, when it is caught like a deer, it can be killed also like it. 93.

अन्तरङ्गस्य यमिनो वाजिनः परिघायते |
नादोपास्ति-रतो नित्यमवधार्या हि योगिना || ९५ ||

antarangghasya yamino vājinaḥ parighāyate |
nādopāsti-rato nityamavadhāryā hi yoghinā || 95 ||

Nâda is the bolt of the stable door for the horse (the minds of the Yogîs). A Yogî should determine to practise constantly in the hearing of the nâda sounds. 94.

बद्धं विमुक्त-छाञ्छल्यं नाद-गन्धक-जारणात |
मनः-पारदमाप्नोति निरालम्बाख्य-खे|अटनम || ९६ ||

baddhaṃ vimukta-chāñchalyaṃ nāda-ghandhaka-jāraṇāt |
manaḥ-pāradamāpnoti nirālambākhya-khe|aṭanam || 96 ||

Mind gets the properties of calcined mercury. When deprived of its unsteadiness it is calcined, combined with the sulphur of nâda, and then it roams like it in tine supportless âkâśa or Brahma. 95.

नाद-शरवणतः कष्हिप्रमन्तरङ्ग-भुजङ्गमम |
विस्मृतय सर्वमेकाग्रः कुत्रछिन्नहि धावति || ९७ ||

nāda-śravaṇataḥ kṣhipramantaranggha-bhujangghamam |
vismṝtaya sarvamekāghraḥ kutrachinnahi dhāvati || 97 ||

The mind is like a serpent, forgetting all its unsteadiness by hearing the nâda, it does not run away anywhere. 96.

काष्ठे परवर्तितो वह्निः काष्ठेन सह शाम्यति |
नादे परवर्तितं छित्तं नादेन सह लीयते || ९८ ||

kāṣhṭhe pravartito vahniḥ kāṣhṭhena saha śāmyati |
nāde pravartitaṃ chittaṃ nādena saha līyate || 98 ||

The fire, catching firewood, is extinguished along with it (after burning it up); and so the mind also, working with the nâda, becomes latent along with it. 97.

घण्टादिनाद-सक्त-सतब्धान्तः-करण-हरिणस्य |
परहरणमपि सुकरं सयाछ्छर-सन्धान-परवीणश्छेत || ९९ ||

ghaṇṭādināda-sakta-stabdhāntaḥ-karaṇa-hariṇasya |
praharaṇamapi sukaraṃ syāchchara-sandhāna-pravīṇaśchet || 99 ||

The antahkaraṇa (mind), like a deer, becomes absorbed and motionless on hearing the sound of hells, etc.; and then it is very easy for an expert archer to kill it. 98.

अनाहतस्य शब्दस्य धवनिर्य उपलभ्यते |
धवनेरन्तर्गतं जञेयं जञेयस्यान्तर्गतं मनः |
मनस्तत्र लयं याति तद्विष्हणोः परमं पदम || १०० ||

anāhatasya śabdasya dhvanirya upalabhyate |
dhvanerantarghataṃ jñeyaṃ jñeyasyāntarghataṃ manaḥ |
manastatra layaṃ yāti tadviṣhṇoḥ paramaṃ padam || 100 ||

The knowable interpenetrates the anâhata sound which is heard, and the mind interpenetrates the knowable. The mind becomes absorbed there, which is the seat of the all-pervading, almighty Lord. 99.

तावदाकाश-सङ्कल्पो यावछ्छब्दः परवर्तते |
निःशब्दं तत-परं बरह्म परमातेति गीयते || १०१ ||

tāvadākāśa-sangkalpo yāvachchabdaḥ pravartate |
niḥśabdaṃ tat-paraṃ brahma paramāteti ghīyate || 101 ||

So long as the sounds continue, there is the idea of âkâśa. When they disappear, then it is called Para Brahma, Paramâtmana. 100.

यत्किंछिन्नाद-रूपेण शरूयते शक्तिरेव सा |
यस्तत्त्वान्तो निराकारः स एव परमेश्वरः || १०२ ||

yatkiṃchinnāda-rūpeṇa śrūyate śaktireva sā |
yastattvānto nirākāraḥ sa eva parameśvaraḥ || 102 ||

Whatever is heard in the form of nâda, is the śakti (power). That which is formless, the final state of the Tatwas, is tile Parameśwara. 101.

इति नादानुसन्धानम
सर्वे हठ-लयोपाया राजयोगस्य सिद्धये |
राज-योग-समारूढः पुरुष्हः काल-वञ्छकः || १०३ ||

iti nādānusandhānam
sarve haṭha-layopāyā rājayoghasya siddhaye |
rāja-yogha-samārūḍhaḥ puruṣhaḥ kāla-vañchakaḥ || 103 ||

All the methods of Haṭha are meant for gaining success in the Raja-Yoga; for, the man, who is well-established in the Raja-Yoga, overcomes death. 102.

तत्त्वं बीजं हठः कष्हेत्रमौदासीन्यं जलं तरिभिः |
उन्मनी कल्प-लतिका सद्य एव परवर्तते || १०४ ||

tattvaṃ bījaṃ haṭhaḥ kṣhetramaudāsīnyaṃ jalaṃ tribhiḥ |
unmanī kalpa-latikā sadya eva pravartate || 104 ||

Tatwa is the seed, Haṭha the field; and Indifference (Vairâgya) the water. By the action of these three, the creeper Unmanî thrives very rapidly. 103.

सदा नादानुसन्धानात्क्ष्हीयन्ते पाप-संछयाः |
निरञ्जने विलीयेते निश्छितं छित्त-मारुतौ || १०५ ||

sadā nādānusandhānātkṣhīyante pāpa-saṃchayāḥ |
nirañjane vilīyete niśchitaṃ chitta-mārutau || 105 ||

All the accumulations of sins are destroyed by practising always with the nâda; and the mind and the airs do certainly become latent in the colorless (Paramâtmana). 104.

शङ्ख-दुन्धुभि-नादं छ न शृणोति कदाछन |
काष्ह्ठवज्जायते देह उन्मन्यावस्थया धरुवम || १०६ ||

śangkha-dundhubhi-nādaṃ cha na śṝṇoti kadāchana |
kāṣhṭhavajjāyate deha unmanyāvasthayā dhruvam || 106 ||

Such a one. does not hear the noise of the conch and Dundubhi. Being in the Unmanî avasthâ, his body becomes like a piece of wood. 105.

सर्वावस्था-विनिर्मुक्तः सर्व-छिन्ता-विवर्जितः |
मृतवत्तिष्ह्ठते योगी स मुक्तो नात्र संशयः || १०७ ||

sarvāvasthā-vinirmuktaḥ sarva-chintā-vivarjitaḥ |
mṝtavattiṣhṭhate yoghī sa mukto nātra saṃśayaḥ || 107 ||

There is no doubt, such a Yogî becomes free from all states, from all cares, and remains like one dead. 106.

खाद्यते न छ कालेन बाध्यते न छ कर्मणा |
साध्यते न स केनापि योगी युक्तः समाधिना || १०८ ||

khādyate na cha kālena bādhyate na cha karmaṇā |
sādhyate na sa kenāpi yoghī yuktaḥ samādhinā || 108 ||

He is not devoured by death, is not bound by his actions. The Yogî who is engaged in Samâdhi is overpowered by none. 107.

न गन्धं न रसं रूपं न छ सपर्शं न निःस्वनम |
नात्मानं न परं वेत्ति योगी युक्तः समाधिना || १०९ ||

na ghandhaṃ na rasaṃ rūpaṃ na cha sparśaṃ na niḥsvanam |
nātmānaṃ na paraṃ vetti yoghī yuktaḥ samādhinā || 109 ||

The Yogî, engaged in Samâdhi, feels neither smell, taste, color, touch, sound, nor is conscious of his own self. 108.

छित्तं न सुप्तं नोजाग्रत्स्मृति-विस्मृति-वर्जितम |
न छास्तमेति नोदेति यस्यासौ मुक्त एव सः || ११० ||

chittaṃ na suptaṃ nojāghratsmṝti-vismṝti-varjitam |
na chāstameti nodeti yasyāsau mukta eva saḥ || 110 ||

He whose mind is neither sleeping, waking, remembering, destitute of memory, disappearing nor appearing, is liberated. 109.

न विजानाति शीतोष्ह्णं न दुःखं न सुखं तथा |
न मानं नोपमानं छ योगी युक्तः समाधिना || १११ ||

na vijānāti śītoṣhṇaṃ na duḥkhaṃ na sukhaṃ tathā |
na mānaṃ nopamānaṃ cha yoghī yuktaḥ samādhinā || 111 ||

He feels neither heat, cold, pain, pleasure, respect nor disrespect. Such a Yogî is absorbed in Samâdhi. 110.

सवस्थो जाग्रदवस्थायां सुप्तवद्यो|अवतिष्ह्ठते |
निःश्वासोछ्छ्वास-हीनश्छ निश्छितं मुक्त एव सः || ११२ ||

svastho jāghradavasthāyāṃ suptavadyo|avatiṣhṭhate |
niḥśvāsochchvāsa-hīnaścha niśchitaṃ mukta eva saḥ || 112 ||

He who, though awake, appears like one sleeping, and is without inspiration and expiration, is certainly free. 111.

अवध्यः सर्व-शस्त्राणामशक्यः सर्व-देहिनाम |
अग्राह्यो मन्त्र-यन्त्राणां योगी युक्तः समाधिना || ११३ ||

avadhyaḥ sarva-śastrāṇāmaśakyaḥ sarva-dehinām |
aghrāhyo mantra-yantrāṇāṃ yoghī yuktaḥ samādhinā || 113 ||

The Yogî, engaged in Samâdhi, cannot be killed by any instrument, and is beyond the controlling power of beings. He is beyond the reach of incantations and charms. 112.

यावद्विदुर्न भवति दृढः पराण-वात-परबन्धात |
यावद्ध्याने सहज-सदृशं जायते नैव तत्त्वं
तावज्ज्ञानं वदति तदिदं दम्भ-मिथ्या-परलापः || ११४ ||

yāvadvidurna bhavati dṝḍhaḥ prāṇa-vāta-prabandhāt |
yāvaddhyāne sahaja-sadṝśaṃ jāyate naiva tattvaṃ
tāvajjñānaṃ vadati tadidaṃ dambha-mithyā-pralāpaḥ || 114 ||

As long as the Prâṇa does not enter and flow in the middle channel and the *vindu* does not become firm by the control of the movements of the Prâṇa; as long as the mind does not assume the form of Brahma without any effort in contemplation, so long all the talk of knowledge and wisdom is merely the nonsensical babbling of a mad man. 113.

THE END.

इति हठ-योग-परदीपिकायां समाधि-लक्ष्हणं नाम छतुर्थोपदेशः |

iti haṭha-yogha-pradīpikāyāṃ samādhi-lakṣhaṇaṃ nāma chaturthopadeśaḥ |

www.ingramcontent.com/pod-product-compliance
Lightning Source LLC
Chambersburg PA
CBHW081343280526
45788CB00009B/2751
9781456467470